# MALARIA IN COLONIAL SOUTH ASIA

This book highlights the role of acute hunger in malaria lethality in colonial South Asia and investigates how this understanding came to be lost in modern medical, epidemic, and historiographic thought.

Using the case studies of colonial Punjab, Sri Lanka, and Bengal, it traces the loss of fundamental concepts and language of hunger in the inter-war period with the reductive application of the new specialisms of nutritional science and immunology, and a parallel loss of the distinction between infection (transmission) and morbid disease. The study locates the final demise of the 'Human Factor' (hunger) in malaria history within pre- and early post-WW2 international health institutions – the International Health Division of the Rockefeller Foundation and the nascent WHO's Expert Committee on Malaria. It examines the implications of this epistemic shift for interpreting South Asian health history, and reclaims a broader understanding of common endemic infection (endemiology) as a prime driver, in the context of subsistence precarity, of epidemic mortality history and demographic change.

This book will be useful to scholars and researchers of public health, social medicine and social epidemiology, imperial history, epidemic and demographic history, history of medicine, medical sociology, and sociology.

**Sheila Zurbrigg** is a physician and independent scholar based in Toronto, Canada. Her health history research investigates rising life expectancy in South Asian history in relation to food security. She has served as Short-Term Epidemiologist for the World Health Organization, Smallpox Eradication Program, Uttar Pradesh, and Coordinator, Village Health Worker Program, Madurai, Tamil Nadu, India. She has held appointments as Adjunct Professor, International Development Studies, Dalhousie University, Halifax, Nova Scotia, Canada; Visiting Scholar, York University, Toronto, Canada; and Visiting Scholar, Jawaharlal Nehru University, New Delhi, India. Her work with traditional village midwives in rural Tamil Nadu (1975–1979) led to the analysis of child survival in contemporary India in relation to food security and conditions of women's work. In 1985, she turned to South Asian health history research, funded by the Social Sciences and Humanities Research Council (Ottawa). Among her published work is the book *Epidemic Malaria and Hunger in Colonial Punjab: 'Weakened by Want'* (2019).

# MALARIA IN COLONIAL SOUTH ASIA

## Uncoupling Disease and Destitution

*Sheila Zurbrigg*

Routledge
Taylor & Francis Group

LONDON AND NEW YORK

First published 2020
by Routledge
2 Park Square, Milton Park, Abingdon, Oxon OX14 4RN

and by Routledge
605 Third Avenue, New York, NY 10017

First issued in paperback 2021

*Routledge is an imprint of the Taylor & Francis Group, an informa business*

*British Library Cataloguing-in-Publication Data*
A catalogue record for this book is available from the British Library

*Library of Congress Cataloging-in-Publication Data*
A catalog record for this book has been requested

Typeset in Sabon
by Apex CoVantage, LLC

ISBN 13: 978-0-367-77769-2 (pbk)
ISBN 13: 978-0-367-27214-2 (hbk)

FOR THE VILLAGE MIDWIVES OF
RAMNAD DISTRICT, REMEMBERED

# CONTENTS

# FIGURES

# TABLES

# ABBREVIATIONS AND ACRONYMS

| | |
|---|---|
| AIIHPH | All-India Institute of Hygiene and Public Health |
| *AJPH* | *American Journal of Public Health* |
| CBR | crude birth rate (annual births per 1,000 population) |
| CDR | crude death rate (annual deaths per 1,000 population) |
| DDT | dichloro-diphenyl-trichloroethane |
| ECM | Expert Committee on Malaria |
| *EPW* | *Economic and Political Weekly* |
| FAO | Food and Agriculture Organization |
| GDP | Gross Domestic Product |
| *GHLC* | *Good Health at Low Cost* |
| GOI | Government of India |
| *GOI-PHC* | *Annual Report of the Public Health Commissioner with the Government of India* [1922–1947] |
| *GOI-SCR* | *Annual Report of the Sanitary Commissioner with the Government of India* [1868–1921] |
| GoP | Government of Punjab |
| HMSO | Her Majesty's Stationery Office |
| IC | Interim Commission (WHO) |
| ICMR | Indian Council of Medical Research |
| *IJMR* | *Indian Journal of Medical Research* |
| *IESHR* | *Indian Economic and Social History Review* |
| IHB | International Health Board (Rockefeller Foundation) |
| IHD | International Health Division (Rockefeller Foundation) |
| *IJM* | *Indian Journal of Malariology* |
| *IMG* | *Indian Medical Gazette* |
| IMS | Indian Medical Service |

| | |
|---|---|
| IRFA | Indian Research Fund Association |
| *JMII* | *Journal of the Malaria Institute of India* |
| LN | League of Nations |
| LNHO | League of Nations Health Organisation |
| LNMC | League of Nations Malaria Commission |
| LNMC-India report | *Report of the Malaria Commission on its Study Tour of India*, Geneva, 1930 |
| LSHTM | London School of Hygiene and Tropical Medicine |
| MBD | Malaria as a Block to Development |
| *MSCR* | *Report of the Sanitary Commissioner for Madras* |
| NNMB | National Nutrition Monitoring Bureau |
| NNSO | National Sample Survey Organisation |
| PLGP | Proc. of the Lieutenant-Governor of the Punjab, in the Home Dept (Sanitary) |
| *PPHA* | *Report on the Public Health Administration of the Punjab* [1922–47] |
| *PSCR* | *Report on the Sanitary Administration of the Punjab* [1868–1921] |
| *QBHO* | *Quarterly Bulletin of the Health Organisation of the League of Nations* |
| RF | Rockefeller Foundation |
| *RCAI* | *Report of the Royal Commission on Agriculture in India* |
| *RMSI* | *Records of the Malaria Survey of India* |
| *Sci. Mem. Off. Med. San. Dep.* | *Scientific Memoirs by Officers of the Medical and Sanitary Departments of the Government of India* (New Series) |
| *Season and Crops Report* | *Report on the Season and Crops of the Punjab* [1901–1944] |
| *Stat. Abst.* | *Statistical abstract relating to British India* (London: HMSO, 1840–1920) |
| *Trans. Bombay Congress* | *Transactions of the Bombay Medical Congress, 1909* |
| UNRRA | United Nations Relief and Rehabilitation Administration |
| WHO | World Health Organization |

# GLOSSARY

**anthropophilic**   propensity of the female mosquito to seek blood meals from humans rather than animals

**basal metabolic rate**   that level of caloric intake required for all internal metabolic and physiological functions in a state of complete rest

**bonification**   a term applied by early twentieth-century Italian malaria workers for agricultural improvement programs in malarious regions

**case fatality rate**   the proportion of deaths within a designated population of 'cases' (people with a medical condition) over the course of the disease

**crore**   ten million

**crude death rate**   annual number of deaths from all causes in a given year per 1,000 population

*dalit*   term for the lowest ('out-caste') level in the Hindu social hierarchy

**exophily**   the mosquito habit of resting outdoors after a human blood meal rather than inside

**gametocyte**   the reproductive stage of the malaria parasite, transmitted from the human host to the female vector mosquito during its blood meal

**holoendemic**   a state of near year-round malaria transmission resulting in high levels of acquired immunity in the local population such that clinical symptoms of infection are minimal amongst all but young children

**hyperendemic**   highly intense but seasonal malaria transmission, associated with high parasite and spleen (splenomegaly) rates (> 50%), with acquired immunity levels sufficient to keep regular re-infection largely asymptomatic in adults and older children

**infant mortality rate**   number of infant deaths in the first year of life, per 1,000 live born

**parasite rate**   that proportion of persons found with microscopically confirmed parasites in the bloodstream (parasitemia)

**premunity**   a sufficient level of naturally acquired immunity where clinical symptoms from continuing re-infection are limited or nil

**protozoa**   a single-celled microscopic animal with a defined nucleus

**species sanitation**   the targeting of anti-mosquito operations specifically to those anopheline species responsible for transmission in a region

**spleen rate**   generally considered the per cent of children under the age of 10 years in a population with an enlarged spleen (splenomegaly)

**splenomegaly**   enlargement of the spleen sufficient to be palpable below the left rib cage

**sporozoite**   the infective stage of the malaria parasite that is passed to the human host from the salivary glands of the female mosquito during a blood meal

*thana*   subdivision of a rural district, under a subinspector of police

*zamindar*   landowner who leases land for cultivation by tenant farmers

**zoophilic**   propensity of the female mosquito to seek blood meals from animals rather than humans

**zymotic**   a nineteenth-century term for acute febrile infectious diseases believed to be caused by atmospheric vapours (miasma) resulting from fermentation of organic matter

# PREFACE AND ACKNOWLEDGMENTS

This exploration into the loss in understanding of hunger in South Asian malaria history could not have been completed without the support and experience of many people, as was the case with the first stage of this health history project, published as *Epidemic Malaria and Hunger in Colonial Punjab: 'Weakened by Want.'* The origins of the study lie in five years of privileged acquaintance with many of the traditional village midwives of Tiruppuvanam Block, Ramnad district in southern Tamil Nadu, women who allowed me a glimpse into their midwifery skills and their lives as daily-wage agricultural labourers. Returning to Canada in 1980, I found development literatures where mortality decline in the 'global south' was interpreted largely in terms of the transfer of modern medical techniques. From the perspective of these women's lives and the general inaccessibility of rural health services still apparent in the late 1970s, this reading was unconvincing. In time, the question led me to explore the historical experience of mortality decline in South Asia through the lens of malaria as pre-eminent trigger of mortality across much of the period of British rule. I was surprised to find how clearly the hunger-malaria lethality relationship had been documented in the colonial records. But also by how fully this understanding seemed to have been lost by the mid-twentieth century. This left me puzzled in turn by the many larger epistemic questions as to *how*.

I am indebted first of all to the late Prof Biswamoy Pati for his immediate, encouraging response to the proposed publication of this study – though my gratitude is accompanied by deep regret that I was unable to convey this in person before his untimely death. For financial support in the early years of this research as a private scholar I remain grateful to the Social Sciences and Humanities Research Council of Canada. Throughout, scholarly support has come from many people. For their interest, expressed in the earliest days of this exploration into South Asian health history, I am grateful to the late Ian Catanach, Nigel Crook, Bill Owen, and John Farley, who gave crucial support along the way, and in John's case, invaluable commentary on first drafts of many chapters. Feedback from Neeladri Bhattacharya on my initial writing was invaluable, as was generous encouragement mid-way from

José-Antonio Ortega Osona. I thank them greatly. My gratitude to Douglas Hay, Jim Phillips, and Paul Antze is enormous for their painstaking commentary on the study overview, and for their insistent assurance of its coherence. In all respects, the critical contemporary health analysis of Imrana Qadeer, Mohan Rao, and Debabar Banerji at the Centre for Social Medicine and Community Health, Jawaharlal Nehru University, New Delhi, has been, and remains, an important touchstone.

For many Madurai friends who made possible my introduction to the subsistence realities of rural Tamil Nadu, my respect and gratitude are abiding. Among them, the late Prof K.A. Krishnamurthy, Mrs Janaki Ramaswamy, her elder brother, Dr G. Venkataswamy, and their extended family are remembered fondly. The practical experience of those years was made possible through the dedication, daily support, and treasured friendship of Anusuya Andichamy and Shahnawaz Ghouse. Personal funding support during these years came from the Canadian International Development Agency and the remarkable Head of its Health Division, the late Dr Bill Jeanes. For onerous editing support for my early efforts in putting pen to paper I remain profoundly indebted to John Desrochers and the late John Maliekal of the Bangalore Social Action Trust. It was their encouragement that convinced me to pursue the Ramnad midwives' insights into an understanding of the broader determinants of health.

The published work of many historians provided essential stepping stones as I sought to place the expanding questions and historical subdisciplines into a larger whole. Central to comprehending the demise in understanding of the 'Human Factor' in malaria historiography has been Christopher Hamlin's 1998 analysis of the wider epistemic content of Edwin Chadwick's 1842 Sanitary Report. It is a story with close parallels a century later to that of malaria in South Asia, and his insights into this earlier stage of the 'uncoupling of disease and destitution' in nineteenth-century Britain have provided critical context to this study. Important also has been the work of Randall Packard, John Farley, and Socrates Litsios on the role of malaria in the shaping of the nascent World Health Organization and related influence of the Rockefeller Foundation.

Much of this study however has necessarily been a solitary journey because so much of the extensive colonial South Asian malaria research literature and records at the time had yet to be explored. Inevitably, there will be many aspects that have been left incomplete, and I look forward to critical commentary and additions to this work.

Once again, I thank the librarian staff of Dalhousie University in Halifax, Nova Scotia – Gwyn Pace, Joe Wickens, Kellie Hawley, Marlyn McCann, and Catherine Pickett – for their painstaking work in locating obscure documents. For many summers of assistance, I thank as well the staff of the India Office Library, now housed within the British Library, and also the National Archives of India, and York University, Toronto.

Throughout, the support of Heidi Williams, Barbara Lent, Sandi Witherspoon, Paul and Sandra Odegaard, Christine Davidson, Jeanette Neeson, Betty Peterson, Fatima and Ismail Cajee, and Carolyn van Gurp have sustained me through the toughest writing times.

Especially, I thank Daniel and Gabe, for their confidence, their indispensable computer skills, and the joy they give. For Philip's editorial and moral support that has never wavered through this project, and for much more, I thank my lucky stars.

# INTRODUCTION

In September 1952, a leading British malaria researcher completed an analysis of epidemic malaria in the Punjab plains of British India by concluding that the 'notorious' epidemics of the colonial period 'were associated with certain rainfall characteristics and with an inadequate immunity in the local population.'[1] Referencing a 1911 enquiry report entitled *Malaria in the Punjab*, commissioned by the then colonial Government of India, George Macdonald noted that the earlier study's quantitative correlations between monsoon rainfall and autumn malaria mortality were 'so close that they formed an obvious basis for forecasting future epidemics.'[2] Here, by periodic epidemics Macdonald was addressing the marked surges in malaria deaths that episodically afflicted the malaria-endemic Punjab region. And by 'inadequate immunity' he was referring to insufficient acquired (malaria-specific) immunity.[3] Wide annual variation in rainfall and malaria transmission in the region, he reasoned, led to varying numbers of 'non-immunes' among the population, and in turn to a corresponding fluctuation in susceptibility of the population to the infection.

If a seemingly small and unremarkable detail in the overall body of research conducted on malaria by the mid-twentieth century, this reading of Punjab malaria history nonetheless revealed a fundamental shift in understanding of the region's epidemic history. More broadly, it exemplified the epistemic transformation in Western epidemic thought that had taken place over the preceding century. The original study to which Macdonald referred had pointed to quite a different factor underlying malaria mortality patterns in colonial Punjab. What distinguished 'fulminant' malaria years, its author, S.R. Christophers (1873–1978), had concluded, was markedly increased human destitution, a condition that he referred to in his 1911 enquiry report as the 'Human Factor.' The vast regional epidemics of malaria mortality that afflicted the Punjab plains across the first half of the colonial period, Christophers had shown, were correlated with preceding harvest failure, soaring foodgrain prices ('scarcity') and, in particular years, overt conditions of famine, a relationship he metaphorically encapsulated as malaria 'merely reap[ing] a harvest prepared for it by the famine.'[4]

1

In detailed *thana*-level mapping of several major epidemics over the 1868–1908 period, Christophers had demonstrated that the epidemics were not spatially related to varying malaria endemicity in the province. Rather, the distinctive geographic distribution of mortality in each case suggested instead a pattern of harvest failure (acute hunger) across the province, destitution often compounded by flooding with return of the rains.[5] Adequate rainfall was a necessary factor for widespread transmission of malaria infection in the province: failure of the annual monsoon rains limited malaria incidence in any given year.[6] But preceding economic stress predicted where, when good rains ultimately returned, lethality of malaria infection would soar to 'disastrous' epidemic proportions. Acute hunger then was an essential predisposing factor underlying malaria's 'fulminant' or 'exalted' form in the region.[7] As the 1911 report also noted, a determining role for semi- or frank starvation in the region's recurring malaria epidemics was a commonplace in the nineteenth-century sanitary records, not only in Punjab but more widely in British India, as well as in popular experience.[8]

Between the 1952 Macdonald reading of Punjab malaria history and the original 1911 report lay an epistemic chasm. By the mid-twentieth century, understanding of the 'Human Factor' in malaria epidemicity in South Asia had come to be transformed from a condition of the human host – acute hunger that undermined general immune *capacity* to mount a successful response to future infection[9] – to one of vector transmission: limited previous exposure to malaria and thus a lack of *acquired*, or specific, immunity. In the process, malaria in the general medical literature had also come to be considered a primary *cause* of hunger and underdevelopment: the nature of the relationship documented in 1911 had been narrowed and in effect turned upside down.[10]

This study explores how understanding of the role of acute hunger in South Asian malaria mortality history came to be lost in modern medical thought. It examines the conceptual consequences of this loss for interpreting the region's health history, and considers the larger epistemic implications for the study of mortality decline in history more generally.

In earlier work, I have explored, and corroborated, the conclusions of Christophers's 1911 study that causally linked epidemic malaria in colonial Punjab to acute hunger.[11] In the process of quantitatively testing Christophers's thesis, it became clear as well that malaria death rates in the province fell very substantially after 1920, a decline that predated by more than three decades the 1950s DDT-based control of malaria transmission in the region (Figure 0.1). Yet there was little evidence of a decrease in malaria transmission or severity of flooding in the province between 1920 and 1950, or shifts in acquired immunity, to explain this decline. Nor does there appear to have been substantial improvement in rural access to treatment (quinine). The conquest of 'fulminant' malaria in the region thus appears to have been temporally associated instead with the control of epidemic destitution ('famine').[12]

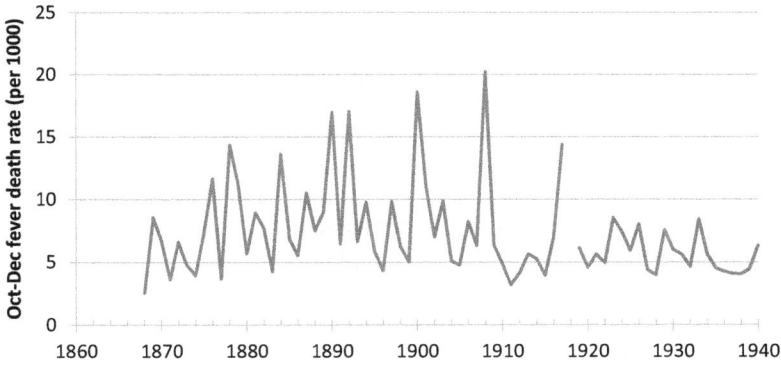

*Figure 0.1* Mean annual Oct.–Dec. fever death rate (per 1,000), 1868–1940, 23 plains districts, Punjab

*Source*: PSCR, 1868–1921; PPHA, 1922–40. See S. Zurbrigg, *Epidemic Malaria and Hunger in Colonial Punjab*, Fig. 4.1, p. 124. For an explanation of the Oct.–Dec. fever death rate as an approximate measure of annual malaria mortality in Punjab, see ibid., pp. 10, 55–56, 200.

*Note*: 1918 omitted due to confounding influenza deaths.

In reinterpreting epidemic malaria patterns in South Asia in terms of acquired immunity, Macdonald was hardly alone among malaria researchers of the period. Immunological aspects to infectious disease epidemicity were at the forefront of medical and public health research from the final decades of the nineteenth century, an interest evident also in British Indian sanitary deliberations by the turn of the century.[13] Macdonald's particular focus on the germ-transmission side of the 'epidemic equation' in analyzing South Asian malaria epidemicity thus reflected a more general narrowing framework in Western epidemic thought, a process already well in train when Christophers penned his enquiry report in 1911. What was anomalous at this point, then, was the latter's detailed attention to conditions of the human 'host' in his interpretation of malaria lethality.

In his efforts to explain the historical patterns of malaria mortality in South Asia, Christophers had found himself plumbing terminology belonging to a much earlier, pre-sanitationist body of medical theory, epidemiological concepts that by the early 1900s had faded from academic medical discourse. In speaking of the 'Human Factor' as 'physiological poverty,' he was applying an earlier medical framework of epidemic causation in which the relationship between infection (exposure to a specific microbe) and disease (clinical morbidity and associated mortality) was understood as often mediated by predisposing factors.[14] Paramount among such factors were conditions of physical exhaustion in the human host through insufficient food: in the words of the 1884 *Gazetteer* of Gurgaon district, 'weakened by want.'[15] *Malaria in the Punjab* was quietly inserting the human host back into the epidemic equation, the enquiry report a meeting ground in effect

3

between the modern biomedical and the pre-germ theory eras of epidemic thought. Christophers, himself a leading Indian Medical Service epidemiologist and entomologist in the emerging field of vector-borne disease, was straddling both, demonstrating there was no contradiction between them: indeed, that both were essential to understanding patterns and determinants of malaria's mortality burden in South Asia.

If reclaimed in the 1911 Punjab study, and administratively acknowledged in fundamental famine relief policy reforms at the time, recognition of this larger predispositionist framework to the phenomenon of 'fulminant' malaria would not be sustained. To the limited extent that the 1911 malaria enquiry report appears in modern medical literature, its conclusions continue to be interpreted in immuno-entomological terms, with epidemic malaria understood as a function of decline in acquired immunity: in other words, in terms of vector transmission.[16] Indeed, by the late twentieth century, malaria had come to be categorized within the historiographic literature as belonging to that group of inherently virulent epidemic diseases such as bubonic plague for which 'nutrition' played little role in their historical mortality patterns,[17] a view that continues to inform historical demographic and health analysis.[18]

The demise of the 'Human Factor' as a central epidemiological concept in malaria research is remarkable in light of the professional stature of the scientist who confirmed its importance in South Asia. But it is equally so in light of the work of the League of Nations Malaria Commission, where leading researchers in the 1920s studied and ultimately concurred with the view arrived at by malaria workers both in India and in much of still malaria-endemic regions of Europe[19] as to the central role of improved economic conditions in markedly reducing malaria's mortality burden.

The question of how earlier insights into the role of acute hunger in malaria history came to be lost is thus a compelling one. Given the prominence of malaria as a leading trigger of historical mortality in South Asia, the loss is unfortunate also in its larger consequences for understanding the region's health history. But the epistemic significance of the question for health historiography arguably extends well beyond South Asia to other once malaria-endemic regions of the world, and as well, potentially to endemic infective diseases other than malaria.[20]

How this understanding was lost is explored in this study. It attempts to trace the conceptual steps involved in the eclipse of acute hunger in malaria mortality historiography. In this endeavour, the period of Britain's colonial rule (1858–1947) offers a particularly important 'window,' provided by the relative wealth and span of available administrative, medical, vital registration, and malaria research records. The book's primary focus is the interwar and immediate post-WW2 years during which understanding of the malaria-hunger relationship came to be inverted.[21] It explores the impact in these years of the emerging subdisciplines of immunology and nutritional science on medical thought within British India, and in twentieth-century institutions of international health, as key intellectual loci of this epistemic shift. Across this period these medical specialisms offered new channels of laboratory research and intriguing theoretic possibilities for interpreting epidemic patterns in the microbiologic realm, an influence that extended well beyond Punjab malaria analysis.

As elsewhere, the impact of the new science of nutrition was particularly marked, as medical attention in British India rapidly shifted in the early twentieth century from hunger – staple foods and their (in)sufficiency – to micronutrient deficiency states in the wake of the discovery of vitamins in the 1910s and 1920s. By the 1930s, the term 'malnutrition' (nutrient *imbalance*) had come increasingly to dominate medical discussion and interest,[22] and hunger as a public health issue receded both conceptually and investigationally. One thus sees the remarkable juxtaposition of a colonial medical literature increasingly directed to questions of 'hidden hunger' (subclinical micronutrient deficiencies) with annual public health reports still prefaced as they had been from the late 1860s with observations on harvest conditions and foodgrain prices, data still considered by local public health officials as central to anticipating mortality conditions in any given year. Those medical colleagues on the 'frontlines' of public health practice in India and those within medical research and academia were now speaking two quite different languages, and practising in effect two quite different preventive medicines.

Beyond the general terminology of hunger, what was being lost in the final decades of colonial rule was a way of thinking about human subsistence in concrete, epidemiological terms: an understanding of hunger as expressed historically in terms of meals per day. Here, two meals a day reflected consumption of staple foods 'sufficient to satisfy hunger'; one, indicated undernourishment ('chronic' hunger); and zero, acute hunger (semi- or frank starvation). As detailed in an earlier work, and summarized in Appendix II below, such categories encompass in general terms the relative prevalence of acute and 'chronic' hunger in populations over time – the term 'prevalence' here being used in its epidemiological sense of frequency, duration, and social extent.

Along with micronutrient discoveries, the inter-war years in British India also witnessed severe imperial retrenchment, creating a climate where to maintain minimum research funding many malaria workers found themselves pushed to 'sell' aggressively the importance of malaria transmission control for the Indian economy: malaria as a cause of India's poverty. Advocates of vector transmission control turned to increasingly hyperbolic arguments for vector control programs, with malaria now framed as a primary 'block' to economic development in the subcontinent, what in contemporary public health analysis has come to be referred to as the 'malaria-as-a-block-to-development' (MBD) thesis.[23] These fiscal pressures in turn fed aspirations for external philanthropic sources of funding for medical research, opportunities that appeared to be at hand through the recently established International Health Board of the Rockefeller Foundation, itself founded with a pedagogical mandate premised on a unifocal view of disease as the cause of world poverty.

At the international level, fundamental divisions within the League of Nations Malaria Commission had arisen between those malaria workers who sought to control malaria transmission *per se*, and those who saw malaria *mortality* as the pressing priority, a public health problem amenable to basic agricultural improvements, reforms, and assured access to treatment. These divisions threatened to undermine the work of the Malaria Commission and the League's larger Health Organisation as well, and appear to have led to a notable muting of discussions of the broader economic dimensions to health. Moreover, by the early 1930s, malaria concerns were being overshadowed by the global economic Depression. 'Nutrition' would soon be at the forefront of the work of the League's Health Organisation. But here, analysis was increasingly directed to issues of dietary quality – declining consumption of 'protective' foods among Anglo-European populations – and attention to global hunger and its structural causes receded. Research on methods of vector transmission control however continued to be initiated and funded by the International Health Division of the Rockefeller Foundation, work that would soon culminate in the international sphere in the post-WW2 prioritisation of global malaria transmission control by the World Health Organization (WHO). Here, India also figures prominently, if somewhat ironically. For it would be Paul F. Russell, Rockefeller Foundation consultant, who would carry the mantle of South Asian malaria expertise into the nascent WHO on the basis of his several years of vector control trials in southern India in the dying days of British rule. Under Russell's unofficial leadership of the WHO's Expert Committee on Malaria,[24] the previous four decades of epidemiological analysis of malaria in relation to hunger, both in India and in the 1920s work of the League of Nations Malaria Commission, were set aside.

The demise of the 'Human Factor' in international malaria deliberations is an important institutional story in its own right. But it is significant for health historiography also because malaria was one of the few major endemic diseases, alongside tuberculosis, for which extensive evidence of its socio-economic determinants was readily at hand in the post-war lead-up to the creation of the World Health Organization. Much of this documentation derived from research conducted in the Indian subcontinent. Indeed, of any global region, it was the early twentieth-century epidemiological studies of malaria in India that challenged the thesis of malaria as a major cause of global poverty, the central argument that would be offered for proceeding with the 1950s global malaria eradication program. In effect, the colonial experience in the Indian subcontinent would be appropriated to underwrite a fundamentally inverted interpretation of the malaria-hunger relationship, one that would manifest in the singular germ-transmission framework of much of the early years of the World Health Organization's work.

Within recent international health historiography, the epistemic impact of the new subdiscipline of nutritional science has been explored by Michael Worboys in his analysis of the 'discovery of malnutrition' in the inter-war period in British colonies in Africa: how, in its application, the new science of nutrition was allowed to overshadow central realities of hunger.[25] In the case of British India, the emergence of nutritional science between the wars has also been explored by V.R. Muraleedharan and David Arnold[26] in accounts of research undertaken into the prevalence of micronutrient deficiencies and 'unbalanced' dietaries. Their work also notes several 1930s household income surveys that indicated grossly insufficient calorie consumption levels (undernourishment) among major portions of the population, both rural and urban. Less explored in this important work however is the extent to which the new nutritional science's focus on dietary quality (micronutrients and 'protective' foods) came to supplant that on quantitative sufficiency and ultimately divert academic and administrative attention away from hunger and subsistence precarity, realities so starkly highlighted in the household income studies. This question has been explored more recently by C. Sathyamala in relation to the post-colonial legacy of the new 'dietary' science.[27]

Important historiographic research has also been undertaken in recent years into the emergence of the League of Nations Health Organisation in the early inter-war period as the first major international health agency with a mandate that extended beyond international epidemic surveillance. This work has cast a renewed spotlight upon the inter-war 'contest' between European and Anglo-American members of the Malaria Commission of the League of Nations Health Organisation in approaches to the global 'malaria problem,' a debate that appeared to pit vector-control techniques against socio-economic measures in the route to malaria mortality control.[28] It has highlighted as well the seminal role malaria continued to play in the shaping of the nascent World Health Organization following the Second World War, and the role of the Rockefeller Foundation in the organization's prioritizing of global malaria control.[29]

Less explored in this literature, however, has been the question of *how*, institutionally, this shift came about – beyond, that is, the ideational power of the paradigm itself and general scientific 'optimism' of the period. For, as will be seen in Chapter 4, the reductive rewriting of disease theory did not proceed unopposed. While the complex interplay among actors within and without the League of Nations Malaria Commission and nascent WHO agencies has begun to be explored,[30] only limited historiographic attention has been directed to the underlying economic claims for malaria eradication: how the malaria 'burden' itself came to be redefined solely in terms of malaria transmission in the days immediately following the close of WW2.[31]

Most importantly, what remains unaddressed in the current historiography is what was set aside in the post-WW2 embrace of the 'malaria as obstacle to development' thesis: which is to say, the extensive empirical and narrative experience underlying interpretation of malaria as a 'social disease' in much of the world, its burden to a large extent a function of intense poverty. Largely invisible have been the detailed accounts of malaria in relation to hunger, a relationship traced in the early years of work of the League of

Nations Malaria Commission, and in greater epidemiological detail before that in the South Asian sanitary records. The colonial public health administration and malaria research records of British India make it possible to analyze with considerable clarity how this broader understanding was lost. They offer critical insights into twentieth-century medical, intellectual, and geopolitical history across a period that represents a final stage in the 'uncoupling' of disease and destitution, one that saw a fundamental transformation in epidemiological concepts, language, and understanding of human subsistence (daily 'bread'), health and disease, and their once-manifest interrelationship.

How specific application of the new medical specialisms of entomology, immunology, and nutritional science research in this period contributed to the academic sidelining of subsistence precarity in malaria analysis takes us beyond any single technology to consider broader spheres of cultural, institutional, and political history of this period, what Worboys has termed, in relation to similar developments in British colonies in Africa, an era of the 'scientizing' or 'medicalizing' of social problems.[32] The consequences for South Asian malaria historiography have been considerable. With central concepts and language of hunger largely superceded, its incorporation within epidemic analysis became increasingly difficult in academic deliberations, and in turn in discussions of malaria mortality.

An important inter-war example of the waning visibility of hunger in modern malaria analysis can be seen in relation to Sri Lankan malaria historiography. Here, too, Western medical analysis has figured largely in this epistemic loss: both in the interpretation of the factors underlying the malaria epidemic of 1934–1935 in Sri Lanka (colonial Ceylon) where famine conditions generally were sidelined;[33] and conversely, one decade later where improvements in food security were overlooked in the interpretation of post-WW2 mortality decline in favour of DDT-based control of malaria transmission, despite Sri Lankan analysts' questioning of such a reading.[34] The 1934–1935 Ceylon epidemic takes on added historiographic significance for being a temporal meeting point between the modern and historical malaria literatures: modern medical analysis of epidemic malaria reaches back to the 1934–1935 epidemic but little further; and historical South Asian malaria research generally extends little beyond. In both cases, the significance of malaria mortality decline in the region between 1920 and 1950 has generally been unrecognized – the period, in a sense, bifurcated and unexplored. It is the continuing prominence of a vector transmission–based reading of modern Sri Lankan malaria history that makes consideration of the epidemic experience of India's southeastern neighbour an important aspect to this larger study.

Without in any way gainsaying the mortality risk inherent to malarial infection, falciparum malaria in particular,[35] one can point to limited appreciation within the historiographic literature of the wide range in disease lethality associated with seasonal malaria transmission.[36] This spectrum varies from a week or so of intermittent fever, on the one hand – 'ordinary' post-monsoon malarial fever with a relatively low mortality rate in historical terms – to extreme prostration and death, on the other. In years of good rains in Punjab, falciparum malaria was widespread. But it was markedly more lethal only in particular circumstances. These, Christophers concluded, related directly to subsistence conditions of the human host, the 'Human Factor,' and indirectly through consequent possible dose effects.[37]

In the absence of this broader perspective, South Asian malaria historiography has been limited largely to the domain of vector *transmission*, the disease's historical mortality burden presumed, it seems, primarily a function of the plasmodial parasite. One example of the epistemic consequences is seen in the view that little was achieved in the realm of 'malaria control' through the colonial period.[38] Save for desultory quinine distribution, the malaria problem is seen as having remained largely unchanged to the end of British rule[39] – even though the 1920–1950 period saw 'fulminant' malaria epidemics decline dramatically in Punjab, and quite possibly elsewhere in the subcontinent. What stands out, then, in much of the historiographic literature is an inadvertent conflation of malaria infection (transmission) and malarial disease (mortality).

The interpretative consequences of this conflation can be seen in the attention directed to the 'malariogenic' effects of canal irrigation.[40] While there is little question that irrigation channels offered highly favourable sites for larval development of *Anopheles culicifacies* – the principal rural malaria vector in the plains of the subcontinent – malaria was endemic to all of rural Punjab quite independent of the vast canal irrigation systems engineered under the British Raj, and indeed across the vast plains of the Indian subcontinent.[41] Unfortunately, with attention directed primarily toward malaria transmission, patterns of actual mortality from the disease have remained unexamined, indeed largely invisible. In this sense, the conflation of the two has served to foreclose essential avenues for incorporating the overall impacts of colonial canal irrigation projects into analysis of historical mortality trends in the region, or indeed for understanding post-1920 mortality decline in Punjab and South Asia more widely.

Profound ecological problems unquestionably were associated with canal irrigation.[42] The detrimental effects of soil alkalization and impact of canal embankments on rural drainage patterns in the province were real, extensive, and in the case of surface drainage obstruction, often preventable.[43] But where malaria developed as a major *mortality* problem in the canal tracts, it was related to the economic effects of waterlogging rather than entomological conditions: underlying decline in agricultural productivity and marked impoverishment. Here, failure to differentiate malaria infection from malaria mortality epidemiologically has left the region's malaria historiography at an impasse, with seemingly little to study regarding malaria's burden under colonial rule until the arrival of the powerful residual insecticides in the 1950s period – and little also, it seems, thereafter.

The current 'malariogenic' critique of canal irrigation stands in notable contrast to earlier colonial-period understanding of malaria's mortality burden in South Asia, and mirrors a narrowed framework to malaria analysis across the final years of British rule. This reductive trajectory was challenged in the inter-war period, both by public figures and by several leading researchers. Yet South Asian epidemic historiography still remains constrained in important areas by the limitations of the modern germ-paradigm, despite what the region's ample historical resources reveal to the contrary. This book attempts to reclaim that earlier understanding of the relationship between hunger and disease through a study of how it was lost.

## This study

It is at the moment of formal acknowledgement by the colonial administration of the role of hunger in the malaria mortality burden of British India that this study begins. Chapter 1 explores the extent to which the economic conclusions to Christophers's *Malaria in the Punjab* report, publicly released in 1911, had come to be taken seriously by the colonial Government of India and, subsequently, by the League of Nations Malaria Commission in the inter-war period. It then identifies and traces the conceptual shifts that took place in the 1930s colonial malaria literature that underlay reinterpretation of Christophers's 'Human Factor' in immunological terms: from hunger-induced weakened immune *capacity* in the human host, to fluctuating levels of *acquired* immunity – now a function of vector transmission. This shift took prominent expression in Western medical commentary on the 1934–1935 malaria epidemic in Sri Lanka (colonial Ceylon), an epidemic that is examined in Chapter 2. Here the central role of famine conditions[44] underlying the epidemic of malaria deaths is analyzed; then, their subsequent omission in expatriate academic interpretations, an omission to which Christophers would call attention in ensuing Royal Society deliberations.

Chapter 3 then traces a parallel inter-war shift in medical attention from quantitative to qualitative (micronutrient) hunger in medical research and writing with the emergence of nutritional science in 1920s South Asia. The epistemic impact of the new dietary science is traced in key government documents through the Bengal Famine Commission (1945) and Bhore Committee (1946) reports,[45] and at the international level within the League of Nations Health Organisation. Highlighted, as well, are the contemporaneous efforts of nascent trade unions, members of the Indian public, and a handful of medical workers – largely 'unsung' figures, South Asian and Anglo-Indian[46] – who queried what they saw as increasingly reductive trends in the application of the new biomedical subdisciplines and who strove to document the commonplace relationship between malaria lethality and human destitution.

These medical subdisciplinary developments are then placed in the broader context of nineteenth-century sanitationist and bacteriological developments in the metropole and their impact on medical thought in colonial South Asia (chapter four). The chapter draws on the work of Christopher Hamlin, who has traced the efforts of leading medical figures in industrializing Britain who challenged the 1842 Sanitary Report's selective focus on 'environmental' filth as the cause of recurring typhus epidemics to the exclusion of predisposing conditions of 'physiological poverty' (destitution).[47] The pages of the annual Punjab sanitary and public health reports reveal a similarly reasoned reluctance on the part of nineteenth-century health officials to embrace an exclusivist germ-transmission theory of epidemic causation; and resistance in the early twentieth century to the inverted thesis of malaria as *cause* of India's poverty.

Such questioning, however, would be overshadowed by the more immediate challenges presented by post-WWI fiscal retrenchment to all aspects of medical research in India, the constraints and consequences of which are explored in Chapter 5. Growing aspirations on the part of colonial researchers for alternate sources of funding would be accompanied by the expanding influence of the Rockefeller Foundation's International Health Rural Division on public health deliberations in South Asia, ultimately leading to vector control trials in southern India in 1938–1941 undertaken by Rockefeller consultant Paul F. Russell – work that would facilitate Russell's rapid rise to prominence as an authority on global malaria.

The influence of the Rockefeller Foundation in shaping an exclusively transmission-based (vector control) framework for the subsequent WHO malaria control program is traced in Chapter 6. Russell's early and preeminent membership on the organization's Expert Committee on Malaria would underlie the designation of malaria transmission control as a global health priority in the earliest deliberations of the nascent WHO's Interim Commission in 1946. This decision, leveraged through UNRRA funding conditionalities (United Nations Relief and Rehabilitation Administration), was accompanied by the sidelining of the extensive South Asian epidemiological malaria research from discussion of the nature of the global malaria *mortality* problem, and the final eclipse of hunger (the 'Human Factor') in understanding of its epidemiology.

Chapter 7 examines the allure of a germ model of malaria shorn of considerations of the human host; the varied professional and often political conveniences of a purely technical approach to vector transmission control in the case of malaria; and the model's ongoing legacy in modern malaria historiography – a legacy evident in the limited visibility of subsistence precarity in modern global mortality decline analysis. As one illustration, the contested assessment of the mortality impact of post-WW2 insecticide-based malaria eradication in Sri Lanka (colonial Ceylon) is revisited.

Chapter 8 considers the on-going legacy of the narrowed epidemic paradigm, seen in the relative invisibility of hunger that continues in modern health historiography. It examines a prominent 1985 study of rapid mortality decline in several low-income countries and queries the limited attention directed to the role of shifts in food security underlying these achievements.[48]

Finally, the study draws attention to the exceptional discerning powers of medical observers in nineteenth-century Britain[49] and early twentieth-century South Asia[50] who challenged the reductive trend in health analysis and sought to re-incorporate subsistence conditions of the human host in interpreting mortality patterns of common endemic diseases in their societies. For them, a reclaiming of this broader 'endemiology' was not a dismissal of science itself. Indeed, many were pre-eminent medical researchers themselves. Their advocacy thus powerfully reminds us, as does Roy Macleod, that '[i]t is clearly possible to examine the culture of western medicine without questioning the benefits of modern [medical] science.'[51]

# Notes

1  G. Macdonald, 'The Analysis of Equilibrium in Malaria,' *Tropical Diseases Bulletin*, 49, 1952, 814, 819–828; reprinted in L. Bruce-Chwatt, and V.J. Glanville, eds., *Dynamics of Tropical Diseases: The Late George Macdonald* (London: Oxford University Press, 1973), 132.
2  Ibid.
3  See ch. 1, text accompanying note 84.
4  S.R. Christophers, 'Malaria in the Punjab,' *Scientific Memoirs by Officers of the Medical and Sanitary Departments of the Government of India* (New Series), No. 46 (Calcutta: Superintendent Govt Printing, 1911), 109.
5  For details, see S. Zurbrigg, *Epidemic Malaria and Hunger in Colonial Punjab* (London and New Delhi: Routledge, 2019), ch. 2.
6  For a summary of malaria transmission bionomics in Punjab, see Appendix I.
7  Christophers, 'Malaria in the Punjab,' 113, 127, 133; S.R. Christophers, and C.A. Bentley, *Malaria in the Duars. Being the Second Report to the Advisory Committee Appointed by the Government of India to Conduct an Enquiry Regarding Blackwater and Other Fevers Prevalent in the Duars* (Simla: Government Monotype Press, 1909), 5, 7.
8  The distinction between acute hunger and lesser degrees of undernourishment ('chronic' hunger) is discussed in Appendix II; as well, in Zurbrigg, *Epidemic Malaria and Hunger*, chs.1, 3. Malaria lethality in South Asia appears to have been heightened mainly by acute hunger and less so by lesser degrees of undernourishment, the latter affecting mortality rates from a range of other common endemic infections; ibid. To this extent, malaria mortality history offers only a partial 'window' on the role of hunger underlying very high pre-modern mortality levels. Nonetheless, because of its historical prevalence in much of the world, malaria figures prominently in human health history.
9  Malaria mortality 'was increased by the enfeeblement of health which a prolonged period of privation had produced'; Christophers, 'Malaria in the Punjab,' 108–109.
10  P. Russell, L.S. West, and R.D. Manwell, *Practical Malariology* (Philadelphia: W.B. Saunders, 1946), 375; J.A. Sinton, 'What Malaria Costs India, Nationally, Socially and Economically,' *Records of the Malaria Survey of India*, 5, 3, Sept. 1935, 223–264; Sinton, 'What Malaria Costs India,' 5, 4, Dec. 1935, 413–489; Sinton, 'What Malaria Costs India,' 6, 1, Mar. 1936, 92–169 [hereafter *RMSI*]; I.A. McGregor, 'Malaria and Nutrition,' in W.H. Wernsdorfer, and I.A. McGregor, eds., *Malaria: Principles and Practice of Malariology* (Edinburgh: Churchill Livingstone, 1988), 754–777, at 754.
11  Zurbrigg, *Epidemic Malaria and Hunger*, ch. 4.

12  Ibid., chs. 12, 9–11.
13  E.L. Perry, *Recent Additions to Our Knowledge of Malaria in the Punjab*. A paper read before the Punjab Branch of the British Medical Association at Simla, on Jul. 17, 1914 (Simla: Thacker, Spink & Co, 1914); C.A. Gill, 'Epidemic or Fulminant Malaria Together with a Preliminary Study of the Part Played by Immunity in Malaria', *Indian Journal of Medical Research*, 2, 1, Jul. 1914, 268–314 [hereafter, *IJMR*]. See ch. 2, below.
14  'Physiological concepts of disease imply that a disease cannot be understood apart from a particular individual suffering from it. . . . [Whereas w]ithin the ontological tradition, disease is posited to be some sort of entity which befalls a previously healthy person'; W. Bynum, 'Nosology,' in W. Bynum, and R. Porter, *Companion Encyclopedia of the History of Medicine* (London: Routledge, 1993), 335–356.
15  Punjab Govt, *Gazetteer of the Gurgaon District, 1883–1884* (Lahore: Government Press, 1884), 131–132.
16  In 1967, Emilio Pampana, former permanent member of the early WHO Secretariat and secretary to the Malaria Committee advised, 'epidemics can take place only in populations without malaria or malaria endemicity at a very low level. . . .[I]f this large proportion of non-immunes does not exist the epidemic cannot materialize'; E. Pampana, and E.J. Pampana, *A Textbook of Malaria Eradication* (London: Oxford University Press, 1969), 92–93. See also M.J. Bouma, and H. van der Kaay, 'The El Niño Southern Oscillation and the historical malaria epidemics on the Indian subcontinent and Sri Lanka: An early warning system for future epidemics?,' *Tropical Medicine and International Health*, 1, 1, Feb. 1996, 86–96. The phenomenon of fluctuating acquired immunity levels in a population and suggested epidemic propensity would come to be denoted as 'unstable' malaria.
17  R.I. Rotberg, 'Nutrition and History,' *Journal of Interdisciplinary History*, 14, 3, 1983, 199–204.
18  S.J. Kunitz, 'Mortality since Malthus,' in R. Scofield, and D. Coleman, *The State of Population Theory: Forward from Malthus* (Oxford: Basil Blackwell, 1986), 279–302; T. Bengtsson, C. Campbell, J.Z. Lee, et al., eds., *Life Under Pressure: Mortality and Living Standards in Europe and Asia, 1700–1900* (Cambridge, MA: MIT Press, 2004), 42–44.
19  See, e.g., A. Celli, 'The Restriction of Malaria in Italy,' in *Transactions of the Fifteenth International Congress on Hygiene and Demography, Washington, September 23–28, 1912* (Washington, D.C., 1913), 516–531.
20  Here, the term 'infective' is used to include those microbial infections that are not primarily communicable (i.e., 'infectious'), such as many forms of pneumonia, where heightened mortality risk is seen particularly among the immune-compromised.
21  For analysis of the evolution of colonial malaria control policy leading up to, and following, the 1909 Imperial Malaria Conference at Simla, see Zurbrigg, *Epidemic Malaria and Hunger*, chs. 7–8.
22  R. McCarrison, *Studies in Deficiency Diseases* (London: Henry Frowde, Hodder & Stoughton, 1921); S.C. Seal, 'Diet and the Incidence of Disease in India,' *Indian Medical Gazette*, May 1938, 291–301.
23  P.J. Brown, 'Malaria, Miseria, and Underpopulation in Sardinia: The "Malaria Blocks Development" Cultural Model,' *Medical Anthropology*, 17, 3, May 1997, 239–254.
24  Expert Committee on Malaria, 'Summary Minutes of the First Session,' 22–25 April 1947, WHO.IC/Mal./6, 1–45 [hereafter, ECM]; ECM, 'Report on the First Session,' Geneva, 22–25 April 1947, WHO.IC/Mal./4, 3.

25  M. Worboys, 'The Discovery of Colonial Malnutrition Between the Wars,' in D. Arnold, *Imperial Medicine and Indigenous Societies* (Manchester: Manchester University Press, 1988), 208–225. The interpretative power of the microbiologic framework in modern epidemic analysis has been explored as well in relation to the 1970s thesis of 'refeeding malaria' in which starvation is considered to protect from malaria. For a critique, see S. Zurbrigg, 'Did Starvation Protect from Malaria? Distinguishing Between Severity and Lethality of Infectious Disease in Colonial India,' *Social Science History*, 21, 1, 1997, 27–58.

26  V.R. Muraleedharan, 'Diet, Disease and Death in Colonial South India,' *Economic and Political Weekly*, Jan. 1–8, 1994, 55–63; D. Arnold, 'The "Discovery" of Malnutrition and Diet in Colonial India,' *Indian Economic and Social History Review*, 31, 1, 1994, 1–26 [hereafter, *IESHR*].

27  C. Sathyamala, 'Nutrition as a Public Health Problem (1990–1947),' International Institute of Social Studies, Working Paper No. 510, Dec. 2010.

28  J.A. Nájera aptly refers to the 'two schools' as the 'anti-parasite' group and the 'anti-disease' group, highlighting the central distinction between infection (transmission) and disease ('pernicious' morbidity and mortality); in 'The control of tropical diseases and socio-economic development (with special reference to malaria and its control),' *Parassitologia*, 36, 17–33, 1994. See also S. Litsios, 'Malaria Control, the Cold War, and the Postwar Reorganization of International Assistance,' *Medical Anthropology*, 17, 1997, 255–278; J. Farley, *Brock Chisholm, the World Health Organization, and the Cold War* (Vancouver: University of British Columbia Press, 2008); H. Evans, 'European Malaria Policy in the 1920s and 1930s: The Epidemiology of Minutiae,' *Isis*, 80, 1, Mar. 1989, 40–59.

29  See, J. Gillespie, 'Europe, America, and the Space of International Health,' in S. Gross Solomon, L. Murand, and P. Zylberman, eds., *Shifting Boundaries in Public Health: Europe in the Twentieth Century* (Rochester: University of Rochester Press, 2008), 114–137; J. Gillespie, 'Social Medicine, Social Security and International Health, 1940–60,' in Esteban Rodriguez-Ocana, ed., *The Politics of the Healthy Life: An International Perspective* (Sheffield: European Association for the History of Medicine and Health, 2002), 219–253; S. Amrith, *Decolonizing International Health: India and Southeast Asia, 1930–65* (Basingstoke: Palgrave Macmillan, 2006); J. Farley, *To Cast Out Disease: A History of the International Health Division of the Rockefeller Foundation (1913–1951)* (New York: Oxford University Press, 2004). See also, I. Borowy, 'International Social Medicine between the Wars: Positioning a Volatile Concept,' *Hygiea Internationalis*, 6, 2, 2007, 13–35, at 29–30.

30  With regard to the challenges faced by Ludwik Rajchman, LNHO Director, and Andrija Stampar as prominent 'social medicine' advocates in the LNHO, see Farley, *Brock Chisholm*; P. Weindling, 'Philanthropy and World Health: The Rockefeller Foundation and the League of Nations Health Organisation,' *Minerva*, 35, 3, 1997, 269–281; Gillespie, 'Social Medicine, Social Security and International Health,' 219–253.

31  Packard points out how weak the evidence was for the original premise of MBD, in R.M. Packard, 'Malaria Dreams: Postwar Visions of Health and Development in the Third World,' *Medical Anthropology*, 17, 1997, 279–296, at 284–286; R.M. Packard, ' "Roll Back Malaria"? Reassessing the Economic Burden of Malaria,' *Population and Development Review*, 35, 1, Mar. 2009, 53–87.

32  M. Worboys, 'The Discovery of Colonial Malnutrition Between the Wars,' in D. Arnold, ed., *Imperial Medicine and Indigenous Societies* (Manchester: Manchester University Press, 1988), 208–225.

33 P.F. Russell, *Malaria: Basic Principles Briefly Stated* (Oxford: Blackwell Scientific Publs, 1952), 100; G. Macdonald, 'The Analysis of Equilibrium in Malaria,' in L. Bruce-Chwatt, and V.J. Glanville, eds., *Dynamics of Tropical Diseases: The Late George Macdonald* (London: Oxford University Press, 1973), 132; C.L. Dunn, *Malaria in Ceylon: An Enquiry into its Causes* (London: Bailliere, Tindall and Cox, 1936).

34 K.N. Sarkar, *The Demography of Ceylon* (Colombo: Govt Press, 1958), 123; S.A. Meegama, 'The Decline in Maternal and Infant Mortality and its relation to Malaria Eradication,' *Population Studies*, 23, 2, 1969, 289–302.

35 The two main malaria species transmitted in Punjab were *P. vivax* ('benign tertian') and *P. falciparum* ('malignant' or 'sub-tertian' malaria), the latter associated with greater morbidity and mortality related to greater parasitization of red blood cells in the human host, potentially causing cerebral malaria also among the well-nourished. Even in falciparum infections, however, historical lethality (case fatality rate) varied greatly depending on previous exposure ('acquired' immunity); immuno-competence (factors affecting general immune *capacity* or its suppression); strain of plasmodium; and possibly, dose of infection. The latter may have contributed to the lethality of infection among Europeans in their exposure to transmission conditions in holoendemic regions of sub-Saharan west Africa, where the prime vector (*Anopheles gambiae*) is a highly anthropophilic species resulting in extreme inoculation rates and high levels of protective *acquired* immunity among the adult population but intense infection rates in the as yet non-immune.

36 Variation in lethality of microbial infections is acknowledged theoretically in modern epidemiology in the concepts of 'case fatality rate' and 'epidemic *equation*', the latter expressing the interplay between germ (pathogen) exposure and human host response or resistance. Marked differentials in child survival rates in relation to undernourishment have been documented in R. Martorell, and T.J. Ho, 'Malnutrition, Morbidity and Mortality,' in H. Mosley, and L. Chen, eds., *Child Survival: Strategies for Research,* Supplement to vol. 10, *Population and Development Review*, 1984, 49–68. Historians generally acknowledge a hunger-infection lethality link, but the question is rarely pursued for paucity of mortality and infection incidence data. An important exception is the field of historical nutritional anthropometry: undernourishment prevalence tracked through historical trends in mean adult stature; see, e.g., R. Floud, R. Fogel, B. Harris, and Sok Chul Hong, eds., *The Changing Body: Health, Nutrition, and Human Development in the Western World since 1700* (Cambridge: Cambridge University Press, 2011). Awareness of the wide range in lethality of common endemic infections in the pre-modern era centrally informed Thomas McKeown's exploration of the determinants of mortality decline in England and Wales; *The Modern Rise of Population* (London: Edward Arnold, 1976), 73.

37 Based on his sparrow experiments, Christophers considered 'dose' of infection to be the number of sporozoites injected by an infected mosquito during a human blood meal. He appears to have hypothesized that immune-suppression among the famished led to higher parasite levels in vector mosquitoes and in turn in the dose of subsequent human infections. On this, see Zurbrigg, *Epidemic Malaria and Hunger*, 78–82, 192–194.

38 W. Bynum, 'Malaria in inter-war British India,' *Parassitologia*, 42, 2000, 25–31; M. Harrison, ' "Hot Beds of Disease": Malaria and Civilization in Nineteenth-Century British India,' *Parassitologia*, 40, 1998, 11–18; S. Polu, *Infectious Disease in India, 1892–1940: Policy-Making and the Perceptions of Risk* (London: Palgrave Macmillan, 2012); D. Arnold, 'Crisis and Contradiction in India's

Public Health,' in D. Porter, ed., *The History of Public Health and the Modern State* (Amsterdam: Rodopi, 1994), 335–355; V.R. Muraleedharan, and D. Veeraraghavan, 'Anti-malaria Policy in the Madras Presidency: An Overview of the Early Decades of the Twentieth Century,' *Medical History*, 36, 1992, 290–305.

39 This assumption appears in much recent writing on the malaria burden, with Sinton's mortality estimates from early twentieth-century experience tending to inform perceptions of the pre-DDT South Asian malaria experience; V.P. Sharma, and K.N. Mehrotra, 'Malaria Resurgence in India: A Critical Study,' *Social Science Medicine*, 22, 1986, 835–845, at 835; V.P. Sharma, 'Battling Malaria Iceberg Incorporating Strategic Reforms in Achieving Millennium Development Goals & Malaria Elimination In India,' *IJMR*, 136, Dec. 2012, 907–925.

40 S. Watts, 'British Development Policies and Malaria in India 1897-c.1929,' *Past and Present*, 165, 1999, 141–181; E. Whitcombe, 'The Environmental Costs of Irrigation in British India: Waterlogging, Salinity, Malaria,' in D. Arnold, and R. Guha, eds., *Nature, Culture, Imperialism: Essays on the Environmental History of South Asia* (New Delhi: Oxford University Press, 1995), 237–259; I. Klein, 'Malaria and Mortality in Bengal,' 1840–1921,' *IESHR*, 9, 2, 1972, 132–160; I. Klein, 'Development and Death: Reinterpreting Malaria, Economics and Ecology in British India,' *IESHR*, 38, 2, 2001, 147–179; K. Wakimura, 'Epidemic Malaria and "Colonial Development": Reconsidering the Cases of Northern and Western India,' Economic History Congress XIII, Buenos Aires, Argentina, July 2002, mimeo.

41 The western canal tracts generally were less affected by the fulminant form of malaria than other regions of the province. Moreover, on-going expansion of the canal networks in the western half of the province in the final decades of the colonial period was associated not with heightened mortality but rather with declining crude death rates, in step with trends across the province; Zurbrigg, *Epidemic Malaria and Hunger*, chs. 2, 4, and 6.

42 See, for example, I. Agnihotri, 'Ecology, Land Use and Colonisation: The Canal Colonies of Punjab,' *IESHR*, 33, 1, 1996, 37–58; I. Stone, *Canal Irrigation in British India: Perspectives on Technological Changes in a Peasant Economy* (Cambridge: Cambridge University Press, 1984); E. Whitcombe, *Agrarian Conditions in Northern India, I, The United Provinces Under British Rule,* 1860–1900 (Berkeley: University of California Press, 1972); E. Whitcombe, 'The Environmental Costs of Irrigation'; Klein, 'Development and Death.'

43 Zurbrigg, *Epidemic Malaria and Hunger*, 282–286. In large tracts of western deltaic Bengal also, the effects of rail and road infrastructure construction on agriculture productivity were catastrophic, heightened malaria intensity following in train; C.A Bentley, 'Some Economic Aspects of Bengal Malaria,' *IMG*, Sept. 1922, 321–326; C.A Bentley, in *Report of the Royal Commission on Agriculture in India*, vol. IV, Bengal Evidence (London: HMSO, 1928), 240–247. Nor is it suggested that criticism of the colonial government's inaction on malaria 'control' is unwarranted. Even in highly localised urban malarious areas, such as Bombay municipality, feasible transmission-control efforts were underfunded, at best erratic, and frequently abandoned. See also Muraleedharan and Veeraraghavan, 'Anti-malaria policy in the Madras Presidency.'

44 R. Briercliffe, *The Ceylon Malaria Epidemic, 1934–35. Report by the Director of Medical and Sanitary Service* (Colombo: Ceylon Govt Press, Sept. 1935), 27, 43.

45 Famine Inquiry Commission, India, *Report on Bengal*, (New Delhi: GOI, 1945); *Report of the Health Survey and Development Committee* (New Delhi: GOI, 1946).

46 See ch. 3, 114.
47 C. Hamlin, 'Predisposing Causes and Public Health in Early Nineteenth-Century Medical Thought,' *Society for the Social History of Medicine*, 5, 1, Apr. 1992, 43–70; C. Hamlin, *Public Health and Social Justice in the Age of Chadwick* (Cambridge: Cambridge University Press, 1998). Similar concerns emerged among early twentieth-century analysts in the industrialized West who also recognized the limitations of a public health mandate selectively directed to germ-transmission control and elimination of micronutrient deficiencies; I. Galdston, 'Humanism and Public Health,' *Bulletin of the History of Medicine*, Jan. 1940, 1032–1039; E. Ackerknecht, 'Hygiene in France, 1815–1848,' *Bulletin of the History of Medicine*, 22, 1948, 117–155. For analysis of the continued dominance of biomedical theories of disease, and of broader social epidemiological frameworks that have emerged in response, see for example, T.K.S. Ravindran, and R. Gaitonde, eds., *Health Inequities in India: A Synthesis of Recent Evidence* (Singapore: Springer, 2018); N. Krieger, *Epidemiology and the People's Health: Theory and Context* (Oxford: Oxford University Press, 2011); A.-E. Birn, Y. Pillay, and T.H. Holtz, *Textbook of Global Health*, 4th ed. (Oxford: Oxford University Press, 2017); I. Qadeer, K. Sen, and K.R. Nayar, eds., *Public Health and the Poverty of Reforms* (New Delhi: Sage, 2001).
48 S.B. Halstead, J.A. Walsh, and K.S. Warren, *Good Health at Low Cost* (New York: Rockefeller Foundation, 1985); D. Balabanova, M. McKee, and A. Mills, eds., *'Good Health at Low Cost': Twenty Years On* (London: London School of Hygiene and Tropical Medicine, 2011).
49 C. Hamlin, 'William Pulteney Alison, the Scottish Philosophy, and the Making of a Political Medicine,' *Journal of the History of Medicine and Allied Sciences*, 61, 2, 2006, 144–186.
50 N. Gangulee, *Health and Nutrition in India* (London: Faber and Faber, 1939); S.R. Christophers, and C.A. Bentley, 'The Human Factor: An Extension of our Knowledge regarding the Epidemiology of Malarial Disease,' in W.E. Jennings, ed., *Transactions of the Bombay Medical Congress, 1909*, (Bombay: Bennett, Coleman & Co., 1910), 78–83.
51 R. Macleod, 'Introduction,' in R. Macleod, and M. Lewis, eds., *Disease, Medicine and Empire* (London: Routledge, 1988), 12.

# 1

# THE 'HUMAN FACTOR' TRANSFORMED

Certainly by 1908 with the commissioning of the Punjab malaria enquiry report,[1] the colonial administration in India was taking seriously the growing notoriety associated with the 'exalted' form of malaria in the country, and was attempting to decipher, and at some level grapple with, the spectrum of causal factors underlying that lethality. Here, by way of context to the Human Factor's ultimate demise, the circumstances leading up to the 1911 enquiry report, and the remarkable (if brief) period of transparency thereafter regarding the hunger-malaria relationship, are outlined.

The preceding decade had been one in which the British Raj was coming to terms with mounting expectations for vector 'extirpation' from both the colonial and metropolitan medical professions, expectations triggered in 1897–1898 by Ross's confirmation of mosquitoes as malaria vector. A six-year trial program of intensive mosquito destruction operations (1902–1908) at the Mian Mir rural cantonment in central Punjab, however, had manifestly failed to eliminate malaria. The severe epidemic in the autumn of 1908 had swept through the cantonment as dramatically as elsewhere in the province and made it clear that there was no ready 'fix' on the horizon for the control of malaria transmission in the vast rural areas of the subcontinent where the disease took its principal toll. Adding to the administration's malaria policy predicament, professional and public concerns about the safety of quinine were compounding the crisis of sanitary legitimacy already made acute with the outbreak of plague a decade earlier.

Mounting public calls in the British and Indian medical press for mosquito extirpation had left the colonial administration little choice but to take into confidence senior medical, sanitary, and military officials regarding the broader economic dimensions to the malaria problem in the subcontinent. It did so through two detailed epidemiological studies of malaria mortality in relation to mass destitution, the findings of which were presented at two medical conferences: the Bombay Medical Congress in February 1909[2] where the conclusions of a recent enquiry into the extreme malaria lethality on the Duars tea plantations were presented (*Malaria in the Duars*, 1909);[3] and the October 1909 Imperial Malaria conference at Simla[4] where S.R.

Christophers's findings regarding the 'disastrous' 1908 malaria epidemic in Punjab framed the proceedings.[5]

The emergence of a concerted malaria policy in colonial South Asia can be traced in large part to the epidemiological findings presented at these two medical gatherings. Though subject to undoubted editing, published proceedings from these meetings open up for historians much more complex aspects to the malaria deliberations taking place within the administration at this point than the vector extirpationist 'versus' ameliorationist ('quininist') framework that had come to characterize public malaria policy discussion in the immediate post-1897 years. They provide, in turn, essential context for interpreting the impact of malaria policy across the final decades of colonial rule, policy directed primarily to reducing malaria's *mortality* burden.

At the Bombay Medical Congress, a report on the disconcerting results of the Mian Mir trial[6] was followed by a paper entitled 'The Human Factor: An Extension of our Knowledge regarding the Epidemiology of Malarial Disease,' co-authored by Christophers and C.A. Bentley (1873–1949), former chief medical officer of the Empire of India and Ceylon Tea Company.[7] The paper summarized the findings of their recent investigation into blackwater fever on the northeastern Duars tea plantations, and their wider implications. Blackwater fever was a generally uncommon but serious medical syndrome associated with malaria involving sudden red blood cell destruction (hemolysis). Considered to be triggered by repeated, often irregular, quinine use, it was seen typically in areas of very high malaria endemicity among those with ready access to the drug. More problematic for the administration, the increasing notoriety associated with blackwater fever on the Duars estates was rapidly undermining medical and public confidence in the therapeutic safety of quinine – and by extension, the principal anti-malarial policy that the government then had at hand.

The Duars enquiry examined two questions. First, the pathophysiology of the syndrome and its relationship to quinine consumption, findings that were immediately published in the prestigious *Scientific Memoirs* series as an official report.[8] And second, analysis of the factors underlying the peculiarly intense ('exalted') form of malaria observed among the Duars plantations' labour population. This second report was a scathing account of conditions of frank destitution among this group, and the role of the labour recruitment system under prevailing indentured labour law in creating and perpetuating such conditions.[9] 'Physiologic misery,'[10] the two investigators had concluded, played an overriding role in the 'intense' form of malaria seen on the Duars estates, the effects of which were spilling over to the non-immune European managerial staff in the form of inordinate quinine use and cases of blackwater fever in turn. Their conclusions, in other words, extended far beyond questions of quinine safety and bore profound implications for understanding malaria mortality patterns more generally in the subcontinent.

Not surprisingly, this latter portion of the enquiry, entitled *Malaria in the Duars*, was left unpublished until its tabling as an unheralded one-off document in 1911. Its conclusions however would thoroughly inform the 'Human Factor' paper presented at the Bombay Congress in February 1909. There, the two investigators articulated a more general relationship between economic hardship and malaria lethality, pointing to endemic destitution among indentured workers in labour camps and industrial sites across much of the subcontinent, also expressed in an intense ('exalted') form of malaria.

The politically incriminating questions raised in Bombay by the second Duars report, and by the 'fulminant' malaria epidemic in Punjab in the autumn of 1908, would form the backdrop eight months later to the Imperial Malaria Conference at Simla in October 1909. The six-day conference attended by leading medical, sanitary, military, and administrative officials was framed by Christophers's findings that identified harvest failure and 'scarcity' (famine-level foodgrain prices) as underlying the 1908 epidemic's severe lethality.[11] Together, the two enquiry reports directly implicated not just epidemic destitution ('famine'), but endemic immiseration in British India as well, conditions related in no small part to indentured labour legislation dating from the mid-nineteenth century. The goal of the Simla conference was to produce consensus on where government priorities should lie: the directing of public effort and resources preferentially to areas of 'intense' malaria, and to their underlying causes, rather than to malaria transmission *per se*. 'If we could prevent the mortality from epidemic fulminant malaria,' Christophers urged, 'we should have removed the most urgent and distressing effects of this disease and those manifestations which the people themselves are most impressed by.'[12]

Formal acknowledgement at Simla of the role of acute hunger in the malaria mortality burden, and subsequent publication of the Punjab enquiry report in late 1911, appear to have succeeded to some considerable extent in quelling public calls by members of the sanitary administration and Indian Medical Service for large-scale expenditure on mosquito control.[13] It also opened up permissible space to voice concern over the larger economic dimensions underlying the malaria mortality problem in the subcontinent.

## The 'Human Factor' within colonial malaria discourse

In the years immediately following the official release of Christophers's Punjab report in late 1911, hunger overtly framed public health analysis of the malaria problem at many levels. In his annual report as Special Malaria Officer for Punjab, C.A. Gill in 1914 would describe conditions in the canal colonies as 'unfavourable to malaria, in so far as the people are well fed and have consequently a high resisting power. A well-nourished man may contract malaria, but he very rarely dies of it.'[14] Attention to the human 'host' in predicting malaria lethality patterns took practical expression as well in the routines of provincial public health administrations. Through the final decades of the colonial period Punjab officials continued to track weekly rainfall and foodgrain prices to predict autumn epidemic potential in the province, predictions upon which food and quinine distribution efforts were based.[15]

Attention to the 'Human Factor' in malaria lethality during these years extended to the formal academic literature as well. 'Christophers has shown very clearly,' a prominent tropical medicine text would point out in 1922, '[that] in malarious localities people of low social status suffer more than the well-to-do and has called attention to the direct and indirect action of various economic factors which influence the spread and intensity of the disease.'[16] Similar views found echo that same year in the *Indian Medical Gazette (IMG)* in a special issue devoted to the 'Economic Factor in Tropical Diseases.'[17] Where 'many millions of the poorer population live on a minimum of food in India,' the lead editorial urged, the medical community needed to take into account 'the play of economic factors in inducing endemic and epidemic disease,' including malaria. '[P]revalence of anopheline carriers is but one factor in the origin of such terrible epidemics [as that in 1908]. . . . Food prices are just as important. A lowered and impoverished diet diminishes body resistance.'[18] Here, as at Simla earlier, concern for hunger extended beyond famine, to endemic 'semi-starvation.' 'Dr. Bentley's statistics for malaria in Bengal,' the editorial pointed out, 'find a parallel in Colonel Christophers' important work on epidemic malaria in the Punjab (1911).' Nor, the *IMG* editorial insisted, was the importance of hunger limited to its effect on malaria. Poverty and economic conditions were now being seen to be of 'immense importance' to a range of infectious diseases.[19]

Timing of the 1922 editorial may well have been prompted by a recently completed study of lathyrism by a senior pathologist at the Calcutta Medical College. A summary of H.W. Acton's findings was published in the same September issue of the *Indian Medical Gazette* and illustrated the stark economic dimensions to the disease: the desperation of labourers forced by destitution to accept wages paid in *kesari dal*, a legume well known to cause permanent neuro-paralysis.[20] In his research into the syndrome, Acton had identified the triggering agent as a specific neurotoxin. But he concluded that the underlying cause was economic, and suggested that the solution to lathyrism had to be 'a sociological one,' starting with abolition of the rural debt-slavery that forced workers to accept *kesari dal* as their wages. His second recommendation was directed to more effective famine relief 'during the years of a bad monsoon, as well as controlling the price of wheat, rice, and *dal*, so that the poor can afford to buy these articles of food.'[21]

Other papers in the September 1922 special issue of the *Indian Medical Gazette* addressed economic factors at a broader level. A detailed report by Bentley on 'Economic Aspects of Bengal Malaria' critiqued land tenure policy in the province and urged government economic development

21

(agricultural 'bonification').[22] Citing parallels with Christophers's Punjab conclusions, the *IMG* editorial argued that 'the study of economics should be part of the medical curriculum, at least in India.'[23]

The first major colonial textbook on malaria, published in India in 1910, also pointed unequivocally to 'impoverishment' as an important 'personal predisposing cause' of malaria mortality. 'There is no doubt,' Patrick Hehir would write, 'that persons in good health are capable of throwing off a mild infection of malaria, . . . [whereas] all conditions enfeebling the body increase the susceptibility to malarial infection.'[24] As with Christophers and Bentley, Hehir's concern was also grounded in economic pragmatism: residual infection among the impoverished in mass labour camps led to wider dissemination of the disease and increased labour costs. Much of Hehir's malaria textbook dealt with anti-mosquito and anti-larval techniques for interrupting transmission and malaria chemotherapeutics. But adequate remedies, he clearly also was saying, lay not just in medical and entomological measures but in the legislative sphere as well. Malaria control policy ought to extend to economic measures that ensured 'a sufficient quantity of wholesome food' such as 'enforcement of a minimum wage for all labourers on all contractors and other employers of coolie labour . . . [a policy] deserving all possible attention.'[25]

This level of frankness in public discussion of hunger in British India was unprecedented. The phrase the 'Human Factor' itself was of course a euphemism. Nonetheless, the Simla proceedings had endowed the subject with legitimacy both as a medical diagnosis and as a leading public health issue. Two decades later, the second edition of Patrick Hehir's *Prophylaxis of Malaria in India* continued to point to 'impoverishment' as a key factor underlying severity of malarial infection, if such references were now tucked amidst the vastly expanded microbiological and entomological sections of updated research. Indeed, in the final pages of the 490-page 1927 edition, Hehir returned, with some 'melancholy,' to the subject of socio-economic conditions. 'Effective dealing with malaria is not simply a matter of doing away with collections of water, filling up or draining borrow-pits and distributing a limited amount of quinine,' he urged. 'A progressive anti-malaria policy in rural areas would . . . attach the greatest importance to the economic and social factor.'[26]

What also distinguished this period was the clarity with which medical figures stressed the distinction between infection and disease (mortality). In its same September editorial, the 1922 *Indian Medical Gazette* stressed that '[w]hat may be merely hookworm *infection* in a well nourished individual passes into hookworm *disease* in states of malnutrition.'[27] It was a distinction articulated a decade earlier by Bentley at the Third Meeting of the General Malaria Committee in November 1912 in relation to the 'moribund' river tracts of lower Bengal:

> the occurrence of epidemics of malarial *disease* among the usu-
> ally tolerant or partially tolerant races, indigenous to malarious

country, signifies something beyond the *mere presence of infection and anopheles*, . . . and it is just that '*something*' which requires to be investigated by malariologists in India.[28]

'[A]lthough the brilliant discoveries of Laveran and Ross have extended our knowledge of the parasitology of malaria,' he continued,

> we are still ignorant of many of the factors responsible for the occurrence of malaria disease, more especially when it appears in epidemic form. . . . [T]he infection index of a population may remain almost stationary although at one time disease might be prevalent and another time almost absent. Unfortunately the significance of these observations has been largely overlooked and the word 'malaria' is almost invariably applied to describe both the conditions of infection and the state of disease which may be associated with it.[29]

By calling attention to this distinction, Bentley was not suggesting the seasonal appearance of malarial fever was innocuous, but highlighting instead the profound contrast in morbid consequence under conditions of economic hardship.

The impetus at this point behind such transparency clearly lay beyond the medical realm, in the strategic need to counter the arguments of those within the sanitary administration advocating 'mosquito extirpation' as a general sanitary policy. But the stimulus had broader origins as well. In the wake of the Boer War–era scandal of physical 'degeneracy' amongst British recruits, medical and public attention in Britain too had returned to poverty to account for the continuing high prevalence of tuberculosis and nutritional stunting among the poorer classes. There was growing recognition of the insufficiency of sanitationist public health interventions in remedying such conditions, which at their root lay in poverty. As delegates were gathering at Simla in October 1909, for example, James Niven, Medical Officer of Health for Manchester, was preparing his Presidential Address, 'Poverty and Disease,' for presentation to the Epidemiological Section of the Royal Society of Medicine in London. In his talk he urged that economic insecurity – irregular employment, livelihood, and time available to women for the feeding and care of children – still determined much of the excess mortality amongst the poor in Britain, and that tuberculosis remained 'the most convenient mirror of [this] poverty.'[30]

It was this period as well in Britain that saw the emergence of significant 'social welfare' policies, measures in no small part adopted in response to testimony of medical officials who explicitly linked disease and physical degeneracy. Such legislation included a Workmen's Compensation Act, provision of school meals in 1906, and two years later, a Mines Act and initiation of old age pensions. Growing pressure in the international sphere for further labour reforms culminated in 1919 in the formation of the International Labour Organization (ILO) with the aim that all states should have standard labour legislation to ensure 'there was no unfair competition' amongst industrialized countries.[31] Though yet modest in scope, legislation on conditions and hours of work held major implications for bare subsistence precarity. The emergence of the ILO itself was an expression of growing political pressure – in Britain with the emergence of trade unions and the Labour Party – to address the economic determinants of health.

In India, this period corresponds to a beginning move away from the expendability of labour ('using up coolies'[32]) with legislation that began the process of ultimately dismantling indentured labour laws. Changes to the Labour Code date, hardly coincidentally, from the 1908 *Malaria in the Duars* enquiry, amendments that would see planters' power of 'private arrest' abolished.[33] Final abolition of the Indentured Labour Act would not come for another twelve years, with the colonial government in 1920 facing increasing international opprobrium after India joined the newly instituted International Labour Organization.[34] Indentured labour contracts were phased out over the following five years, although penal convictions continued to be registered under the old Act for some years.[35] Abolition in 1920 nonetheless marked the beginning of rudimentary public oversight over conditions of work on the tea estates. A 1922 Enquiry Committee for the first time sought to investigate levels of food consumption and individual and family budgets of tea plantation labour on some estates.[36]

## Malaria as a 'Social Disease': the League of Nations Malaria Commission

Alongside its industrial-scale military slaughter, the 1914–1918 war would offer an equally stark demonstration of the relationship between hunger and epidemic disease. By the end of the war, mass destitution in Russia and eastern Europe had spawned widespread and highly lethal typhus and malaria epidemics, a mortality toll that helped spur the creation in 1922 of a Health Organisation within the newly formed League of Nations. Its initial mandate was global epidemiological surveillance, and here the recently created Rockefeller Foundation responded immediately as a major financial contributor.[37] Interest soon expanded however to the investigation of broader socioeconomic conditions underlying epidemic mortality patterns. With respect to malaria, S.P. James, an earlier research colleague of Christophers in the Indian Medical Service, recounted that at this point '[f]aith in the efficacy of every prophylactic and therapeutic measure had fallen almost to zero.'

> Everyone who had actually taken part in efforts to deal with malaria in different parts of the world during the War came home with the

24

uncomfortable feeling that we know much less about the disease than we thought we did. . . . Malaria was everywhere prevalent and severe . . . [raising] the old question whether malaria among poor illiterate people should be dealt with as an isolated problem separate from the general medical and public health problems of the country concerned.[38]

Researchers in Europe were arriving at similar economic conclusions to those of Bentley in Bengal a continent away, concluding that agricultural development and prosperity were a pre-condition for solving the malaria problem.

By 1924, a specially dedicated Malaria Commission (LNMC) had been established within the League of Nations Health Organisation. Within its first year it had embarked upon a series of study tours undertaken in the still malarious regions of eastern and southern Europe and the southern United States, to observe and collate the varying experience of control efforts. One of the first countries included was Italy where intensive malaria control work had been going on since the turn of the century under the energetic guidance of Angelo Celli. Although Italian scientists had been at the forefront of efforts to unravel the microbiological and entomological intricacies underlying malaria transmission, anti-malaria policies had not been directed primarily to vector control but rather to ensuring access to treatment (quinine) and promoting agricultural improvement. The approach, referred to as 'bonificazione,'[39] involved land reclamation that made possible intensive agricultural production on previously waste or abandoned land, with permanent settlement of the labourers who were guaranteed a portion of the produce.

Such efforts, Celli explained in a 1912 address, were not limited to drainage. 'We are now directing our attention to new laws to make those lands remunerative . . . [by providing] loans to labourers in addition to landowners, inexpensive credit with interest redirected back into farms.'[40] The goal, the Malaria Commission would later observe, was one of changing 'a swampy region with a poor, scattered, often semi-nomadic population into a settled well-to-do one. . . . Now that villages have been formed, the poor law can come into action; sick-clubs are formed to bring medical assistance to those unable to pay for it.'[41] Malaria deaths in the country over this initial period of Celli's efforts had declined dramatically, from an estimated 16,000 per year, a rate of 0.49 per 1,000 in 1900, to 2,045 in 1914 (0.057 per 1,000).[42]

In its 1924 overview of anti-malarial measures in Europe, the Malaria Commission pointed out that land reclamation efforts in malarious tracts of Europe likewise often had had little impact on rates of malaria transmission.[43] Improved economic conditions however, N.H. Swellengrebel concluded in an appended report on malaria in Italy, meant 'the disease, although still present, had lost much of its terrors.'[44] Land reclamation in Italy, he stressed,

> has been closely connected with anti-malarial measures [n]ot because these 'bonifications' were supposed to have any immediate beneficial effect in reducing the incidence of malaria, even when complete, but because they were rightly supposed to enrich the population, the enhanced well-being reflecting favourably on the resistance of the population against various diseases and against malaria in particular. The argument in favour of encouraging 'bonifications' was an economic one: to gain sanitary ends by economic means.[45]

Coming from a researcher highly regarded for his work on 'species sanitation' (the targeting of anti-mosquito operations specifically to those anopheline species responsible for transmission in a region), Swellengrebel could hardly be accused of being biased against mosquito control.[46]

Three years later, in a report on 'Antimalarial Measures in Europe,' the Malaria Commission acknowledged that despite many experimental programs in Malaria Commission member countries directed at vector 'sanitation,' there were in fact few examples of successful rural control of malaria transmission.[47] It concluded that the painstaking and costly work of anti-mosquito measures as a general approach to malaria control was unaffordable even in Europe; their costs, moreover, put at risk adequate funding of agricultural improvements.[48] Though not ruling out the importance of local anti-larval measures where financially and technically feasible, the Commission urged that the benefits of such programs had to be assessed in relation to their financial costs, and not undertaken at the expense of economic and therapeutic measures. 'Since the advent of the new knowledge of the transmission of malaria by mosquitoes,' it warned, 'there has been a tendency to forget that there are many methods of dealing with the disease.'[49] As Bentley had done two decades earlier in Bengal, the Commission urged that 'a sharp distinction should be made between reduction of mortality and morbidity, two results of antimalarial activity which need by no means run a parallel course.'[50]

## The Malaria Commission's study tour in India

It would be to India that the Commission turned in 1929 for extensive experience of 'malaria among poor illiterate people . . . in the tropics.'[51] The four-month India tour led by W.A.C. Schüffner, Director of the Section of Tropical Hygiene of the Royal Colonial Institute, Amsterdam,[52] studied malaria conditions and control efforts in three major malarial regions of the subcontinent: Bengal, Punjab, and the hyperendemic hill tracts in the Himalayan foothills and the Deccan peninsula. For all three regions the study group ultimately came to concur with local malaria researchers regarding the centrality of underlying economic conditions in determining the illness and mortality burden of the disease. Several Commission members had expressed initial scepticism over Bentley's interpretation of the malaria problem in the 'dying river' tracts of lower Bengal, in the 1860s and 1870s referred to as 'Burdwan fever,' views which 'were so contrary to all our own experiences.'[53] However by the close of the eight-day tour of Bengal, Schüffner had come to agree with Bentley: what was needed in Bengal was more irrigation, not less. Re-establishing inundation irrigation and agricultural prosperity, it concluded, was the key to the malaria problem in the 'unhealthy' dying-rivers districts of Bengal.

> No special anti-larval measures are needed: merely the re-establishment of the old system of irrigation by dredging the canals and improving embankments, roads, railways and bridges, so that they no longer obstruct the free flow of water. It is an economic and agricultural measure, which will not prevent anopheles breeding, but which will render them harmless.[54]

The Malaria Commission's report went further, pointing to broader political conditions of land tenure in Bengal under colonial rule as instrumental in undermining agricultural productivity. At the time of the 1793 Permanent Settlement Act,[55] it noted, special local taxes used to maintain the canals for irrigation had been abolished, thus depriving the traditional irrigation system of its financial base. In a scarcely disguised reference to the zamindari system of absentee landlords established under East India Company rule, the Commission pointed out, the Permanent Settlement compounded the problem by 'prevent[ing] the deterioration of the soil being noticed, except by the actual tiller of the soil.'[56] The malaria problems in Bengal bore obvious parallels to conditions of intense malaria in the Italian latifundia and demonstrated equally the limitations of anti-larval work in isolation from such larger determinants.

With respect to Punjab, the Malaria Commission concurred with Christophers's conclusions as to the key role of economic conditions underlying the phenomenon of fulminant epidemics in the province:

> Excessive rainfall, causing adverse economic conditions by flooding and water-logging, especially if these conditions were already bad owing to a number of dry years, predicts the advent of an epidemic outbreak of malaria. . . . The duty of the public health officer is . . . what Colonel Gill is doing. . . '[taking] measures to assure prompt treatment . . . and to improve, by supplying food, clothing, housing and other means, the physical conditions of the population.'[57]

In major industrial mining, rail and plantation enclave regions, efforts directed to vector control had been employed with some success, the report detailed. Criticism, however, was directed to urban vector control efforts, where 'much still remain[ed] to be done' in Bombay and Delhi.[58] In the Bombay municipality, vector control was considered both technically possible and financially feasible, involving anti-larval measures of public and private cisterns and wells, the chief sites of *An. stephensi* breeding.[59] But the municipal Malaria Department had been disbanded in 1918 and malaria reappeared episodically in Bombay thereafter. Elsewhere, however, the Study Tour report noted approvingly that malaria control activities had been directed primarily to broader economic measures rather than vector control, and to improved quinine access. Even in the Rohilkand Terai – the poorly drained sub-Himalayan hill tract of the United Provinces where highly anthropophilic malaria vectors and plantation in-migration made for intensive transmission rates – the report concurred that '[c]onditions greatly improve if the immigrant population is well-housed, well-fed, well-cared for medically and sanitarily, even without any special anti-malarial precautions.'[60] These observations closely mirrored those from the earlier Malaria Commission study tours in Europe.

Well into the 1930s, then, a role for human destitution in malaria epidemiology and lethality was documented and taken seriously by public health officials and malaria researchers within India and internationally, a view that informed malaria control policy at a number of levels. Where then did this understanding go?

## Hunger eclipsed

Within South Asian malaria literature, it is difficult to identify a discrete moment or debate where the role of human destitution in the mortality burden of malaria was questioned. Instead, a role for hunger in malaria lethality seems simply to have been set aside. A range of factors contributed. Among them was the decline after 1908 in the fulminant form of malaria itself, certainly in Punjab, with the control of famine. In the wake of the two 'great' famines at the turn of the twentieth century, famine relief policy was transformed over the ensuing two decades from palliative relief of 'established' famine to early, pre-emptive support of the agricultural economy *before* frank famine 'had declared itself.' This support included, but was not limited to, agriculture taxation (land revenue) relief. In Punjab, relief measures after 1920 also began to be sanctioned for crop losses due to flooding; and ultimately, on the basis of 'scarcity' (foodgrain prices more than 40 per cent above normal levels) alone, without famine ever being declared.[61] Moreover, drought relief after 1908 increasingly became a policy of routine application in response to local harvest shortfall, in contrast to the 1880 policy which restricted relief to years of widespread, severe harvest failure. These changes held major implications for human survival across periods of acute harvest failure. And as overt famine increasingly was brought under control after 1908, so too were the most dramatic examples of the link between starvation and epidemic malaria mortality. Thus with each new cohort of younger malaria researchers, fewer among them had direct experience of the phenomenon of fulminant malaria.

Meanwhile, public health administrators in the post-famine era would find it increasingly difficult to incorporate economic conditions into practical ways of measuring such stress. Gill's efforts, for example, to take price data into account in his annual predictions of expected autumn epidemic severity were frustrated by the fact that price swings after the first decade of the twentieth century were determined less by local harvest conditions and more by international events: two world wars and the global Depression. Without a statistical vehicle for measuring local economic conditions, malaria research by default shifted to measures that *could* be readily measured: human spleen and parasite rates, and infected mosquitoes, *viz.*, measures of malaria transmission (infection).

Even so, malaria would reappear in fulminant form in 1934–1935 in South Asia in concert with famine in neighbouring Ceylon (Sri Lanka), and again a decade later both in Bengal and in 1942 Punjab,[62] each a stark reminder of the powerful relationship between epidemic starvation and epidemic malaria mortality. Clearly then, there were factors other than lack of examples of 'fulminant' malaria conditions at play in the fading visibility of the 'Human Factor' in academic epidemic analysis.

Among them, microbiologic advances in the emerging medical subdisciplines of medical entomology and immunology in the early decades of the twentieth century were accentuating a narrow focus on disease transmission, offering competing hypotheses of epidemic patterns. Already, there was intense interest within the Indian Medical Service in immunological approaches to the control of infective diseases with the development of vaccines against cholera, plague, and typhoid fever, as well as rabies antivenin, many produced locally in the early twentieth century at Pasteur institutes in India.[63] Developments in the field of immunology held particular sway in malaria analysis with what came to be referred to as the 'theory of non-immunes.' The significance of acquired immunity had long been apparent to imperial administrations in relation to holoendemic malaria conditions in West Africa, a region where differences in susceptibility to clinical illness between newcomers to an endemic area and the indigenous population were marked.[64] Differences in malaria susceptibility were apparent also in relation to the hyperendemic hill tracts of South Asia, and assumed by the early twentieth century to be related to acquired immunity. Such interest in the protective effect of malaria-specific immunity soon took more systematic form, spurred in part by observations on spleen rate patterns in Punjab in the wake of the 1908 epidemic.

## Punjab and the theory of non-immunes

In 1914, immunological interpretation of malaria epidemicity received a fillip in the writing of E.L. Perry, an IMS officer then on special duty investigating malaria in the hyperendemic Jeypore hills of the Madras Presidency. In July of that year, Perry read a paper before the Punjab Branch of the British Medical Association in which he reported 'startling' observations on spleen rates in the Gujrat district of Punjab province in the years following the 1908 epidemic.[65] The spleen rate, a measure of spleen enlargement prevalence in a population, was considered a general indicator of malaria transmission in a population.[66] Surveys he had conducted in Khatala village showed continuing high child spleen rates of 75 per cent in 1909 and 1910. By 1912 however the rate had fallen to 21 per cent.[67] Perry was struck by the 'enormous degree of fluctuation' in spleen rate, contrasting this with conditions in the Jeypore hills, a hyperendemic region where spleen rates were high but not subject to major variation year to year, nor apparently to severe epidemics.[68] He went on in his paper to infer a causal relationship between fluctuating levels of acquired immunity (as reflected by spleen rate levels) in Punjab and the region's vulnerability to 'fulminant' malaria.

To medical scientists already intrigued by ongoing developments in the emerging field of immunology, the 1914 Perry paper appeared to offer the compelling prospect of being able to predict epidemic patterns.[69] That same year provincial public health authorities instituted province-wide biannual spleen surveys of young school children, a program recommended by Perry and initiated under C.A. Gill as special malaria officer in the province. In an article published in the *Indian Journal of Medical Research* earlier that year, Gill himself had proposed that 'when a period of low immunity is associated with a sudden great increase in the amount of infection, the unprotected population will suffer from a severe epidemic.'[70]

In subsequent years Gill pursued the waning-immunity hypothesis further, attempting to test the thesis in Punjab by employing Christophers's rain-price epidemic model to analyze malaria mortality patterns in the city of Amritsar for the period 1870–1913.[71] Gill's choice of Amritsar city as test locality is puzzling. In a major urban setting, grain prices would be expected to reflect less closely economic stress than for the rural areas where both employment livelihood and foodgrain price levels were directly determined by harvest conditions. But it was curious also because only two of the city's four major epidemic years over the 43-year period had been preceded by drought and thus held the possibility of testing decline in acquired immunity as a factor in epidemic etiology.[72] Nevertheless, employing similar quantitative measures as in Christophers's 1911 study, he calculated a correlation coefficient of 0.57 between fever mortality, rainfall, and foodgrain prices. Viewing his statistical results as 'still incomplete,' he went on to postulate – with no empirical data on spleen rate levels available – the 'missing' variable to be acquired immunity.[73]

Gill's hypothesis was questionable in many respects, making application of the waning-immunity thesis of malaria epidemicity to Punjab province manifestly premature. But Perry's observations had also been premature, limited to only three years' observations in a single village area.[74] Rainfall levels in Gujrat district in 1911 had been in marked deficit, and in 1912 were also below normal, conditions that likely contributed to the marked fall in spleen rate in the study village.[75] Yet fulminant malaria did not follow in 1913 with the return of good rains,[76] the autumn fever death rate recorded as 5.3 deaths per 1,000 for the district compared to 27.0 per 1,000 in 1908. In other words, there was little empirical evidence that supported Perry's hypothesis of a link between fluctuating acquired immunity levels and fulminant malaria mortality.

To be clear, in pursuing a role for acquired immunity in malaria epidemicity in the province, neither Gill nor Perry was rejecting Christophers's economic 1911 conclusions: both emphasized 'scarcity' and 'disastrous floods' as 'predisposing' factors in the 1908 epidemic. Nevertheless, the Perry paper would come to be cited in subsequent malaria literature in support of the waning-immunity thesis of Punjab malaria epidemicity.[77] It would take three more decades before district spleen rate data were analyzed by Punjab public health officials. M. Yacob and S. Swaroop would find no significant correlation between June spleen rates and subsequent autumn malaria mortality for the period 1914–1943, analysis that suggested little empirical support for the thesis.[78] Well before, however, malaria researchers in the province had begun to modify the non-immune thesis, based in part on the results of a study by Christophers of hyperendemic malaria conditions in the iron mine labour camps of Singhbhum district, southwest Bengal (what is now western Bihar state).

### Singhbhum

The Singhbhum study, conducted in 1923, was one of the first field studies in India to provide extensive data on malaria infection rates over time among an entire population.[79] The study confirmed what Christophers earlier had observed in Sierra Leone under conditions of extremely high malaria transmission rates:[80] that gametocyte levels, the sexual form of the malaria parasite transmitted from infected humans to the anopheline vector during the mosquito's blood meal,[81] were highest among very young children undergoing initial 'acute [malaria] infestation.'[82] Through meticulous observations on parasite rates and gametocyte counts, Christophers estimated that over two-thirds of the gametocyte 'load' of the labour camp population occurred among children under 2 years of age. Near-continuous re-infection through much of the year (hyperendemicity) induced rapid development of acquired immunity in all but the youngest children, a state termed 'premunity' where clinical symptoms are negligible and parasite levels, including gametocytes, are low despite high re-infection rates.

31

Christophers's findings confirmed the key role of young, non-immune, children in the chain of malaria transmission in hyperendemic populations. Malaria workers began to ask to what extent fluctuations in numbers of non-immune infants in Punjab province might account for epidemicity there, a region where rainfall and malaria transmission was highly variable from year to year. A single year of drought and negligible transmission, it was suggested, could add an entire additional year's cohort of newborns to the non-immune child population.[83]

## The Karnal Research Station, 1929–1936

Through the late 1920s and 1930s intensive epidemiological studies were conducted in six villages in the southeastern district of Karnal to explore 'the mechanism of the production of epidemics of malaria in the Punjab.' In 1931, a 28-year-old George Macdonald and colleague, J. Abdul Majid, published the results of two years' observations that included extensive entomological data on vectors, breeding sites, seasonal profile of vivax and falciparum parasite rates, and spleen rates, data that would contribute to subsequent theoretical modelling of malaria transmission.[84] Unfortunately for the investigative purposes of the study, the two consecutive study years (1929–1930) were marked by below normal rainfall, which meant there was little opportunity to observe malaria under epidemic conditions.

Despite the deficit in precipitation however, little decline was observed in spleen rate levels. Those villages subject to more severe epidemic malaria conditions in the recent past continued to show higher rates of transmission, even when rainfall was low.[85] Further, they observed, villages worst affected in recent severe epidemics were those most vulnerable to higher fever mortality during the study years. Evidently the persistence of higher endemic levels of malaria transmission in the study villages overrode any protective effect of acquired immunity in the population derived from previous epidemic conditions. These observations were generally consistent with what Christophers had recorded two decades earlier for the province more broadly. The northern submontane districts with generally higher endemic levels of transmission, he showed, were at least as prone to fulminant epidemics as the north-central and southeast districts.[86]

Macdonald offered the hypothesis that in regions of what he termed 'unstable' malaria such as Punjab, where active transmission was highly variable year to year, epidemicity did not depend primarily upon waning levels of acquired immunity levels among the general population,[87] but instead upon fluctuations in numbers of non-immune infants born since the previous severe epidemic, among whom gametocytes rates could be expected to be much higher.

[T]he fact that we are able to demonstrate marked signs of immunity in the older children in Karnal, even after four successive years of deficient rainfall, makes us believe that the effect of a series of years of low rainfall is not so much to lessen the immunity of the general population as to allow of the growth of an infant population, the larger part of which has never been infected with malaria and is consequently non-immune.[88]

In closing remarks, however, he went further to suggest that '[i]f the period of transmission is sufficiently long, and there is a suitable non-immune infant population, this will culminate in a fulminant epidemic at the end of the malaria season.'[89] The assumption here, if not articulated precisely, was that episodic low-transmission years and corresponding rise in non-immune young children underlay a population's vulnerability to epidemic malaria conditions.

Yet the study period did not encompass an epidemic in the sense of 'fulminancy' as addressed in Christophers's 1911 study. With monsoon rainfall for the two study years (1929–1930) well below average levels, there had been little opportunity to actually test the non-immune hypothesis of epidemicity. Nor had the study investigated mortality rates. It appears, then, that the investigators's closing statement linking non-immune infants and fulminant malaria was offered rather as a tentative hypothesis, in anticipation of ongoing research.

Research did continue at the Karnal research station for another five years. Conducted now by E.P. Hicks and J. Abdul Majid, these later efforts included tracking gametocyte and spleen rates by year of age among village children in relation to rainfall, conditions of atmospheric humidity, and in addition, accompanying malaria mortality rates through the pre-monsoon and malarial seasons. Unlike in the hyperendemic regions of Singhbhum, however, infectivity of children at Karnal (in terms of numbers of gametocytes) was found to decline much later in childhood than observed at Singhbhum, children above the age of five years showing high levels of gametocytes.[90] This much wider age group of heavy gametocyte carriers appeared to suggest that adding one year's cohort of non-immune infants (induced by a preceding year of drought and low transmission) was unlikely to be a factor in explaining epidemicity.

The single factor that *was* observed to influence malaria transmission rates year to year was continuity of monsoon rainfall. Fluctuations in levels of malaria infection between 1932 and 1935 were found to be 'almost entirely' due to variation in amount of rainfall and its even distribution across the monsoon period. Adequate atmospheric humidity, where levels were continuously above 60 per cent, was key to vector longevity, Hicks and Majid concluded.[91] It ensured that those adult anopheline mosquitoes, infected at the beginning of the transmission season from the few gametocyte carriers left in the population from the previous year, survived long enough to transmit infection in each subsequent 30-day round of vector-host transmission.

In 1933 and 1935, both years of above average rainfall, July–September atmospheric humidity never fell below 60 per cent and falciparum parasite rates were observed to increase from very low (6 to 7 per cent) to levels above 40 per cent, a level considered to indicate near-universal infection prevalence in the population.[92] Hicks and Majid concluded that

> fluctuations in the malaria of the Karnal district are almost entirely due to fluctuations in the dose of infection, and that the dose of infection is determined chiefly by the length of the period of low saturation deficiency [*viz.* high atmospheric humidity]. The latter depends rather on an even distribution of rainfall than on the total amount of rain.[93]

The observed importance of continuous adequate humidity helped, in turn, to explain the epidemic-facilitating impact of flooding.

Here, the investigators' use of the term 'dose' of infection was as a measure of malaria transmission in a population: the percentage of gametocyte carriers among children under 10 years multiplied by the mean number of *An. culicifacies* identified in sample sites for each month of July, August, September. This was a different meaning to the term than that explored by Christophers in his earlier sparrow experiments, where 'dose' was considered the number of sporozoites injected by an infected mosquito with each blood meal.[94] But Hicks and Majid were employing a different meaning to the term 'epidemic' as well, one based on levels of *infection* in the village community, rather than malaria *mortality* as had framed Christophers's 1911 study. Though a central purpose to the study as set out in the 1937 paper's introduction was ostensibly one of investigating the 'severe epidemic[s]' of Punjab[95] – severity measured by malaria mortality – most of the analysis presented was directed instead to levels of malaria transmission.

Did geometric increase in malaria infection rates (incidence) in itself explain fulminancy, *viz.*, soaring malaria death rates? The Hicks and Majid study did record autumn child mortality (< 10 yrs of age) across the 1929–1935 study period, converting autumn fever deaths into 'epidemic figures,' as employed by Christophers in 1911.[96] Here, autumn death rates (Sept.–Dec.) were found to correspond to levels of malaria transmission: the years 1933 and 1935 showing the highest Epidemic Figures, 2.21 and 1.99, respectively. Yet these levels of mortality were hardly representative of the epidemics of the pre-1909 period. By comparison, the 1908 epidemic had seen entire *thanas* (100 or more villages) with Epidemic Figures of 11, some as high as 30: autumn mortality reaching 30 times that of non-epidemic years.[97] By contrast, the highest mortality recorded in the study villages in 1933 and 1935 were at a level Christophers had considered to be the 'normal' endemic autumnal increase in the province – an Epidemic Figure of 1.0 indicating no autumn rise in fever deaths above the April–July rate. In other words, favourable atmospheric humidity conditions could explain year-to-year fluctuation in malaria transmission, but not the soaring mortality witnessed in 'fulminant' epidemics such as that in 1908.

One final comment on the Karnal Research Station results relates to a 'missing' epidemic. Though not remarked upon in either of the major scientific papers coming out of the 1929–1935 Karnal research period, the two initial study years (1929–1930), as years of drought, presented the investigators in effect with a non-immune 'scenario.' Third-quarter rainfall was nine inches in 1929 compared to a mean for the district of 20 inches, with 'extremely few cases of "fever"' that year. The year 1930 was also one of relative drought, with monsoon rainfall at 13.8 inches. Presumably these conditions produced several years' cohorts of lesser- or non-exposed (non-immune) infants. Yet malaria conditions did not take on epidemic proportions with the return of good rains in 1931 (at 23.6 inches, slightly above normal level). The recorded Epidemic Figure in the study villages was 1.34, again a tiny fraction of that recorded in epidemic tracts in 1908.[98]

In sum, extremely valuable observations had come out of these years of field research at the Karnal Research Station between 1929 and 1935. But the work offered little support for the thesis that an expanded cohort of never-exposed infants was a key factor underlying variation in malaria transmission year to year, let alone an explanation of fulminancy (greatly heightened malaria lethality). Efforts to explain malaria epidemicity in terms of waning acquired immunity appeared to be at an impasse.

## Acquired immunity and immune capacity conflated

In the meantime, another development relating to the non-immune thesis of malaria epidemicity had emerged. In his 1928 *Genesis of Epidemics* text – an ambitious overview of existing epidemiological understanding of major epidemic diseases including malaria – Gill would propose the term 'communal immunity' to encompass both spleen rate and economic conditions together as an index of a population's vulnerability, or resistance, to epidemic malaria.[99] Though offered perhaps as a shorthand in annual epidemic forecasting discussion, the combining of the two phenomena arguably helped set the stage for the conflation of the two concepts of immune *capacity* and *acquired* immunity.[100]

The distinction between the two concepts was of course a central one. The former reflected immunological potential, the human host's physiological ability to mount an adequate immunological response to future infection. Acquired immunity, on the other hand, referred to specific antibodies already present, stimulated by previous infection. The contrast was *current* immune-competence versus *past* exposure, the former encompassing Christophers's 'Human Factor' and representing the host side of the epidemic equation; the latter, a function of prevailing levels of malaria transmission, the germ side of the epidemic equation. Though fundamentally different, in the heady enthusiasm for immunological developments of this period, it was a distinction that would inadvertently come to be blurred with Gill's term, 'communal immunity.'

Despite the unpromising findings of the Karnal research regarding the influence of 'non-immunity' in malaria epidemicity, medical interest in immunological factors as contributing to epidemic malaria behaviour continued, with the concept of 'communal immunity' framing academic malaria discussion through the 1930s. The phrase increasingly would be employed, however, not in Gill's original sense of combined immune capacity and acquired immunity, but to the effective exclusion of the former, and with it conditions of the human host.[101] In the meantime, too, the meaning of 'epidemic,' itself, was also becoming blurred, as malaria infection (transmission) was increasingly conflated with malaria mortality.

It was in the final years of the Karnal field research work that genuinely 'fulminant' malaria conditions re-appeared in South Asia – not in Punjab, but in an opposite corner of the region, also under British colonial rule. The Ceylon epidemic of 1934–1935 would be one of the last highly lethal regional malaria epidemics to occur in South Asia (save for the war-time epidemics of 1942 and 1943). Because of its timing in the 1930s, it attracted exceptional attention from the now-burgeoning community of Western malariologists, and in its wake, numerous academic articles appeared offering unofficial commentary and analysis. These accounts largely interpreted the epidemic in entomological and related immunological terms, a view that has predominated through to the post-colonial period.[102] In effect, the 1934–1935 Ceylon epidemic marked the final stage in the demise of the 'Human Factor' as a central concept in understanding malaria lethality historically as articulated in Christophers's 1911 Punjab study – an epidemic to which we now turn.

## Notes

1  S.R. Christophers, 'Malaria in the Punjab,' *Scientific Memoirs by Officers of the Medical and Sanitary Departments of the Government of India* (New Series), No. 46 (Calcutta: Superintendent Govt Printing, 1911).

2  W.E. Jennings, ed., *Transactions of the Bombay Medical Congress, 1909* (Bombay: Bennett, Coleman & Co., 1910) [hereafter, *Trans. Bombay Congress*].

3  S.R. Christophers, and C.A. Bentley, 'The Human Factor: An Extension of our Knowledge regarding the Epidemiology of Malarial Disease,' in Jennings, ed., *Trans. Bombay Congress*, 78–83; S.R. Christophers, and C.A. Bentley, *Malaria in the Duars. Being the Second Report to the Advisory Committee Appointed by the Government of India to Conduct an Enquiry Regarding Blackwater and Other Fevers Prevalent in the Duars* (Simla: Government Monotype Press, 1909).

4 GOI, *Proceedings of the Imperial Malaria Conference held at Simla in October 1909* (Simla: Government Central Branch Press, 1910) [hereafter, Simla Conf.].
5 Christophers, 'Malaria in the Punjab,' 127, 133.
6 S.P. James, 'Malaria in Mian Mir,' in Jennings, ed., *Trans. Bombay Congress*, 84–93.
7 Christophers and Bentley, 'The Human Factor.'
8 S.R. Christophers, and C.A. Bentley, 'Black-water Fever: Being the First Report to the Advisory Committee Appointed by the Government of India to Conduct an Enquiry Regarding Black-Water and Other Fevers Prevalent in the Duars,' *Sci. Mem. Med. Sanit. Dep.*, no. 35, 1908.
9 Christophers and Bentley, '*Malaria in the Duars*, 5.
10 Christophers and Bentley, 'The Human Factor,' 83; Christophers and Bentley, *Malaria in the Duars*, 5.
11 S.R. Christophers, 'On Malaria in the Punjab,' Simla Conf., 29–47.
12 Ibid., 43.
13 S. Zurbrigg, *Epidemic Malaria and Hunger in Colonial Punjab* (London: Routledge, 2019), ch. 8.
14 *Report on Malaria in the Punjab During the Year 1914* (Lahore: Punjab Medical Dept), 2.
15 For details, see Zurbrigg, *Epidemic Malaria and Hunger*, ch. 9.
16 S.P. James, and S.R. Christophers, 'Malaria. General Etiology,' in W. Byam, and R.G. Archibald, eds., *The Practice of Medicine in the Tropics* (London: Henry Frowde and Hodder and Stoughton, 1922), vol. 2, 1509–1515, at 1514.
17 Editorial, 'The Economic Factor in Tropical Disease,' *Indian Medical Gazette*, 57, Sept. 1922, 341–343 [hereafter *IMG*].
18 Ibid.
19 Ibid. In an article entitled 'Malnutrition and Malaria,' the August 1921 issue of *The Modern Review* (Calcutta) also highlighted Bentley's Bengal findings, suggesting that 'the conditions which produce malarial fever are the self-same conditions which produce poverty by causing agricultural deterioration'; 266.
20 H.W. Acton, 'An Investigation into the Causation of Lathyrism in Man,' *IMG*, July 1922, 241–247.
21 Ibid., 247.
22 C.A Bentley, 'Some Economic Aspects of Bengal Malaria,' *IMG*, Sept. 1922, 321–326.
23 Editorial, 'The Economic Factor,' 343.
24 P. Hehir, *Prophylaxis of Malaria in India* (Allahabad: Pioneer Press, 1910), 33, 30.
25 Ibid., 31, 33.
26 P. Hehir, *Malaria in India* (Bombay: Humphrey Milford, 1927), 434–435. See also C.A. Gill, *The Genesis of Epidemics* (London: Bailliere, Tindall and Cox, 1928), 208–210.
27 Editorial, 'The Economic Factor,' 343 [emphasis added].
28 C.A. Bentley, 'A New Conception Regarding Malaria,' *Proceedings, 3rd Meeting of the General Malaria Committee, Nov. 18–20, 1912, held at Madras* (Simla: Govt. Monotype Press, 1913), 61–84, at 62 [emphasis in the original].
29 Ibid., 61.
30 J. Niven, 'Poverty and Disease,' Presidential Address, Epidemiology Section, Oct. 22, 1909, *Proceedings of the Royal Society of Medicine*, 3, 1910, 1–44, at 11.
31 P. Weindling, 'Social Medicine at the League of Nations Health Organisation and the International Labour Office compared,' in P. Weindling, ed., *International*

*Health Organisations and Movements, 1918–1939* (New York: Cambridge University Press, 1995), 134–153, at 138.

32  R. Senior White, *Studies in Malaria as It Affect Indian Railways*, Indian Research Fund Association, Technical Paper, 258 (Calcutta: Central Publications Branch, 1928), 7, 1.

33  R.P. Behal, and P. Mohapatra, 'Tea and Money Versus Human Life: The Rise and Fall of the Indenture System in the Assam Tea Plantations 1840–1908,' *Journal of Peasant Studies*, 19, 3/4, 1992, 142–172, at 167. Whether draft amendments to the Labour Act were already in process during the course of the Duars enquiry is unclear. It is perhaps safe to assume by the scope of the study that its conclusions were scarcely in doubt from its earliest stages.

34  M. Anderson, 'India, 1858–1930: The Illusion of Free Labour,' in D. Hay, and P. Craven, eds., *Masters, Servants and Magistrates in Britain and the Empire, 1562–1955* (Chapel Hill/London: University of North Carolina Press, 2004), 433–454, at 448. In part this reflected a change in politics in the metropole, where the momentum of the labour movement in the wake of the 1901 Taff Vale decision heightened political and social attention to labour conditions; ibid., 447. In India, growing labour militancy and more organised forms of labour resistance emerged after 1920; R.P. Behal, 'Power Structure, Discipline, and Labour in Assam Tea Plantations under Colonial Rule,' *International Review of Social History*, 51, 2006, Supplement, 143–172, at 168–169; P. Mohapatra, 'Assam and the West Indies, 1860–1920: Immobilizing Plantation Labour,' in D. Hay and P. Craven, *Masters, Servants*, 455–480, at 478. For treatment of post-war labour reforms motivated by fears of Russian Bolshevism, see D. Chakrabarty, 'Conditions for Knowledge of Working-Class Conditions: Employers, Government and the Jute Workers of Calcutta, 1890–1940,' in R. Guha, ed. *Subaltern Studies II, Writings on South Asian History and Society* (Delhi: Oxford University Press, 1983), 259–310, at 266.

35  'The penal legislation may have been abolished, but the huge unrelenting apparatus of surveillance and detention, carefully crafted since 1860, remained,' what Mohapatra refers to as 'the power behind the shadow'; 'Assam and the West Indies,' 478–480.

36  *Report of the Assam Labour Enquiry Committee, 1921–22*, 35; cited in R.P. Behal, *Wage Structure and Labour: Assam valley tea plantations, 1900–1947* (New Delhi: V.V. Giri National Labour Institute, 2003).

37  Through the 1920s, the Foundation contributed over one-third of the finances of the League of Nation's Health Organisation; P. Weindling, 'American Foundations and the Internationalizing of Public Health,' in S.G. Solomon, L. Murard, and P. Zylberman, eds., *Shifting Boundaries of Public Health: Europe in the Twentieth Century* (Rochester: University of Rochester Press, 2008), 63–85, at 75.

38  S.P. James, 'Advances in Knowledge of Malaria Since the War,' *Transactions of the Royal Society of Tropical Medicine and Hygiene*, 31, 1937, 263–280, at 268–269.

39  A. Celli, 'The Restriction of Malaria in Italy,' in *Transactions of the Fifteenth International Congress on Hygiene and Demography, Washington, September 23–28, 1912* (Washington: Govt Publ. Off., 1913) 516–531, at 530. 'Land reclamations' appear to have begun as early as 1901, possibly even before quinine distribution increased in 1904; J.A. Nájera, ' "Malaria Control" Achievements, Problems and Strategies,' *Parassitologia*, 43, 2001, 1–89, at 12.

40  Celli, 'The Restriction of Malaria in Italy,' 530.

41  League of Nations Malaria Commission, *Principles and Methods of Antimalarial Measures in Europe* (Geneva: League of Nations, 1927), 87 [hereafter LNMC].

42 F.L. Snowdon, *The Conquest of Malaria: Italy, 1900–1962* (New Haven: Yale University Press, 2006), 89.

43 LNMC, *Report on its Tour of Investigation in Certain European Countries in 1924* (Geneva: League of Nations, 1925), 59.

44 N.H. Swellengrebel, 'Some Aspects of the Malaria Problem in Italy,' in *Investigation in Certain European Countries*, Annex 11, 168–171, at 171.

45 Ibid., 168–169.

46 S. Litsios, *The Tomorrow of Malaria* (Wellington, NZ: Pacific Press, 1996), 63, 48–49. Similar conclusions would be reached by J.A. Sinton in Spain investigating intense malaria associated with extension of rice cultivation, under conditions of aggregation of migrant labour; 'Rice cultivation in Spain, with special reference to the conditions in the delta of the River Ebro,' *Records of the Malaria Survey of India*, 3, 3, June 1933, 495–506 [hereafter, *RMSI*].

47 The report cited two exceptions, regions in which anti-larval measures had been carried out on a considerable scale 'with definitely successful results': the first was in the Karst Mountains of Dalmatia, 'bare, dry, waterless hills'; and in Palestine where the 'mountains are dry, the valleys easy to drain . . . [and] rainfall is negligible during the malaria season'; LNMC, *Principles and Methods of Anti-malarial Measures in Europe* (Geneva: League of Nations, 1927), 81–82.

48 Ibid., 31, 89.

49 Ibid., 13.

50 Ibid., 86.

51 James, 'Advances in Knowledge of Malaria Since the War,' 264.

52 LNMC, *Report of the Malaria Commission on its Study Tour of India* (Geneva: League of Nations, Aug. 1930), [hereafter, LNMC, India Report] Other study tour members included M. Ciuca, secretary of the Malaria Commission, Prof., Faculty of Medicine in the University of Jassy, Roumania; N.H. Swellengrebel, Chief of Laboratory of the Section of Tropical Hygiene of the Royal Colonial Institute, Amsterdam; Louis Williams, Head of the Anti-Malaria Service, U.S. Public Health Service; Dr S. de Buen, Professor of Parasitology, Institute of Health Madrid; Major M. Peltier, Prof. of Social Hygiene, School of Sanitary Service of Colonial Troops, Marseilles.

53 W. Schüffner, 'Notes on the Indian Tour of the Malaria Commission of the League of Nations,' *RMSI*, 11, 3, Sept. 1931, 337–347, at 340.

54 LNMC, India Report, 43; Schüffner, 'Notes on the Indian Tour,' 340.

55 Under the Permanent Settlement, state demand was fixed at 89 per cent of the rent, with 11 per cent retained by the *Zamindars*.

56 LNMC, India Report, 42–43. Recent analysis of Burdwan fever has taken varied perspectives: cultural, literary, eco-entomological, science-decolonising, in addition to imperial critique. See, e.g., A. Samanta, *Malaria Fever in Colonial Bengal, 1820–1939: Social History of an Epidemic*, (Kolkata: Firma KLM, 2002); I. Kazi, *Historical Study of Malaria in Bengal, 1860–1920* (Dhaka: Pip International Publishers, 2004); R. Deb Roy, *Malarial Subjects: Empire, Medicine and Nonhumans in British India, 1820–1909* (Cambridge: Cambridge University Press, 2017); P.B. Mukharji, 'Verncularizing Political Medicine: Locating the Medical betwixt the Literal and the Literary in Two Texts on the Burdwan Fever, Bengal c. 1870s,' in R. Deb Roy, and G.N.A. Attewell, eds., *Locating the Medical: Explorations in South Asian History* (New Delhi: Oxford University Press, 2018), 235–263. In this work, rural immiseration consequent on interruption of irrigation flows is generally acknowledged, including within a 'political medicine' and 'psychic injuries' critique (Mukharji). The profound implications of abrupt cropping decline on human survival and attendant rending of social relations has perhaps been less explored. For discussion of these immiserating

consequences, see Zurbrigg, *Epidemic Malaria and Hunger*, 274–276, 229–230; also, A. Biswas, 'The Decay of Irrigation and Cropping in West Bengal, 1850–1925,' in B. Chattopadhyay, and P. Spitz, eds., *Food Systems and Society in Eastern India* (Geneva: United Nations Research Institute for Social Development, 1987), 85–131; R. Mukherjee, *Changing Face of Bengal: A Study in Riverine Economy* (Calcutta: University of Calcutta, 1938).

57 LNMC, India Report, 38–39.

58 Ibid., 60–61.

59 C.A. Bentley, *Report of an Investigation into the Causes of Malaria in Bombay* (Bombay: Miscellaneous Official Publications, 1911).

60 LNMC, India Report, 45.

61 For details of these policy changes and discussion of their potential impact, see Zurbrigg, *Epidemic Malaria and Hunger*, chs. 10–11; A. Maharatna, 'The Regional Variation in the Demographic Consequences of Famines in the Late Nineteenth Century,' *Economic and Political Weekly*, 29, 23, 1994, 1399–1410; A. Maharatna, *The Demography of Famines* (Delhi: Oxford University Press, 1996).

62 For details, see Zurbrigg, *Epidemic Malaria and Hunger*, ch. 12. Also, ch. 2, below.

63 P. Chakrabarti, *Bacteriology in British India Laboratory Medicine and the Tropics* (New York: University of Rochester Press, 2012); M. Worboys, *Spreading Germs: Disease Theories and Medical Practice in Britain, 1865–1900* (Cambridge: Cambridge University Press, 2000), 43. For an account of the intense interest in immunology at the Tenth International Congress of Medicine at Berlin in 1890, see P.M.H. Mazumdar, 'Immunity in 1890,' *Journal of the History of Medicine and Allied Sciences,* 27, 3, 1972, 312–324.

64 P. Curtin, 'Malaria Immunities in Nineteenth-Century West Africa and the Caribbean,' *Parassitologia*, 36, 1994, 69–92.

65 E.L. Perry, *Recent Additions to Our Knowledge of Malaria in the Punjab. A paper read before the Punjab Branch of the British Medical Association at Simla, on July 17, 1914* (Simla: Thacker, Spink & Co, 1914), 11.

66 As the principal organ that breaks down malaria parasite–damaged red blood cells, the spleen typically enlarges following malaria infection to be palpable below the left rib cage: the 'spleen rate' is generally defined as the per cent of children under the age of 10 years with an enlarged (palpable) spleen.

67 Ibid., 7. The paper provided a graph but no actual rates. Gill, in an earlier paper, did provide numerical rates in a graph that also included data for December 1913; C.A. Gill, 'Epidemic or Fulminant Malaria Together with a Preliminary Study of the Part Played by Immunity in Malaria,' *Indian Journal of Medical Research*, 2, 2, 1, July 1914, 268–314, Chart II, 294 [hereafter, *IJMR*].

68 Perry, *'Recent Additions,'* 12.

69 Randall Packard documents a similar tendency in this period for colonial officials in Swaziland to interpret malaria epidemicity in entomological terms related to rainfall patterns, despite limited empirical evidence; 'Maize, Cattle and Mosquitoes: The Political Economy of Malaria Epidemic in Colonial Swaziland,' *Journal of African History*, 25, 1984, 189–212, at 193–194.

70 Gill, 'Epidemic or Fulminant Malaria,' 297.

71 C.A. Gill, *Report on Malaria in Amritsar, Together with a Study of Endemic and Epidemic Malaria and an Account of the Measures Necessary to Their Control* (Lahore: Punjab Govt, 1917).

72 Between 1870 and 1913 the town experienced four severe epidemics. Of these, two were preceded by drought, 1908 and 1881; Zurbrigg, *Epidemic Malaria*

*and Hunger*, ch. 5. The 1876 and 1887 epidemics however were not, though both were associated with marked economic stress: export-triggered soaring foodgrain prices in 1887, and severe flood-related crop failure in 1875 preceding the 1876 epidemic.

73  C.A. Gill, 'The Relationship of Malaria and Rainfall, *IJMR*, 7, 3, 1920, 618–632, at 628–629.

74  Perry, 'Recent Additions,' 7.

75  Provincial 1911 third-quarter rain was 6.8 inches compared to a mean of 13.9; for Gujrat district, 8.3 versus 16.4 inches; 1909 and 1910 Gujrat district rain was 21.9 and 19.1 inches, respectively.

76  Perry did not include actual spleen rate data in his July 1914 paper, simply a chart; Perry, 'Recent Additions,' 7. Data appear however in an article published by Gill earlier in the year; 'Epidemic or Fulminant Malaria,' 294.

77  Lewis Hackett, prominent malaria worker with the Rockefeller Foundation, would cite Perry's 1914 paper as support for the waning-immunity thesis, the observed spleen rate decline showing that the study village was 'then ready for an epidemic'; *Malaria in Europe: An Ecological Study* (London: Oxford University Press, 1937), 228–229.

78  M. Yacob, and S. Swaroop, 'Malaria and Spleen Rate in the Punjab,' *Indian Journal of Malariology*, 1, 4, Dec. 1947, 469–489, at 479. The routine spleen surveys involved male school children under the age of 10 years, among whom prevalence of splenic enlargement was considerably lower than rates recorded by Perry. The discrepancy is likely attributable to the older age group of children, cumulative acquired immunity resulting in gradual reduction in spleen size with increasing age. As well, as Yacob and Swaroop pointed out, children attending school were largely from 'well-to-do' classes, whereas spleen rates were notably higher among the poor; ibid., 469.

79  S.R. Christophers, *Enquiry on Malaria, Blackwater-fever and Ankylostomiasis in Singhbhum. Report No. 1* (Govt Publ. Behar and Orissa, 1923), 363–407.

80  J.W.W. Stephens, and S.R. Christophers, 'The Malaria Infection in Native Children,' in *Reports of the Malaria Committee of the Royal Society*, 3rd series (London: Harrison and Sons, 1900).

81  For an overview of the microbiological life cycle of the malaria parasite, its different forms and species, and conditions of transmission in the Punjab plains, see Appendix I.

82  S. Christophers, 'The Mechanism of Immunity against Malaria in Communities Living under Hyper-Endemic Conditions,' *IJMR*, 12, 2, Oct. 1924, 273–294.

83  Growing interest in immunological explanations of epidemic behaviour across this period was reflected in Gill's 1928 text, *The Genesis of Epidemics*.

84  G. Macdonald, and J. Abdul Majid, 'Report on an Intensive Malaria Survey in the Karnal District, Punjab,' *RMSI*, 2, 3, Sep. 1931, 423–477.

85  'This,' the investigators surmised, 'is presumably due to the greater number of gametocyte carriers in the village providing a ready means of infection for the reduced numbers of dangerous anophelines than in the neighbouring villages'; ibid., 435.

86  Christophers, 'Malaria in the Punjab,' 71, 73, 131; Simla Conf., 38. On this, see Zurbrigg, *Epidemic Malaria and Hunger*, ch. 2.

87  For an overview of the early twentieth-century emergence of the concept of 'herd immunity,' see M. Worboys, 'Before McKeown: Explaining the Decline in Tuberculosis in Britain, 1880–1930,' in F. Condrau and M. Worboys, eds., *Tuberculosis Then and Now: Perspectives on the History of an Infectious Disease* (Montreal: McGill-Queen's University Press, 2010), 148–170 at 159–160.

88 Macdonald and Majid, 'Report on an Intensive Malaria Survey,' 466.

89 Ibid., 468.

90 'We have found little evidence of any change in the immunity of the population in the period under review. If the size of the average enlarged spleen is accepted as a valid measurement of immunity, it shows that if there has been any change, it has been unimportant'; E.P. Hicks, and J. Abdul Majid, 'A Study of the Epidemiology of Malaria in a Punjab District,' *RMSI*, 7, 1, Mar. 1937, 1–43, at 33.

91 Rather than atmospheric humidity, the investigators used 'saturation deficiency,' a measure that takes into account additional factors such as temperature affecting the rate of loss of water from insects; Hicks and Majid, 'Malaria in a Punjab district,' 23. See also P.A. Buxton, 'The Effect of Climatic Conditions upon Population of Insects,' *Transactions of the Royal Society of Tropical Medicine and Hygiene*, 28, 4, 1933, 325–256.

92 Given the intermittent nature of malarial parasitemia, a parasite rate of 50 per cent generally was considered to indicate near-universal infection in a population; Hicks and Majid, 'Malaria in a Punjab District,' 40, Appendix 3, 31.

93 Ibid., 34.

94 Zurbrigg, *Epidemic Malaria and Hunger*, 78–82.

95 Ibid., 2, 29.

96 For the purposes of mapping comparative levels of epidemic intensity in 1908, Christophers devised a ratio measure of autumn malaria mortality. For each *thana* he calculated what he termed an 'Epidemic Figure,' derived by dividing the number of deaths recorded in October by the average non-epidemic monthly death rate. The latter was calculated as the previous five-year average of June and July deaths, 'avoiding those years in which plague or cholera disturbed the figures'; Christophers, 'Malaria in the Punjab,' 19. See also, Zurbrigg, *Epidemic Malaria and Hunger*, 66. For discussion of the limitations of the Epidemic Figure, see, ibid., 103.

97 Christophers, 'Malaria in the Punjab,' 21.

98 Hicks and Majid, 'Malaria in a Punjab District,' 7. The epidemic figure employed by Hicks and Majid represents malaria deaths in children less than 10 years whereas Christophers's 1908 figures included all age groups; however, given that the measure is a ratio of non-malaria to malaria deaths, and the fact that malaria mortality affected predominately young children, the two figures can be considered roughly comparable.

99 Gill, *Genesis of Epidemics*, 191.

100 A 1924 report by the newly formed Malaria Commission of the LNHO included an entire section on 'The Human Factor,' considered under three separate headings: 'Immunity,' meaning acquired immunity; 'Increase of Population'; and 'Economic Changes'; N.H. Swellengrebel, *Malaria in the Kingdom of the Netherlands* (Geneva: League of Nations, 1924), 15–17.

101 See, e.g., G. Harrison, *Mosquitoes, Malaria and Man: A History of the Hostilities since 1880* (New York: E.P. Dutton, 1978), 203.

102 Among many examples, see A.T.A. Learmonth, 'Some Contrasts in the Regional Geography of Malaria in India and Pakistan,' *Transactions and Papers (Institute of British Geographers)*, 23, 1957, 37–59, at 48.

# 2

# THE 1934–1935 CEYLON EPIDEMIC AND ITS EPISTEMIC AFTERMATH

> The necessity for ensuring that the population of the affected area has sufficient food is of primary importance as an anti-malarial measure.
> —— R. Briercliffe, *The Ceylon Malaria Epidemic, 1934–35. Report by the Director of Medical and Sanitary Service* (Colombo: Ceylon Govt Press, Sept. 1935), 73

Though important insights into malaria transmission had come out of the field research conducted in Karnal district, this work had not succeeded in explaining fulminant malaria in immunological terms. As the researchers were completing the second phase of their epidemiological studies, a major malaria epidemic, coincidentally, was unfolding on the neighbouring island of Sri Lanka (colonial Ceylon), one that would soon come to be interpreted as offering the entomo-immunological 'test-case' that Karnal had not. 'The great epidemic of 1934–35 was the result of the failure of the South-West Monsoon of 1934,' C.L. Dunn, a former provincial Director of Public Health in India, concluded in a prominent 1936 monograph, conditions that 'caused a great extension in the favourite breeding grounds of the insect carrier (*An. culicifacies*)' in drying river beds, amongst 'a "susceptible" population due to four years of waning immunity.'[1] That same year, researchers with the Malaria Survey of India compared the 1934–1935 Ceylon epidemic to that in 1929 in the western province of Sind (now southern Pakistan) and concluded in similar terms that 'the origin of both these epidemics may be adequately explained by the sudden production of conditions unusually favourable to the propagation, longevity and activity of *An. culicifacies* in an area inhabited by a population in whom the communal immunity is at a low level.'[2]

Interpretation of the 1934–1935 Ceylon epidemic has many other links to the malaria research community in India, in the methodological tools and concepts employed to analyze it and in the investigators directly involved. C.A. Gill, recently retired from the Indian Medical Service and returning to

43

Britain from Burma, on hearing of the epidemic, chose to detour to Ceylon and volunteer his services for the official investigation already underway. His study, conducted in the final months of the epidemic, would be published as a Ceylon Sessional Paper alongside the colonial government's report.[3] S.R. Christophers, now based in London, would also figure in the professional deliberations on the epidemic in a 1936 meeting of the Royal Society of Tropical Medicine and Hygiene.[4] In that role, he would offer key, if characteristically epigrammatic, commentary on the significance of prevailing economic conditions leading up to the epidemic, as he had done a quarter-century earlier in relation to epidemic malaria in Punjab[5] – and as concluded in the official investigation by R. Briercliffe, Director of Medical and Sanitary Services for Ceylon, some months before.[6]

Alongside enhanced malaria transmission, triggered in the case of Ceylon by drought, failure of the 1934 southwest monsoon had brought record crop failure to over half of the country's major districts.[7] Harvest failure however was only the final phase of a period of severe economic hardship, set against a backdrop of four years of plummeting tea and rubber exports triggered by the global Depression. Thus amongst local health officials, widespread destitution was seen as both triggering and fuelling a vicious circle of starvation and disease. Indeed, throughout the epidemic, food and employment provision had been accorded as much prominence as medical treatment (quinine) in government relief efforts.

In subsequent Western malaria literature, however, an entomo-immunological reading of the 1934–1935 epidemic would prevail, one deemed to have become 'classic in malariology' among historians as resolving the larger 'riddle' of malaria epidemicity. 'It now seems so obvious,' Gordon Harrison, concluded in 1978, 'how with a large number of man-biting mosquitoes, a mighty epidemic could grow rapidly from so few carriers . . . [and] spread rapidly among non-immunes.'[8] In epistemic terms, the Sri Lankan malaria epidemic of 1934–1935 can thus also be seen as marking the final stage in the transformation of the 'Human Factor' from a concept of 'physiological poverty' (hunger) to one of microbe transmission. In a very concrete sense, the two epidemics, that in Punjab in 1908 and in Sri Lanka in 1934–1935, represent book-ends to an era of remarkable epidemiological research on malaria mortality bounded on each side, before and after, by a marked narrowing in epidemiological thought. These links to Punjab malaria history, together with its paradigmatic significance in malaria historiography, warrant consideration of the Ceylon epidemic in some detail.

## Sri Lankan malaria endemiology

Malaria in Sri Lanka, as in Punjab and much of the plains of the Indian subcontinent, is transmitted primarily by the mosquito vector, *Anopheles culicifacies.* But despite a common vector, the specific conditions conducive to transmission and epidemicity in Ceylon were generally viewed in the late colonial malaria literature as the inverse of those in the Punjab plains. Where excess rainfall and consequent flooding was the key trigger of severe epidemics in northwest India, many contemporary entomologists considered the prime trigger in Ceylon to be drought: the still, clear pools of drying river beds or irrigation channels acting as major anopheline breeding sites.[9]

This emphasis on river pools derived from well-recognized differences in malaria prevalence rates across the island. In the dryer plains region of the north and northeast, hyperendemic malaria generally prevailed, in contrast to conditions in the hills and mountains of the central and southwest 'wet' zones where malaria prevalence rates were low or negligible. Marked differences in regional rain catchment and topography accounted for this contrast, presenting two distinct ecological zones. The southwest quadrant of the island receives the benefit of both the southwest (May to September) and northeast (October to January) monsoons, with an annual rainfall ranging between 100 to 200 inches, compared to 50 to 75 inches in the northern and eastern regions where rainfall is limited principally to the later northeast monsoon (Figure 2.1).[10]

In the hills and mountains of the southwest and central 'wet zone,' rivers generally were full and fast flowing, the more regular rains tending to wash clear potential riverine *An. culicifacies* breeding sites, and doing so also in the western tracts downstream from the hills.[11] Vector numbers and malaria incidence were considered to vary from low to moderate. By contrast, in the plains of the northern dry zone, rainfall was highly seasonal and malaria transmission was endemic, reflected in much higher spleen rates (Figure 2.2).[12]

Regional contrasts in rainfall predicted large economic differences across the island as well. Except for the coastal areas, agriculture in the northern zone was precarious, with only a single, highly variable period of annual rainfall, and limited irrigation infrastructure. Death rates often exceeded birth rates and the sparse population was maintained only through immigration.[13] In the southwest region of the island with its generous rainfall, agriculture was more secure, double-cropping common, and population density high.

These two major ecological regions were separated by a narrow 'intermediate zone' of malaria prevalence in the central and south-central hills (Figure 2.1), the site of rubber, tea, and coconut plantations dating from the later nineteenth century. By the early twentieth century the plantation estates numbered over 1,400 and were worked primarily by Tamil labourers recruited from southern India. Like the wet zone, the intermediate zone was densely populated, with the majority non-estate Sinhalese

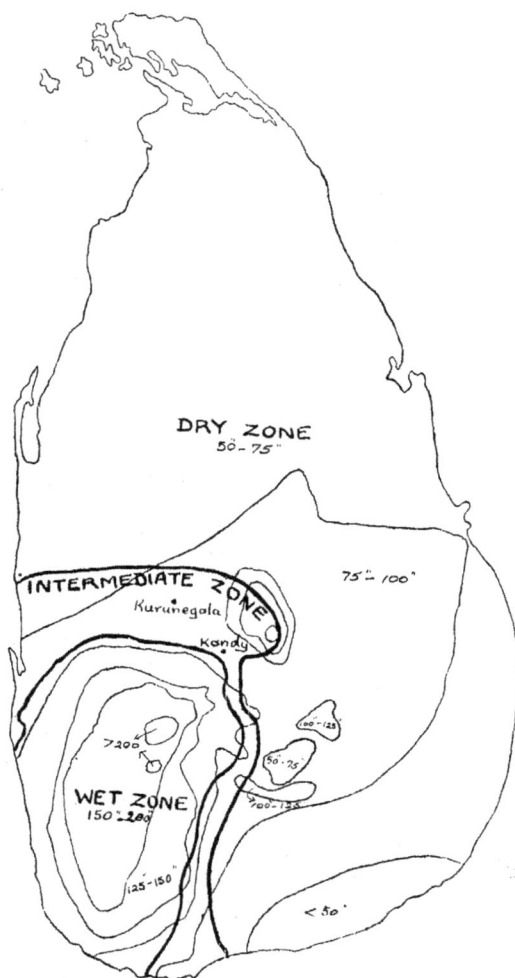

*Figure 2.1* Mean annual rainfall (inches), Ceylon

*Source:* T.W. Tyssul Jones, 'Deforestation and epidemic malaria in the wet and intermediate zones of Ceylon', *Indian Journal of Malariology*, 5, 1, Mar. 1951, 135–161, Map 2, p. 140; reproduced from K.J. Rustomjee, 'Observations on the epidemiology of malaria in Ceylon,' *Sessional Paper XXIV*, 1944, Ceylon Government Press.

population involved in rice cultivation and small-scale rubber and coconut production. By virtue of its dual economy the intermediate region also enjoyed relative economic insulation from the vagaries of the monsoon. However, in years of poor rains, the upper reaches of the streams and rivers tended to dry and form river-bed pools particularly conducive to

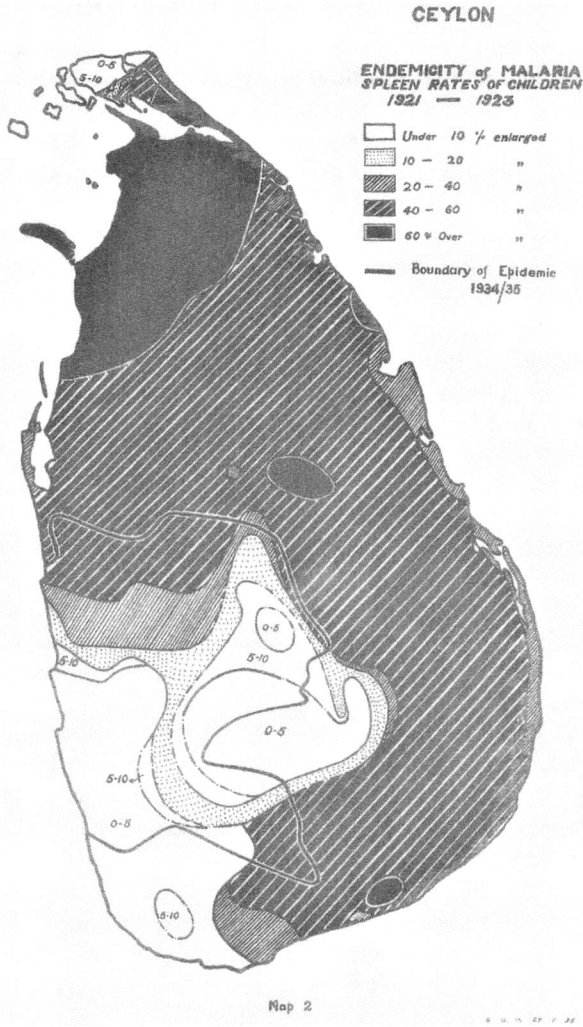

*Figure 2.2* Spleen rate (per cent), Ceylon, 1922–1923

*Source:* R. Briercliffe, *The Ceylon Malaria Epidemic, 1934–35* (Colombo: Ceylon Govt Press, Sept. 1935). Supplement to the *Sessional Paper XXII – 1935*, Map 2.

mosquito breeding, a phenomenon likely enhanced by the deforestation that accompanied establishment of the plantation economy.[14] As in Punjab, however, effective malaria *transmission* awaited rising atmospheric humidity and increased mosquito lifespan with return of the October monsoon rains.

## Portrait of the 1934–1935 malaria epidemic

Record drought conditions on the island in 1934 were broken by heavy rains beginning on October 6, followed by the sudden outbreak of malarial fever amongst all age-groups on October 27.[15] Dispensary attendance and hospital admissions rose simultaneously across much of the island in the early weeks of November, rising exponentially in the early weeks of December. Between November 1934 and April 1935 attendances at government hospitals and dispensaries rose by an estimated 3 million above levels in pre-epidemic years in a total population of 5.5 million.[16] The earliest increase occurred in the plantation-region districts of Kegalle, Kurunegala, and Ratnapura, where mortality, in absolute numbers, ultimately was heaviest.[17]

The focal centre of the 1934–1935 epidemic involved Kurunegala district straddling the intermediate and dry zones, and Kegalla and Kandy districts in the wet and intermediate zones. By January 1935 the spleen rate in Kurunegala district had risen to 71.9 per cent from a pre-epidemic average of 40–60 per cent, whereas the rate in the western coastal district of Colombo rose only to 8.8 per cent.[18] Entomological surveys conducted during the course of the epidemic documented increased numbers of *An. culicifacies* in the river basins of the intermediate zone where river and stream water levels had been reduced to standing pools.[19] The Briercliffe report concluded that many of the severely affected villages bordered rivers, but also noted that 'the breeding places of *An. culicifacies* . . . were by no means confined to pools in the river beds.'[20]

A total of 69,615 excess deaths were recorded for the island as a whole between November 1934 and March 1935, the crude death rate increasing from a preceding quinquennial mean of 23.1 to 36.6 in 1935.[21] Of these deaths, 54.6 per cent were recorded in children under 5 years of age.[22] Deaths among children 5–10 years accounted for a further 7.9 per cent of excess mortality. No systematic surveys of malaria species prevalence were undertaken during the epidemic, but among severe cases admitted to hospital, falciparum infection was as high as 43 per cent at the peak of the epidemic in January 1935. Thus an increase in prevalence of falciparum infection may have been a factor underlying epidemic intensity in the later stages of the epidemic. However, the high prevalence of vivax infection, a species not normally lethal, among severe cases also suggests that species of parasite likely was not the main factor contributing to lethality of infection.[23]

Of the total excess deaths, the large majority (59,144) were recorded in the nine districts encompassing the watershed regions of the four major west-draining rivers of the intermediate and wet zones.[24] Assuming a key etiological role for the drying river-beds of this region, Briercliffe designated this nine-district watershed tract as 'the epidemic area,' indicated on his maps with a black boundary line and there termed the 'epidemic zone' (Figure 2.3).[25]

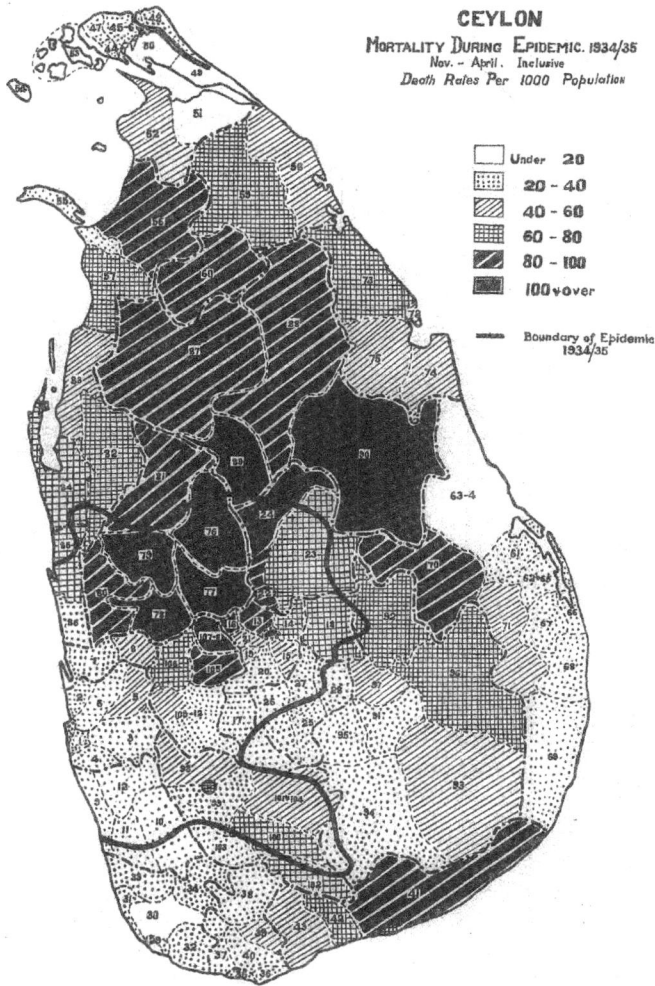

*Figure 2.3* Nov.–Apr. death rate per 1,000, Ceylon, 1934–1935

*Source:* R. Briercliffe, *The Ceylon Malaria Epidemic, 1934–35* (Colombo: Ceylon Govt Press, Sept. 1935). Supplement to the *Sessional Paper XXII* – 1935, Map 18.

*Note*: The four-river watershed 'epidemic area /zone' is designated by a solid black line.

In the worst affected divisions of Kegalla and Kurunegala districts, mortality rates appear to have reached 5 per cent or more of the population.[26] Encompassing much of the intermediate zone and neighbouring wet zone plantation districts, the 'epidemic area /zone' extended southwest to include Colombo as well, together encompassing well over half the entire 5.5 million

49

population of the island. Excess deaths 'outside the epidemic area,' by contrast, numbered 10,471.[27]

Initial mapping of mortality for the epidemic period of November 1934 to April 1935 showed extremely high death rates in much of the northern dry zone in addition to the plantation districts of the intermediate and wet zones (Figure 2.3).[28] Recognizing the dry zone's 'normally excessive' mortality levels, Briercliffe chose an additional measure to convey relative epidemic severity across the island in 1934–1935, calculating for each division (subunits of a district) the per cent *increase* in mortality over non-epidemic year levels (Figure 2.4).[29]

The resulting map indicated that the 'epicentre' of the malaria epidemic – those divisions where mortality increased 400 per cent or more in 1934–1935 – lay in the three intermediate zone and peri-intermediate zone districts of Kegalla, Kurunegala, and Kandy. But it also showed that while the greatest relative increase in mortality occurred within the watershed-defined 'epidemic area /zone,' markedly heightened death rates extended into the northern dry zone districts of Anuradhapura and Puttalam well beyond the catchment area of major intermediate zone rivers.[30]

Briercliffe pointed out this lack of complete congruence between epidemic intensity and the watershed-defined epidemic area/zone, acknowledging that the boundaries of the 'epidemic area' were 'fixed rather arbitrarily and are to some extent artificial.'[31] Nevertheless, he framed much of his mortality analysis on the basis of the 'epidemic area' categorization, presenting and comparing data in the nine districts of the 'epidemic area' versus those districts 'outside the epidemic area.'

Briercliffe's attention perhaps understandably was directed to those districts where excess deaths were geographically concentrated. In the context of near universal malaria infection and plummeting access to basic subsistence, the administrative demands entailed in providing famine relief alongside medical treatment to much of the population were enormous.[32] Deaths in absolute numbers in the sparsely populated dry zone northern districts by comparison were far fewer. Nonetheless, the report's focus on the 'epidemic zone' was problematic interpretatively, conveying a sense of the primacy of dry river beds and lack of previously acquired specific immunity, *viz.*, entomological conditions, underlying epidemic intensity.

However, there also were interpretative problems associated with Briercliffe's proportionate (per cent increase) mortality measure of epidemic intensity. In northern districts, the 'normal' death rate was in the range of 35–40 per 1,000, compared to 20 per 1,000 or less in the intermediate and wet zone districts.[33] Mean infant mortality for the previous decade in Anuradhapura district, for example, was 309 per 1,000 live births; in Puttalam district, 342 per 1,000 live births. With infant deaths a leading component of malaria mortality, such high rates allowed little statistical 'room' for a four-fold increase in overall mortality, as was observed during the epidemic in the normally lower-mortality tracts.[34] A proportionate measure

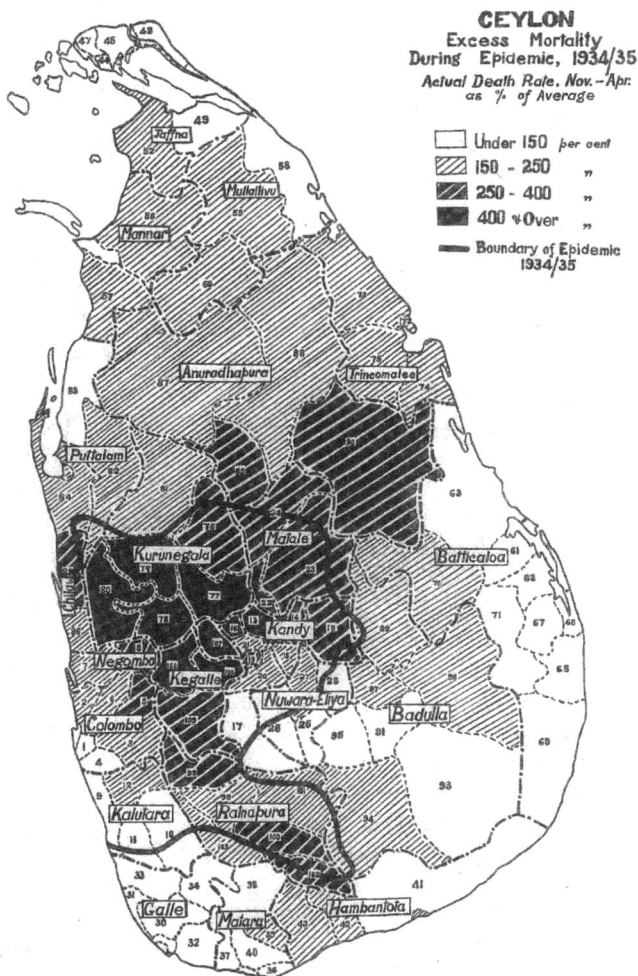

*Figure 2.4* Per cent increase in total mortality, by division, Ceylon, Nov. 1934 to Apr. 1935

*Source:* R. Briercliffe, *The Ceylon Malaria Epidemic, 1934–35* (Colombo: Ceylon Govt Press, Sept. 1935). Supplement to the *Sessional Paper XXII – 1935*, Map 19.

*Note:* The four-river watershed 'epidemic area /zone' is designated by a solid black line.

of epidemic intensity thus tended to underestimate epidemic severity in those regions of the island where death rates were endemically very high before the epidemic.

An alternative measure of epidemic intensity Briercliffe might have used was simply the absolute increase in death rate per mille. Had such figures been used, the northern district of Anuradhapura, for example, would have stood out as one where the epidemic rise approximated that for many of the severely affected districts in the 'epidemic area/zone' (Table 2.1). In other non-'epidemic-area' northern districts also, the 'excess' death rate was moderately severe.

Despite the methodological limitations of Briercliffe's proportionate measure of epidemic intensity, his mapping did provide important epidemiological insights. It suggested that considerable malaria endemicity as judged by 1920s spleen rates did not necessarily offer protection against epidemic mortality in 1934–1935 (Figs. 2.2 and 2.4).[35] In much of Kurunegala district, where mortality increase was greatest, endemic malaria transmission levels in the decade preceding the epidemic appear to have been relatively high, with a spleen rate ranging between 40 and 60 per cent. Moreover, death rates soared in neighbouring dry zone districts like Anuradhapura despite prevailing hyperendemic malaria conditions but where drought-triggered harvest failure had also been severe. Famine relief efforts were in fact already in progress in the dry zone when the malaria epidemic struck in the final months of 1934.[36] Even in the 'intermediate' zone of greatest relative epidemic severity, malaria endemicity likely was not inconsiderable, if spleen rate levels (20–40 per cent) observed in the 1920s can be assumed to have prevailed into the 1930s.

But it also suggests that a purely vector-driven explanation of epidemicity was questionable as well: it is difficult to interpret the epidemic increase in mortality in the northern highly endemic district of Anuradhapura in entomological terms of drying riverbeds when such conditions characterized the region even in non-epidemic years. Entomological factors alone, in other words, appear insufficient to explain why the epidemic in 1934–1935 assumed, in Eric Meyer's terms, 'une forme virulente.'[37] Further, Briercliffe's mortality mapping left unclear was how the entomological effects of drought in the watersheds could be distinguished from the economic consequences.

Briercliffe himself was fully aware of the larger economic backdrop to the epidemic. In a separate section on 'economic factors' he detailed the scale of the impact of the economic recession triggered by the global Depression. Between 1929 and 1933, exports had plummeted, the value of rubber, tea, and coconut exports falling 60 per cent.[38] With 42.1 per cent of the island's GDP based on the export of these products, the impact on livelihood had been severe.[39] H.E. Newnham, Commissioner for Relief during the epidemic, described the consequences:

> The export of tea and rubber was restricted in an endeavour to raise the price of those commodities, and this restriction had caused the closing down of an appreciable acreage of estates, particularly, among the smaller holdings. . . . The effect of the general depression was . . . felt in the villages of the wet zone where most of the

Table 2.1 Crude death rate (per 1,000 population), infant mortality rate (per 1,000 live births), Nov. 1934–Apr. 1935, extent harvest failure, by district, Ceylon [Sri Lanka]

| District | Crude death rate | | | Infant mortality rate | Estimated extent of 1934 crop loss |
|---|---|---|---|---|---|
| | 'Expected' (previous 4-yr. mean) | Actual | Excess | | |
| **Districts 'affected by the epidemic' ("epidemic area")*** | | | | | |
| Kurunegala | 13.4 | 62.3 | 48.9 | 799.9 | 'greatest degree' |
| Matale | 12.8 | 46.0 | 33.2 | 497.1 | 'limited areas' |
| Kegalla | 8.3 | 41.2 | 32.9 | 452.2 | 'greatest degree' |
| Kandy | 10.4 | 28.6 | 18.2 | 310.4 | 'limited areas' |
| Chilaw | 9.0 | 22.6 | 13.7 | 311.2 | 'very limited areas' |
| Negombo | 8.5 | 20.9 | 12.4 | 269.5 | n.a. |
| Ratnapura | 10.4 | 22.6 | 12.2 | 232.8 | 'limited areas' |
| Colombo | 10.2 | 17.2 | 7.0 | 196.4 | 'limited areas' |
| Kalutara | 9.2 | 12.1 | 2.9 | 128.9 | 'very limited areas' |
| **Districts 'outside the "epidemic area"'**** | | | | | |
| North-Central: | | | | | |
| Anuradhapura | 20.7 | 48.2 | 27.5 | 613.0 | 'greatest degree' |
| Puttalam | 18.6 | 33.3 | 14.7 | 512.3 | 'very limited areas' |
| Mullaittivu | 20.4 | 32.6 | 12.2 | 474.3 | 'greatest degree' |
| Mannar | 19.9 | 27.6 | 7.6 | 434.0 | 'greatest degree' |
| Hambantota | 16.2 | 30.9 | 14.7 | 310.8 | 'limited areas' |
| Trincomalee | 15.1 | 25.3 | 10.2 | 285.1 | 'very limited areas' |
| Badulla | 12.5 | 17.6 | 5.0 | 204.2 | 'limited areas' |
| Matara | 10.5 | 14.9 | 4.4 | 142.3 | 'very limited areas' |
| Nuwara Eliya | 9.9 | 13.1 | 3.1 | 195.0 | 'very limited areas' |
| Galle | 10.7 | 12.9 | 2.1 | 136.1 | 'limited areas' |
| Batticaloa | 14.4 | 15.3 | 0.9 | 209.7 | 'limited areas' |
| Jaffna | 14.2 | 14.8 | 0.5 | 222.9 | 'limited areas' |

Source: R. Briercliffe, The Ceylon Malaria Epidemic, 1934–45. Report by the Director of Medical and Sanitary Services, Sessional Paper XXII, (Colombo: Ceylon Govt Press, Sept. 1935), pp. 40, 44, 27.

* For definitions, see text at pages 48–50.

tea, rubber, and coconut plantations are situated. . . . The estates no longer needed the same amount of causal labour for weeding, tapping, and plucking. Contractors no longer needed their services on public and private works. Their coconuts ceased to add to the family income. But in almost every village there are rice fields . . . which provide some degree of insurance against a slump in commercial products.[40]

Superimposed upon four years' economic depression however was the severe 1934 drought, 'the greatest drought on record' for the island.[41] '[W]ith failure of the summer rains,' Newnham continued,

a rice shortage emerged by the second half of 1934, the autumn harvest amounting to 'about a quarter of the normal crop. . . . The peasants of the wet zone, who were formerly better off had lost many of their usual chances of maintaining their higher standard, and had begun to sink towards the level of those in the dry zone.[42]

Data on acreage of failed crops by district apparently were not available to Newnham, but he categorized the 21 districts of the island into three levels of harvest failure severity, detailed in the Briercliffe report.[43] Those districts hardest affected by the drought overlapped both the intermediate zone and the northern dry zone. Only in the southern two districts of Galle and Matara and the northern tip of the Jaffna peninsula had 1934 rainfall been at normal levels, and these districts did not suffer from epidemic malaria.[44]

In other words, there were two major sources of economic hardship leading up to the epidemic in late 1934, each varying in their impact geographically across the island and accounting for quite marked differences in economic stress among regions. Where harvest failure and the effects of the global Depression overlapped in the three hill districts in and bordering the intermediate zone, epidemic intensity was greatest: precisely that area where dependence on the plantation export economy was highest and crop failure most severe. Patterns of economic hardship, then, can be seen to have predicted epidemic severity (increase in death *rate*) at least as closely as entomological conditions and considerably more closely than low immunity (spleen rate).

It appears that the dry zone districts that experienced heightened malaria mortality in 1934–1935 were not considered part of 'the epidemic area' because such increases occurred often, endemically. As Briercliffe explained,

[i]n most parts of the dry zone, increased prevalence of malaria was not considered to be in the nature of an epidemic. In the North-Central Province [in 1934–35] . . . there was an abnormal increase both in the morbidity and mortality due to malaria, but as malaria

in this province is hyper-endemic the increase was attributed to a worse malaria season than usual. If there had been no epidemic else-where conditions in the North-Central Province would have called for little comment since 'bad malaria years' are frequent there.[45]

In effect, as Newnham observed, combined drought- and Depression-unemployment appear to have pushed up destitution (acute hunger) levels in export-dependent districts to those in the dry zone, a 'catching-up' of sorts to conditions normally endemic in the north-central districts.

But there was a further limitation to Briercliffe's mapping of epidemic relative intensity, minor by comparison, but one also with important inter-pretative consequences. Although he employed four categories of mortality severity, the highest level (400 per cent or more above non-epidemic levels) itself included a wide range of severity levels, from 'severe' to extreme. C.A. Gill, working apparently with the same subdistrict (divisional) data, also mapped epidemic intensity patterns. But in doing so, he included an even higher category, 7–12 times 'normal,' a categorization that allowed even greater spatial discernment of epidemic mortality patterns across the island. The significance becomes apparent in comparing Briercliffe's epidemic inten-sity map (Figure 2.4) with that prepared by Gill (Figure 2.5).[46]

As a *ratio* of epidemic to previous years' mortality, Gill's mapping of his 'Epidemic Figures' also tended to underestimate intensity in the higher mor-tality northern dry zone, as did Briercliffe's. Nonetheless, his mapping sug-gests more clearly than do the Briercliffe maps a broad focal character to epidemic mortality in 1934–1935, a pattern reminiscent of Christophers's maps of epidemic mortality in Punjab three decades earlier: that is to say, one of regular mortality increase as the centre of the epidemic region is approached.[47] Thus it suggested a similar 'general determining influence' unlikely to be explained by local entomological factors. Indeed, Christo-phers himself would later describe the Ceylon epidemic of 1934–1935 as 'show[ing] the same focal character which was so conspicuous in the Punjab epidemics,'[48] and which he had concluded in the latter case to be a function of agricultural hardship: harvest failure and associated famishment (acute hunger).

## Mortality differentials within epidemic tracts

The impact of economic conditions (destitution) on malaria lethality was supported as well by mortality differentials observed within the epidemic tracts, differentials that were not readily explained by differences in expo-sure to malarial infection. The increase in death rate amongst the general population, for example, was recorded to be almost three times greater than that observed for the estate population.[49] Mortality in the plantation population rose from 21.1 per 1,000 in the 1924–1933 period, to 26.7 per

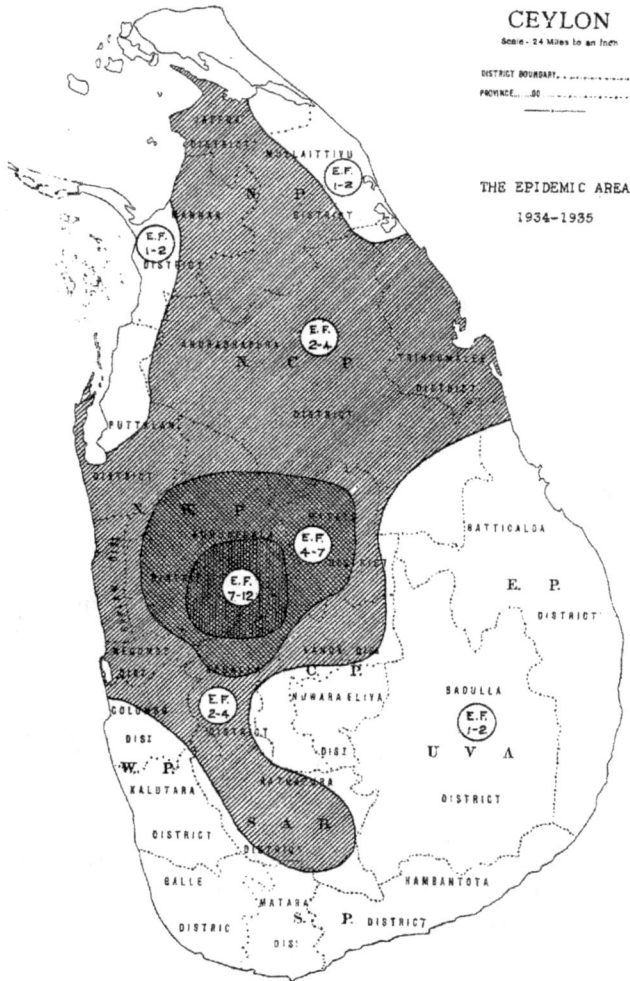

*Figure 2.5* 'Epidemic Figure'* map of 1934–1935 Ceylon malaria epidemic

*Source:* C.A. Gill, *Report on the Malaria Epidemic in Ceylon in 1934–35* (Colombo: Ceylon Govt Press, Sept. 1935), Map IV. *Sessional Paper XXIII – 1935.*

*Calculated by C.A. Gill as the number of times the Nov. 1934–Mar. 1935 mortality rate exceeded that of the same period for the preceding year. See note 46.

1,000 in 1935, an increase of 21 per cent; for Ceylon as a whole, from 23.1 to 36.6 per 1,000, a 58 per cent increase. Direct comparison is somewhat problematic because these rates are not age-adjusted. However, similar differentials are apparent for infant mortality rates, where this is not a concern. In Kegalla district, for example, infant mortality levels in estate and non-estate sectors were at similar levels before 1935, but rose 315 percent in the non-estate population in 1935, from approximately 125 deaths to 515 per 1,000 live births, compared to a 116 percent in the estate population, to 251 deaths per 1,000 live births (Table 2.2).[50]

It seems unlikely these mortality differentials reflected major differences in malaria exposure. 'Looking for an explanation in natural causes,' Meyer notes, 'medical authorities . . . asserted that severity was proportionate to proximity to the rivers.' But there were many settlements, he suggests, citing *Village Expansion Schemes* within Kegalle and Kurunegala districts, seriously affected by the epidemic that were situated far from water courses.[51]

The Kegalla district, Meegama has pointed out,

> can broadly be divided into two sectors, the estate sector with a settled Indian labour force, and in between them a rural peasant sector dependent on paddy cultivation. The drought of 1934–35 led to a failure of crops in the peasant sector where there were famine and distress on an unprecedented scale. The estates, on the other hand, . . . cultivated a perennial like rubber which, in the short term, was not affected by a drought. Thus the estate labourer . . . had stable employment and he lived on imported food [hence] his level of nutrition was unaffected by the drought.[52]

Meegama's observations can be qualified somewhat. Estate labour may have had relatively 'stable employment' for those left on the plantations in 1934–1935. But according to Meyer, as prices and export demand plummeted during the Depression years of 1931–1934, considerable emigration from some estates had taken place.[53] Some labourers no doubt repatriated to India in advance of the epidemic, though under Depression conditions

*Table 2.2* Infant mortality rate, estate and non-estate sectors, Kegalla district, Ceylon [Sri Lanka], 1930–1940

| Year | Estate sector | Non-estate sector |
| --- | --- | --- |
| 1930 | 136 | 133 |
| 1931 | 127 | 126 |
| 1932 | 128 | 114 |
| 1933 | 112 | 123 |
| 1934 | 116 | 136 |
| 1935 | 251 | 515 |
| 1936 | 103 | 132 |
| 1937 | 109 | 118 |
| 1938 | 137 | 124 |
| 1939 | 141 | 159 |
| 1940 | 117 | 113 |

*Source*: S.A. Meegama, 'Malaria Eradication and its Effect on Mortality Levels', *Population Studies*, 21, 3, Nov. 1967, p. 230.

there was perhaps little incentive to do so. Others may well have added to the numbers of destitute labourers in the surrounding non-estate areas, further amplifying estate/non-estate differentials in destitution, and in turn epidemic mortality levels in 1934–1935. Even on the estates, livelihood 'stability' was also relative. In the context of a dramatic fall in estate production, labour households likely accepted having fewer members in employment, and lower wage levels, before abandoning the estates altogether in search of livelihood off the plantation. If relatively protected from the effects of harvest failure, many estate households, in other words, probably were also under considerable economic stress leading up to the epidemic.

At the same time, only a small portion of the population in the 'estate districts' was employed on the estates.[54] Most households were non-estate Sinhalese small peasants, dependent on subsistence rice cultivation and small-scale cash crop cultivation of rubber and coconut. In the economic circumstances of 1934, these non-estate small peasant producers were hit doubly hard: first by the Depression-induced loss of cash crop income since as small independent producers their access to international export markets likely was even more limited than on the estates; and then by crop failure.[55]

Other indicators of a major role for economic hardship in epidemic severity are anecdotal accounts of class and caste differentials within the non-estate village population. Colonial officials were struck by the evident severity of the epidemic amongst the poorest. 'In almost adjacent *wasamas* [groups of villages], one finds surprising differences in the change of the death rate during this year,' Meyer notes, adding that 'the areas most affected were not of the [higher] Goyigama caste.'[56] The 1935 administrative report also noted that '[t]he most affected localities were the poorest and the most depressed.'[57]

The importance of underlying emaciation is suggested in clinical observations as well. Medical officers documented 'a large number' of cases of oedema among malarial patients, particularly among children. Variously attributed to malaria-induced anaemia and hookworm infection, Briercliffe questioned this interpretation, recounting in some detail the findings of a study of 19 severe malaria cases. Vivax malaria (a species generally associated with lower parasite levels) was as common as falciparum malaria, and less than a third were found to have hookworm infection. Among those with anemia there appeared to be 'no correspondence between the degree of anaemia and the severity of the oedema.' Briercliffe's 'personal opinion' was that these were cases of starvation oedema 'of the same category as . . . famine oedema' or 'war oedema,' adding that 'the one feature common to all . . . was repeated attacks of fever.' Good food, enforced rest, and treatment provided in hospital, he noted, effected 'a rapid and striking improvement,' though the overall death rate among young children was 45 per cent.[58]

There was of course a third economic dimension to the epidemic, also dramatically apparent in narrative accounts: that of starvation secondary to malaria debility. '[W]ith whole communities laid low with fever,' local officials observed, 'there was no one to work the *chenas* (village fields) . . . people, weakened by disease and unable to work, were under threat of death through starvation.' In one house

> everyone was down with fever with the exception of a small child eighteen months old. She was sprawling about, howling for food which her mother, in a state of delirium, was unable to give. . . . [F]ew, if any, villagers could provide for themselves or had sufficient food to maintain a livelihood. It was obvious therefore that steps had to be taken to provide not only medical comforts but the ordinary necessities of life.[59]

This level of distress was officially recognized on December 6, a month into the epidemic, and relief was initiated that included school feeding. It was clear to administrators that breaking the circle required food.

Still, the question remained as to how the vicious circle came to be established. Without preceding starvation, would the downward cycle have begun in the first place? Or at least would it have been amenable to interruption? It was a question that Briercliffe also felt compelled to address in the official report on the Ceylon epidemic. 'Even if the masses had been well fed and prosperous,' he concluded, 'there would have been an epidemic of malaria, but the vicious circle of malaria and destitution acting and reacting on one another would not have been established.'[60]

## The non-immune thesis resurgent

Despite the many references to extreme economic hardship in Briercliffe's official report,[61] subsequent writing by Western malaria workers on epidemic causation would focus almost exclusively, as we have seen, on aspects of malaria transmission: a sudden increase in malaria transmission amongst a population with only limited previously acquired specific immunity.[62] These later accounts share several features. First, there is little discussion of the maps that indicated spatial distribution of epidemic mortality, in particular, Gill's 'Epidemic Figure' map. Second, even in those accounts that made reference to economic hardship, such conditions generally were left unexplored and failed to appear in the writers' conclusions.[63]

A further characteristic of the later 'off-shore' accounts is a paucity of historical context. Meyer remarks on the tendency of subsequent analysts to view the 1934–1935 epidemic as exceptional, 'sans précédent.'[64] A largely ahistorical analysis, Meyer suggests, allows the convenience of a manageable, clearly delineated and dramatic epidemic 'story,' the designation 'unprecedented' suggesting that exploration of broader dimensions and patterns is unnecessary.

Curiously also, in a paper on the 1934–1935 epidemic presented to the Royal Society of Medicine in November 1935, Briercliffe and his co-contributor, W. Dalrymple-Champneys, made no mention of famine conditions leading up to the epidemic.[65] Gill, in a presentation to the Royal Society of Tropical Medicine and Hygiene two months later, also dealt solely with microbiological aspects of malaria transmission across the epidemic period,[66] despite having referred to famine 'as an important predisposing cause' of regional epidemics in his initial 1935 report. Indeed, he went on to propose a purely speculative explanation as epidemic 'trigger' – a biologically determined periodic reactivation ('relapse') of the malaria parasite.[67] It would be left up to Dalrymple-Champneys, the Deputy Chief Medical Officer of Health of Ceylon, also in attendance at the January 1936 Royal Society meeting, to remind Gill of 'the important fact that these [Sri Lankan] people were undernourished, very many of them grossly so, owing to the partial failure of the paddy crop.'[68] It was as if an implicit obligation existed to direct analysis for a scientific audience solely to microbiological considerations.

Certainly, increasing political sensitivity would have been a factor in the downplaying or setting aside of the role of starvation in the 1934–1935 epidemic. In the final years of the colonial period, growing anti-colonial movements in South Asia left even less political 'space' for highlighting hunger in published documents in the metropole.[69] At the same time, attraction to entomo-immunological explanations of the Ceylon epidemic reflected burgeoning medical anticipation of tools to predict epidemic events in the microbiologic realm, a pursuit expressed earlier in Gill's efforts to forecast epidemic occurrence in Punjab province. It was an interest that can be traced back to Ross's early efforts at mathematical modelling of malaria transmission in India,[70] work later pursued more intently by G. Macdonald.[71] Mathematical precision conferred an aura of analytic certitude and competency, whereas acknowledgement of social determinants seemed to take control of epidemic malaria out of the hands of the medical profession.

But the retreat from economic dimensions in epidemic causality can be seen to reflect a larger dichotomy in views of epidemic malaria causation in the 1930s. That fault-line had been etched a decade earlier in heated debates within the League of Nations Malaria Commission, with members largely divided between those with extended 'field' experience of malaria – and direct responsibility for its toll, such as Bentley – and those whose expertise lay in vector-control work. In the case of Ceylon, H.E. Newnham, Special Commissioner for the Relief of Distress in 1934–1935 Ceylon, represented the former, who urged – in terms starkly reminiscent of the 1924 and 1927 Malaria Commission reports – a program of complete 'rural reconstruction' to address the 'near starvation of the peasantry' as the only realistic solution to future epidemics.[72]

Yet it would be the entomo-immunological explanations of the Ceylon epidemic that prevailed in subsequent medical literature. 'In Ceylon,' Paul Russell wrote in 1952, 'deficiency in the . . . monsoon rains will result in certain rivers drying to the point where they become series of countless pools of the type favoured by *culicifacies*. In each case an epidemic of fulminant proportions has resulted.'[73] That same year Macdonald again asserted that 'the disastrous Ceylon epidemic of 1934 and 1935 was shown, like the 1908 Punjab epidemic, to be . . . [the result of] the general interplay of interrupted transmission and varying immunity.'[74] Analysis was marked by a 'narrow environmental determinism' that continues to influence, Silva suggests, modern interpretation of malaria history.[75]

Within modern malaria historiography, where economic hardship is recognized in the case of major South Asian epidemics, generally it is so only in passing, the compelling quantifiable micro-dynamics overshadowing conditions of the human host. In his 1978 *Mosquitoes, Man, and Malaria*, Harrison would acknowledge the possibility of 'other conditions' contributing to the 1934–1935 epidemic, including 'general physical well-being.' But attracted, it seems, by the mathematic models of malaria transmission, he concluded that

> [t]he events in Ceylon could be precisely accounted for, Mac-Donald calculated, by an increase of 5.3 times in the numbers of *culicifacies* or equally by a slight increase in longevity. . . . Briefly what happened in 1934–35 was that [following] an extraordinary drought . . . the resultant epidemic swept devastatingly through a non-immune population.[76]

The contribution of prevailing economic hardship, in turn, was deemed 'coincidence,' at best 'suggestive,' unlike the role attributed to factors of transmission: '[t]he coincidence that the people of Ceylon, like those of Sind and Punjab, met their enemy somewhat debilitated by hard times was suggestive if not conclusive that a lowering of general physical resistance played some part.'[77]

## Christophers's query

There is a serious loss here. Harrison was hardly at fault in his reading of the post-1935 secondary literature on the Ceylon epidemic in such terms. The privileging in this period of microbiologic factors in explaining epidemic malaria to the virtual exclusion of conditions of the human host had left the central question of malaria historiography unaddressed: what factors underlay the immense range in historical malaria mortality? A further glimpse into this question appears in brief commentary by Christophers, also in attendance at the January 1936 meeting of the Royal Society of

Tropical Medicine devoted to the Ceylon malaria epidemic. As in his earlier work, the question of malaria intensity was clearly on Christophers's mind, though he would raise the issue in characteristically oblique fashion. It would appear in his response to the relapse hypothesis offered by Gill to explain the initial two-week phase of mild cases documented in October 1934. '[E]vidence of such [initial] mildness,' Christophers observed, 'does not necessarily prove the relapse theory since the mildness of the cases in the beginning might be a result of numerically poor infections in the anophelines.'[78]

Here, by inference, Christophers appears to have been addressing the question of dose of infection, and in turn the possibility of heavy, 'intense' infections arising among subsequent cases. What was significant, he was suggesting, was not the mildness of the early cases, which might be expected in the initial cycle of infections transmitted from those in the population still harbouring sparse gametocytes from the previous year's transmission season. Rather, what was exceptional was the exponential rise in fever death rate (lethality) thereafter. As in *Malaria in the Punjab*, Christophers appears to have interpreted the rapid rise in malaria mortality as suggesting heightened vulnerability among the famished, but possibly also an increased dose of infection being transmitted, by virtue of this famishment.[79]

Interestingly, too, Christophers went on to query the emerging view that the conditions underlying the fulminant form of the malaria in Ceylon were the inverse to those in northern India.

> Emphasis has been laid on the fact that the [Ceylon] epidemic was one occasioned by unusual drought, i.e., conditions quite the opposite to those in *North India*. It is well, however, to note that a preceding period of drought is also seen in the northern epidemics [in India], and the heavy rainfall in October occurring after the drought may have been the actual cause of unusual prevalence of *A. culicifacies*.[80]

The Ceylon epidemic, he emphasized, was preceded by 'the greatest drought on record,' inferring that appreciation of the severity of prevailing economic stress was essential for understanding why the 1934–1935 epidemic assumed such severe proportions. And to press the point, he had come prepared.

Presenting his earlier mortality maps of the 1908 and 1892 Punjab epidemics alongside Gill's Ceylon 'Epidemic Figure' map (Figure 2.5), Christophers indicated the spatial similarities in mortality patterns. That a 'general determining influence' was at work in the Ceylon epidemic was suggested, as in earlier Punjab epidemics, by the broad focal pattern to mortality, one of regular increase as the epicentre of the epidemic is approached. Such a pattern was more likely the result of generalized harvest failure than ecological particularities of dry river-bed catchment areas. 'No one looking at these [Punjab] maps,' he continued,

> or that prepared by Colonel Gill of the Ceylon epidemic, can fail, I think, to be struck by the resemblance to maps of meteorological phenomena. They are, one feels instinctively, maps of 'malaria cyclones.' This resemblance is not merely superficial, but is due to the fact that the fundamental causation of these epidemics is meteorological.[81]

In his 'meteorological' phrasing, was Christophers referring to entomological conditions as the general determining influence? Or related immunological consequences of preceding drought? Or instead the economic impact of preceding drought patterns, as in 1908 Punjab? Or perhaps all three? True to form, he doesn't tell his audience explicitly. Yet in his cartographical comparison of the Ceylon malaria epidemic to fulminant epidemics in Punjab, the intended meaning seems evident – if perhaps clearer to those in attendance already familiar with his 1911 Punjab study.[82]

The distinction between malaria transmission and malaria mortality was crucial in understanding the epidemic of deaths in 1934–1935. Nor was it a new insight, forming the core of the earlier Duars and Punjab analyses. It lay also at the centre of many of the League of Nations Malaria Commission's 1920s study-tour observations, as seen above in Chapter 1. Destitution and starvation ('physiological poverty') triggered and fed the vicious circle between illness, unemployment, and prolonged parasitemia rates ('residual infection'), undermining previously acquired specific immunity and in turn 'profoundly influencing the incidence of malaria.'[83]

The two sides of the epidemic equation – germ transmission and host response – were not mutually exclusive. Yet in medical interpretation after 1935 they had become so. Under the gaze of a new generation of Western malaria researchers the Ceylon epidemic came to be interpreted exclusively in terms of malaria transmission: enhanced transmission in the epidemic year itself, and 'insufficient' transmission levels in the period preceding the epidemic, leaving a non-immune ('little salted') population particularly vulnerable.[84]

But the narrowed framework post-1935 also held a larger significance. For many of the malaria researchers whose work focused primarily on malaria transmission control, the Ceylon epidemic marked a shedding of the so-called pessimistic view that malaria, like tuberculosis, was a 'social disease' requiring broad economic development. An immuno-entomological reading of the 1934–1935 Ceylon epidemic arguably allowed a final jettisoning, in the academic literature that followed, of the brake to the sanitationist (vector control) approach. There was, of course, a deep irony to this 'shedding.' For the 1934–1935 epidemic had also brought open recognition among colonial medical officers of the technical difficulties of controlling malaria transmission on the island under conditions of drought. From the earliest weeks of the epidemic, the public health department had attempted extensive anti-larval measures to control river-bed anopheline larval development – oiling pools, flushing river beds – to little avail. In the aftermath of the epidemic, all involved acknowledged that anti-larval efforts could not hope to alter drought-triggered vector breeding that triggered such epidemics on the island.[85] V.B. Wigglesworth, lecturer at the London School of Hygiene and Tropical Medicine, . . . would conclude that '[f]or the moment, efficient treatment of the disease is all that can be offered to the villager.'[86] In effect, the 'mere-palliation' ghost of Mian Mir had arisen once again.

At the theoretical level, however, interpretation of the 1934–1935 epidemic in entomo-immunological terms rekindled the 'optimistic' view that malaria 'control' need not await economic development, *viz.*, 'control' of destitution. It lay in identifying and altering the weakest link in the fragile chain of vector transmission,[87] in turn pushing malaria analysis even further in the direction of theoretical modelling.

## Post-1935 mathematical modelling

In the aftermath of the 1934–1935 Ceylon epidemic, the 'Human Factor' in its original meaning, as applied to Punjab regional epidemics, largely disappeared from literature on South Asian malaria. Macdonald would go on to formulate mathematical models of malaria transmission, work which helped lay the theoretical basis for malaria eradication programs in the post-WW2 period. At the same time, fiscal retrenchment in India further intensified in all spheres of British colonial governance including public health. To the extent that malaria research continued on the subcontinent, increasingly it was undertaken by malaria workers funded by the International Health Division of the Rockefeller Foundation and the Ross Institute in London, and was directed to anti-vector experimental work and circumscribed control programs in industrial and plantation estates. With European political tensions rising, little in the way of field research into epidemicity continued at the Karnal malaria research station, and British and U.S. malaria researchers were soon reassigned to WW2 military priorities.

In the early post-war period Punjab became the site of residual insecticide (DDT) trials, which brought an end to field research work on the mechanisms of malaria mortality epidemicity. Academic interest in malaria immunity now shifted to another form, channelled into intense debate over the wisdom of extending DDT programs in holoendemic regions of Africa and the possible risks associated with reducing levels of protective immunity in populations.[88] By this time, Yacob and Swaroop had revisited the question of epidemicity and immunity in Punjab by analyzing the almost three decades of spleen rate data collected in the province.[89] Their conclusion that spleen rates failed to predict epidemicity was overshadowed, however, by the immunological view now prevailing in the international literature on South Asian regional ('fulminant') epidemics.[90]

It was in this period that Macdonald would reach back briefly to Christophers's 1911 Punjab study, interpreting its conclusions regarding the region's 'fulminant' epidemics, as we have seen, in terms of 'certain rainfall characteristics and an inadequate immunity in the local population.'[91] Given the context, by 'inadequate immunity' Macdonald almost certainly was referring to acquired (malaria-induced) immunity.[92] Here, the conceptual blurring of general immune capacity and acquired immunity under Gill's term 'communal immunity' had given way to a complete supplanting. In effect, acquired immunity, a function of malaria transmission, had come to be accorded the full mantle of the 'Human Factor' in malaria.

The most important question left unanswered by the theory of non-immunes was explaining the post-1920 decline in South Asian malaria epidemics. Episodic drought continued to afflict Punjab after 1908, as before, with presumably year-to-year fluctuation in the proportion of non-immune infants in the population. Yet fulminant malaria epidemics did not.[93] Writing in the 1920s, at a point when this decline in epidemicity was not yet definitive, Gill's attraction to the non-immunes thesis is perhaps understandable. But by mid-century, with three decades essentially free of 'fulminant' epidemics, commitment to the thesis is more puzzling.[94]

More curious still, in his quantitative modelling of malaria epidemicity, Macdonald never directly incorporated a non-immune factor.[95] Indeed, at one point he would express doubts about the adequacy of the theoretical models for explaining fulminant malaria in South Asia. 'Personal work in two of the great epidemic areas – the Punjab and Ceylon,' he openly acknowledged in the same 1952 paper,

> has left [me] satisfied that the accepted explanation of periodic epidemics is an entirely satisfactory statement of what happens, but completely unsatisfying as a statement of why it happens. . . . [I]t is not clear why small changes in climate should produce such dramatic changes in the *amount of transmission*.[96]

What Macdonald appears to have been puzzled about was not 'dramatic' changes in levels of malaria transmission – the proportion of a population infected – but rather changes in its lethality. The mathematical models could explain how rates of infection could rise rapidly from low to near-universal levels in a given year, but not why soaring malaria lethality was seen in some years of universal infection such as 1908 and not in others. It was as if, Macdonald was suggesting, a key variable was still missing.

Despite offering his mathematical modelling as potentially a 'complete' representation of malaria transmission and epidemicity,[97] in fact a number of factors relating to the human host and 'physiological poverty' were missing from them, which potentially could be important for influencing rates of transmission. Dose of infection was one, and the range of possible factors influencing effective dose. Recovery rate was another, the time required for a person with malaria to throw off infection, or to succumb to it. Any lengthening of the period that gametocytes remained patent in the human host, for example, could potentially amplify the man-mosquito cycle of transmission. In the early years of malaria research in India, such questions relating to 'residual infection' and recovery rate had been assumed to be central for understanding epidemiological patterns of malaria transmission. 'All the circumstances . . . which tend to delay recovery, or to lessen the resisting power of individuals,' a tropical medicine text in 1922 had stressed, 'enhance the prevalence and severity.'[98] Interestingly, at one point Macdonald himself would acknowledge the possibility of variation in recovery rate. But as a factor in the practical workings of his epidemic malaria model, he considered that it was 'not liable to abrupt change . . . and its significance in this context is therefore slight.'[99] In the process, the question as to what could *cause* variation in recovery rate also was left unaddressed.

The 'great epidemics' of Punjab were, above all, epidemics of death. What appears to have been perplexing Macdonald was the enormous variation in mortality from year to year: how 'small changes in rainfall' could explain 10- or 20-fold increases in mortality as seen throughout the first half of the colonial period. But he does not pose the question in these terms; his reference is solely to 'amount of transmission,' in a seeming conflation of the two issues. The analytic difficulties stemming from the conflation appear obvious. But at the time, the transformation in meaning of 'epidemic' – from one of mortality to one of infection (transmission) – appears to have been anything but. What had intervened in the interim was the emergence, unarticulated, of a very different concept of 'epidemic.' No longer viewed as 'epidemics of death,' the term by the 1930s had come to mean primarily increased rates of infection. This narrowed meaning can be seen in the Ceylon colonial literature as well. Briercliffe's designation of 'epidemic zone' was an entomological definition, delineated by watershed boundaries in terms of drying river-bed pools: malaria transmission. The equating of 'epidemic' to infection (transmission) would be articulated even more explicitly in Wigglesworth's assessment of 1934–1935 Ceylon mortality patterns, one in which he excludes the dry-zone northern districts from his analysis on the basis that 'the people are so saturated with the disease that true "epidemics" of malaria [there] are impossible.'[100] Dunn similarly would explain that

[a]s this [northern dry zone] is the hyperendemic area, a rise of this nature, while noteworthy, may be considered to be in the nature of a minor 'localised epidemic' of the kind which often occurs owing to the failure or partial failure of the North-East Monsoon without

any important connection with the chief epidemic, mostly confined to the non-endemic area.[101]

The point here is that this reading was possible because an immunological explanation of epidemicity was already assumed, seemingly internalized, in epidemiological thought: drought and dry river beds may have been widespread across much of the island in the lead-up to the 1934–1935 epidemic, but malaria mortality was presumed to have soared primarily where specific (acquired) immunity was low, despite spleen rate data to the contrary in the case of the northern epidemic areas and much of Kurunegala district.[102]

Of course, one can recognize reasons for attention to specific immunity. Acquired immunity could and did offer relative protection in hyper- and holoendemic regions of the world, including in some areas in South Asia. Indeed, recent epidemiological reports suggest that some degree of 'acquired' protection (immunity) among adults can follow even a limited number of episodes of falciparum malaria infection.[103] What was problematic was preoccupation with the concept in analytic circumstances where a different set of questions – patterns of relative mortality risk – required to be addressed.[104] With epidemicity equated to infection (transmission), other issues previously recognized as key to epidemicity such as recovery rate, dose of infection, and case fatality rate would fade in importance and in investigative attention in turn.

## Epistemic aftermath

This brief sketch of South Asian malaria research through the second half of the colonial period suggests that understanding of the 'Human Factor' in malaria epidemicity dropped out of sight not through empirical refutation, but instead by default. Earlier socio-economic observations, rather than being integrated with new developments in microbiology, immunology, and entomology, were in effect superseded by them.

The supersession, however, was not universal. Christophers would retire from the Indian Medical Service and the Directorship of the Central Research Institute at Kasauli in 1932, and was appointed Professor of Malaria Studies of London University at the London School of Hygiene and Tropical Medicine, a post he held until 1938. In this subsequent work attention to hunger remained peripheral to his continuing entomological writing and research into anti-malarial drugs and their modes of action. But where economic questions arose his analysis remained as meticulous as for parasite and vector investigation. In his 1928 League of Nations Malaria Commission report on 'How to do a malaria survey,' for example, one section included the 'study of the economic, immigration and other human conditions.' Under the heading of 'Food conditions – price of food stuffs [and] wages,' he advised assiduous analysis of '[d]ietary as ascertained by *actual observation and weighment*.'[105] As a scientist, in other words, Christophers had not forgotten the subsistence circumstances of the human host, taking into account hunger as meticulously as entomological, microbiological, and biochemical aspects. There is thus little to suggest that he himself had come to reconsider his earlier conclusions.

True to character he never openly queried the non-immune thesis, respectfully acknowledging the views of colleagues, though in his own 1911 analysis of fulminant epidemics in Punjab he had stressed that more highly endemic tracts in the province were equally vulnerable to fulminant epidemics.[106] Indeed, in all his writing and literature reviews Christophers scrupulously reported the views of his colleagues: quoting verbatim, for example, Macdonald, Gill, and Perry's non-immune conclusions.[107] Yet in addressing specific epidemics he never failed to insert, if undemonstrably, economic dimensions. In 1949, in a chapter on malaria epidemiology and endemiology in M.F. Boyd's *Malariology: A Comprehensive Survey*, the first major compendium of malaria science, he cited once again the statistical results of his 1911 study, *Malaria in the Punjab*, complete with reproductions of his original epidemic maps.[108] He also described Bentley's work on intense malaria in lower Bengal in relation to agricultural decline and 'decay in human prosperity': 'physical changes in the land' that had transformed once 'prosperous communities . . . [into] decayed and poverty stricken' regions;[109] elsewhere lauding Bentley's 'bonification' efforts.[110] Addressing the significance of 'tropical aggregation of labour,' he highlighted – in addition to the potential mixture of non-immunes with those already infected – the likelihood of 'much private hardship' in labour camps, 'especially when sickness breaks out and families become broken up.'[111]

Nor had his earlier studies been forgotten among Indian Medical Service colleagues. In his 1926 testimony to the Royal Commission on Agriculture in India, J.D. Graham, Public Health Commission for the GOI, would cite Christophers and Bentley's *Malaria in the Duars* as a 'very interesting [report] . . . work[ing] out . . . the economic side of the labour wage' by addressing 'questions of food, housing, social conditions and standards of comfort of labour in this intensely malarious area.'[112] Christophers's 1911 economic conclusions continued to be cited in scientific papers throughout the 1930s.[113] Yet despite continuing acknowledgement, and apparent regard, few papers actually attempted to incorporate economic factors in interpreting the results of their own studies. The earlier 'Human Factor' research remained in full view as historical documents, but as an investigative subject it did not.[114]

The non-immune thesis, in Gill's hands, did not start off as a rival theory of fulminant malaria. But it quickly became so. By the 1930s, the focus in research and theoretical interest now lay elsewhere, and Christophers's earlier research came to be read through very different conceptual lenses. In a highly laudatory 12-page bibliographic memoir of Christophers's scientific accomplishments following his death in 1977, both the Punjab and Duars malaria studies were cited among his 215 published scientific papers, reports, and texts. Yet Punjab epidemic causality would be interpreted solely in terms of disease transmission: flooding and 'practically absent immunity.' More puzzling still, *Malaria in the Duars* would be grouped among a number of studies of hyperendemic malaria in 'population[s] saturated with infection, [where] pathogenicity was low.'[115]

Beyond absorption with immunological theory, however, there was an additional source of conceptual loss at play in the demise of the 'Human Factor' within academic malaria thought through the final years of the colonial period. Already by the 1930s, practical comprehension of 'predisposition' to disease rapidly was fading as the subject of hunger came to be reformulated under the influence of another new medical subdiscipline, that of nutritional science. In place of hunger, qualitative 'dietary' issues increasingly would come to dominate medical discussion, overshadowing quantitative issues of not enough of any food to eat.

The analytic impact of this parallel development can be glimpsed in a 1941 address delivered to the Rotary Club of the Nilgiris in southern India by Paul F. Russell on deputation from the Rockefeller Foundation's International Health Division for experimental mosquito control measures in southern India. We will meet up with Russell again in his central role in post-WW2 malaria eradication policy. Here, however, his 1941 talk sheds light on the conceptual shift already well underway in medical understanding of human hunger. In the epidemiology of malaria in the Indian subcontinent, Russell argued, there was 'not the slightest evidence that better food will help either to prevent infection or to produce a milder attack. Well fed soldiers in perfect physical condition go down with malaria as rapidly and as seriously, with as high a death rate as average villagers.'[116]

In this dismissal of nutritional factors in South Asian malaria lethality Russell was probably correct, if in relation to 'better' food he had in mind issues of micronutrient deficiency: there was little evidence that a qualitatively 'better' diet offered protection from fulminant malaria.[117] But here he would have been speaking to a very different meaning of 'nutrition' than that expressed in the term the 'Human Factor' in earlier malaria literature: the latter denoting acute hunger (semi- and frank starvation). In interpreting past epidemic experience in India, malaria workers by mid-twentieth century, in other words, were working with concepts of hunger fundamentally different than those addressed by researchers and public health officials in colonial service a generation earlier. That Russell's dismissal of hunger in relation to malaria mortality stood uncontested in 1941 speaks to a fundamental transformation in understanding of human subsistence which had taken place in the intervening decades since publication of *Malaria in the Punjab*.

However anodyne the term 'Human Factor' had been in the earlier malaria literature, the designation nevertheless had conferred scientific prominence and legitimacy, if fleetingly, on the issue of human hunger within the emerging discipline of malaria studies. Now stripped of its formal designation, acute hunger (semi-/frank starvation) as a causal agent in malaria epidemicity no longer belonged within medical discourse. The demise of hunger as a medical category in epidemic history is a central question for health historiography. In the chapter that follows, one key stage in this loss is explored in the emergence of nutritional science as it took disciplinary shape in early twentieth-century colonial India.

## Notes

1 C.L. Dunn, *Malaria in Ceylon: An Enquiry into its Causes* (London: Bailliere, Tindall and Cox, 1936), 54.

2 G. Covell, and J.D. Baily, 'Further Observations on a Regional Epidemic of malaria in Northern Sind,' *Records of the Malaria Survey of India*, 6, 3, Sept. 1936, 411–437, at 426.

3 C.A. Gill, *Report on the Malaria Epidemic in Ceylon in 1934–35* (Colombo: Ceylon Govt Press, 1935).

4 S.R. Christophers, 'Commentary,' in C.A. Gill, 'Some Points in the Epidemiology of Malaria Arising out of the Study of the Malaria Epidemic in Ceylon in 1934–35,' *Transactions of the Royal Society of Tropical Medicine and Hygiene*, 29, 5, Feb. 1936, 427–480, at 466–469.

5 S.R. Christophers, 'Malaria in the Punjab,' *Scientific Memoirs by Officers of the Medical and Sanitary Departments of the Government of India* (New Series), No. 46 (Calcutta: Superintendent Govt Printing, 1911).

6 R. Briercliffe, *The Ceylon Malaria Epidemic, 1934–35. Report by the Director of Medical and Sanitary Services* (Colombo: Ceylon Govt Press, 1935), 26–27. Briercliffe's maps and charts were published separately as a Supplement to his main 1935 report.

7 Ibid., 27.

8 G. Harrison, *Mosquitoes, Malaria and Man: A History of the Hostilities since 1880* (New York: E.P. Dutton, 1978), 203.

9 V.B. Wigglesworth, 'Malaria in Ceylon,' *Asiatic Review*, 32, 1936, 611–619, at 613; Dunn, *Malaria in Ceylon*, 5; Harrison, *Mosquitoes, Malaria and Man*, 205.

10 T.W. Tyssul Jones, 'Deforestation and Epidemic Malaria in the Wet and Intermediate Zones of Ceylon,' *Indian Journal of Malariology*, 5, 1, Mar. 1951, 135–161, Map 2 at 140 [hereafter, *IJM*].

11 S. Rajendram, and S.H. Jayewickreme, 'Malaria in Ceylon,' *IJM*, 5, 1, Pt. 1, Mar. 1951, 1–73.

12 For the definition of spleen rate, see ch. 1, note 66.

13 Agricultural impoverishment was not inevitable in the dry zone; historically, the northern half of Ceylon supported a vibrant canal irrigation rural economy; T.W. Tyssul Jones, 'Malaria and the Ancient Cities of Ceylon,' *IJM*, 5, 1, Mar. 1951, 125–133; Briercliffe, *The Ceylon Malaria Epidemic*, 43.

14 Tyssul Jones, 'Deforestation and Epidemic Malaria; Briercliffe, *The Ceylon Malaria Epidemic*, 23–26; H.F. Carter, and W.P. Jacocks, 'Observations on the Transmission of Malaria by Anopheline Mosquitoes in Ceylon,' *Ceylon Journal of Science*, Section D, Pt. 2, 1929, 67–86.

15 Gill, *Report on the Malaria Epidemic in Ceylon,* 19. Dunn reports '11.3 inches of rain between October 6 and October 30. . . rain [that] partially flushed the river breeding grounds of the mosquito . . . but the relative humidity rose from 51 per cent before the rain to 72 per cent after'; *Malaria in Ceylon,* 22.

16 Briercliffe, *The Ceylon Malaria Epidemic,* 35.

17 Ibid., 28, 41–42, Chart 7.

18 Gill, *Report on the Malaria Epidemic in Ceylon,* 17.

19 Ibid., 16.

20 Briercliffe, *The Ceylon Malaria Epidemic,* 26. Gill summarized earlier entomological findings by H.F. Carter as showing that 'although *An. culicifacies* exhibits a predilection for sun-lit pools in river beds, it also breeds freely and frequently in many other situations, more especially in wells, . . . borrow pits, quarries, drains, and pools and sheets of water formed during the rains'; Gill, *Report on the Malaria Epidemic in Ceylon,* 15; H.F. Carter, 'Report on Malaria and Anopheline Mosquitoes in Ceylon.' Sessional Paper VII. (Colombo: Ceylon Govt Press, 1927); H.F. Carter, and W.P. Jacocks, 'Observations on the Transmission of Malaria by Anopheline Mosquitoes in Ceylon,' *Ceylon Journal of Science,* 2, Pt. 4, 1930.

21 Briercliffe, *The Ceylon Malaria Epidemic,* 39; S. Rajendram and Jayewickreme, 'Malaria in Ceylon,' 54.

22 Briercliffe, *The Ceylon Malaria Epidemic,* 44–46. Deaths recorded among children under 5 years of age in 1908 Punjab ranged from 47 per cent in Amritsar city to 60–80 per cent in smaller rural towns where age distribution was less likely affected by adult male migration; S. Zurbrigg, *Epidemic Malaria and Hunger in Colonial Punjab: 'Weakened by Want'* (London and New Delhi: Routledge, 2019), 62.

23 The proportion of falciparum infections increased over the course of the epidemic, from 24.7 per cent in November to 43.7 per cent in January; Briercliffe, *The Ceylon Malaria Epidemic,* 46–48.

24 Ibid., 39.

25 Ibid., Map 18. Rather confusingly, Briercliffe uses the term 'epidemic *zone*' on a contour map (Map 6) and in a subheading (p. 21); otherwise, he refers to the 'epidemic *area*' (or 'districts affected by the epidemic') throughout the text, in contrast to districts 'outside the epidemic area.' The demarcating line based on the four-river watershed is referred to on Maps 18 and 19 as the 'Boundary of Epidemic 1934–35.'

26 Ibid., 40.

27 Ibid., 39.

28 Briercliffe, *The Ceylon Malaria Epidemic,* 43, Map 18.

29 Ibid., Map 19.

30 Ibid., 40, 43.

31 Ibid., 18.

32 Ibid., 21, Table 9; R.M. Dickson, 'The Malaria Epidemic in Ceylon, 1934–35,' *Journal of the Royal Army Medical Corps,* 1935, 85–90.

33 Briercliffe, *The Ceylon Malaria Epidemic,* 46, Table 24(b).

34 Ibid., 44.

35 The highest 'Epidemic Figure' area (7–12 times 'normal') appears to have extended beyond the 'intermediate zone' of 20–40 per cent spleen rates to slightly overlap the neighbouring dry zone divisions of 40–60 per cent spleen rate; the second highest 'Epidemic Figure' area (4–7) extended well into the northern 40–60 per cent region.

36 Briercliffe, *The Ceylon Malaria Epidemic,* 43. In a 1929 report, Carter described 'great hardships' for the dry north-central population, 'the people are in a

continual state of ill-health through malarial infections and lack of food. . . . [I]t
is scarcely surprising that many of the villages in the interior of the dry zone are
poverty stricken, that malaria and other disease are prevalent'; Carter, 'Report
on Malaria and Anopheline Mosquitoes in Ceylon,' 8, as cited in Briercliffe, *The
Ceylon Malaria Epidemic*, 43.

37  E. Meyer, 'L'Épidémie de malaria de 1934–1935 à Sri-Lanka: fluctuations
économiques et fluctuations climatiques,' *Cultures et Développement*, 14, 2–3,
1982, 183–226, at 186; ibid., 14, 4, 589–638.
38  Briercliffe, *The Ceylon Malaria Epidemic*, Supplement, Chart 3.
39  World Bank, *The Economic Development of Ceylon* (Baltimore: Johns Hopkins
Press, 1952), 12.
40  H.E. Newnham, *Report on the Relief of Distress due to Sickness and Shortage of
Food, September 1934 to December 1935* (Colombo: Ceylon Government Press,
1936), 6–7.
41  Ibid., 7; S.R. Christophers, 'Endemic and Epidemic Prevalence,' in M.F. Boyd,
ed., *Malariology* (Philadelphia: W.B. Saunders, 1949), 698–721, at 712.
42  Newnham, *Report on the Relief of Distress*, 7.
43  Briercliffe, *The Ceylon Malaria Epidemic*, 27. Briercliffe mapped 1934 South-
West Monsoon (May–Sept.) deficit levels using absolute rainfall figures rather
than proportionate decline, the resulting map failing to convey *relative* severity
of the drought in the normally low-rainfall (dry) zone; Briercliffe, *The Ceylon
Malaria Epidemic*, Map 13; R. Briercliffe, and W. Dalrymple-Champneys, 'Discussion on the Malaria Epidemic in Ceylon, 1934–35,' *Proceedings of the Royal
Society of Medicine*, 29, 1936, 543, Fig. 5.
44  Briercliffe, *The Ceylon Malaria Epidemic*, 27, 68.
45  Ibid., 20.
46  Gill employed subdistrict (division) mortality data from 130 registration circles,
as had Christophers with Punjab *thana*-level data, to map epidemic intensity spatially across the island. His 'normal' comparative rate, however, was the mean
Nov. 1933–Mar. 1934 death rate rather than a quinquennial mean 'because the
statistical data for a longer period could not be obtained without undue delay';
*Report on the Malaria Epidemic in Ceylon*, 11–12, Map IV.
47  Christophers, *Malaria in the Punjab*, Maps 1 and 3; reproduced in Zurbrigg,
*Epidemic Malaria and Hunger*, 67, 69.
48  Christophers, 'Endemic and Epidemic Prevalence,' 712. On the etiological significance of the focal mortality pattern, see Zurbrigg, *Epidemic Malaria and
Hunger*, 68–69.
49  Ceylon, *Administrative Report*, Commissioner of Labour, 1935, 24; as cited in
Meyer, 'L'Épidémie de malaria,' 195; S.A. Meegama, 'Malaria Eradication and its
Effect on Mortality Levels,' *Population Studies*, 21, 3, Nov. 1967, 207–237, at 230.
50  Meegama, 'Malaria Eradication,' 230.
51  Meyer, 'L'Épidémie de malaria,' 194.
52  Meegama, 'Malaria Eradication,' 229.
53  Meyer, 'L'Épidémie de malaria,' 194. Meyer questions the strict 'enclave' notion
of the estate economy, suggesting considerable interflow; ' "Enclave" Plantations, "Hemmed-In" Villages and Dualistic Representations in Colonial Ceylon,'
*Journal of Peasant Studies*, 19, 3/4, 1992, 199–228, at 194.
54  Dunn's figures suggest one-eighth of the population of the estate districts constituted estate labour households; *Malaria in Ceylon*, Graph 2.
55  Meyer, 'L'Épidémie de malaria,' 213.
56  '[I]l existe une corrélation spatiale précise entre la localisation de l'épicentre du
fléau et celle de nombreuses communautés non-Goyigama'; Meyer, 'L'Épidémie
de malaria,' 198–199.

57 *Administrative Report*, Western Province (Colombo, Kalutara), 1935, A5; *Administrative Report*, Sabaragamuwa Province (Ratnapura, Kegalle), 14; as cited in Meyer, 'L'Épidémie de malaria,' 194, 198–200.

58 Briercliffe, *The Ceylon Malaria Epidemic*, 51.

59 Newnham, *Report on the Relief of Distress*, 45–46; cited in Meegama, 'Malaria Eradication,' 230.

60 Briercliffe, *The Ceylon Malaria Epidemic*, 27.

61 In his review of earlier epidemics, Briercliffe pointed to co-existing conditions of famine or aggregation of migrant labour. An 1894 epidemic was 'attributed to "the opening of tea estates on new land in the district aggravated by scarcity of food and bad water from long continued drought.". . . . The following year, 1895, fever was . . . attributed to the disturbance of the soil when cutting the railway from Galle to Matara.' A major epidemic in 1906 occurred in 'those parts of the country where large tracts of land were being cleared for the extension of rubber cultivation, there the fever was most virulent and widely prevalent'; *The Ceylon Malaria Epidemic*, 66. On the heightened malaria lethality related to 'aggregation of tropical labour' in British India, see Zurbrigg, *Epidemic Malaria and Hunger*, 228–231.

62 Dunn, *Malaria in Ceylon*, 54l; Wigglesworth, 'Malaria in Ceylon,' 617.

63 Dunn, *Malaria in Ceylon*, Appendix, 'Graph 2.' Dunn, too, noted large mortality differentials within the epicentre districts – indeed, went to the trouble of graphing death rate differentials between the estate and non-estate (general) population for each of the six estate districts. But these apparent anomalies were set aside in his conclusions, leaving the impression that local differences in transmission and non-immunes were sufficient to explain the epidemic of deaths.

64 He describes 'un intéressant phénomène *d'amnésie collective*, chacune des épidémies qui se sont succédées depuis le milieu du XIXème siécle ont été qualifiées par les contemporains de sans précédent'; Meyer, 'L'Épidémie de malaria,' 205 [emphasis added]; as noted in R. Briercliffe, and W. Dalrymple-Champneys, 'Discussion on the malaria epidemic in Ceylon, 1934–35,' *Proceedings of the Royal Society of Medicine*, 29, 1936, 537–562, at 547.

65 Briercliffe and Dalrymple-Champneys, 'Discussion on the Malaria Epidemic.'

66 Gill, 'Some Points in the Epidemiology of Malaria,' 458.

67 Ibid., 460–465.

68 Ibid., 477.

69 In their account of the Ceylon epidemic to the Royal Society of Medicine three months earlier in November 1935, Briercliffe and Dalrymple-Champneys prefaced their presentation by pointing to 'the misleading and inaccurate accounts [of the epidemic] in the lay press of many countries . . . render[ing] it particularly desirable that a clear account of the chief events and circumstances should be given to the medical profession'; Briercliffe and Dalrymple, 'Discussion on the Malaria Epidemic,' 537.

70 Ross, in admonishing Christophers and colleagues in 1904 for the 'failure' of malaria control at Mian Mir, Punjab, had faulted them for inadequate quantitative assessment of vector numbers, and urged analysis 'prefaced by a mathematical inquiry'; R. Ross, 'The Anti-Malarial Experiment at Mian Mir, Punjab, India,' *Journal of Tropical Medicine*, Aug. 15, 1904, 255.

71 L. Bruce-Chwatt, and V.J. Glanville, eds., *Dynamics of Tropical Diseases: The Late George Macdonald* (London: Oxford University Press, 1973).

72 Interestingly, it would be Newnham, a non-medical official, who cited the socioeconomic conclusions of the earlier League of Nations Malaria Commission reports; Newnham, *Report on the Relief of Distress*, 42, as noted by M. Jones in her overview of the 1934–1935 epidemic and relief measures; *Health Policy*

*in Britain's Model Colony, Ceylon (1900–1948)* (New Delhi: Orient Longman, 2004), 187–203.

73  P.F. Russell, *Malaria: Basic Principles Briefly Stated* (Oxford: Blackwell Scientific Publs, 1952), 100.

74  G. Macdonald, 'The Analysis of Equilibrium in Malaria,' in Bruce-Chwatt and Glanville, eds., *Dynamics of Tropical Diseases*, 132 [emphasis added].

75  K.T. Silva, 'Malaria Eradication as a Legacy of Colonial Discourse: The Case of Sri Lanka,' *Parassitologia*, 36, 1994, 149–163.

76  Harrison, *Mosquitoes, Malaria and Man*, 202–206. For continuing focus on acquired immunity in contemporary epidemic malaria analysis, see M.J. Bouma, and H. van der Kaay, 'The El Niño Southern Oscillation and the Historical Malaria Epidemics on the Indian Subcontinent and Sri Lanka: An Early Warning System for Future Epidemics?,' *Tropical Medicine and International Health*, 1, 1, Feb. 1996, 86–96. For a critique of mathematical modelling in malaria work, see J.A. Nájera, 'A Critical Review of the Field Application of a Mathematical Model of Malaria Eradication,' *Bulletin of the World Health Organization*, 50, 1974, 449–457.

77  Harrison, *Mosquitoes, Malaria and Man*, 205.

78  Christophers, 'Commentary,' in Gill, 'Some Points in the Epidemiology of Malaria,' 469.

79  Harrison notices Christophers's attention to dose of infection. But he appears to interpret increased dose simply as a function of exponential increase in transmission and infection prevalence, assuming that a 'snowballing' in human and/or vector infection rate (prevalence) is accompanied necessarily by a parallel increase in the *amount* of infection (numbers of sporozoites) inoculated per infected mosquito bite; *Mosquitoes, Malaria and Man*, 207.

80  Christophers, 'Endemic and Epidemic Prevalence,' 712.

81  Christophers, 'Commentary,' in Gill, 'Some Points in the Epidemiology of Malaria,' 467–469.

82  Christophers, *Malaria in the Punjab*.

83  S.R Christophers, and C.A. Bentley, *Malaria in the Duars: Being the second report to the Advisory Committee Appointed by the Government of India to Conduct an Enquiry Regarding Black-water and Other Fevers Prevalent in the Duars* (Simla: Government Monotype Press, 1911), 7, 51.

84  Russell, *Malaria: Basic Principles Briefly Stated*, 100; Macdonald, 'Analysis of Equilibrium in Malaria,' 132; W. Dalrymple-Champneys, 'Commentary,' in Gill, 'Some Points in the Epidemiology of Malaria,' 477.

85  Briercliffe, *The Ceylon Malaria Epidemic*, 64; Rajendram and Jayewickreme, 'Malaria in Ceylon,' 21.

86  Wigglesworth, 'Malaria in Ceylon,' 619.

87  Packard and Gadelha also suggest that in the wake of the LNMC's emphasis on malaria as a 'social disease,' the highly publicized Rockefeller campaign to eradicate *An. gambiae* (recently identified as *An. arabiensis*) in northwest Brazil was key to the 'resuscitation of the vector centred approach' in the late 1930s; 'A Land Filled with Mosquitoes: Fred L. Soper, the Rockefeller Foundation, and the Anopheles Gambiae Invasion of Brazil,' *Medical Anthropology*, 17, 1997, 215–238.

88  M.J. Dobson, M. Malowany, and R.W. Snow, 'Malaria Control in East Africa: The Kampala Conference and the Pare-Taveta Scheme: A Meeting of Common and High Ground,' *Parassitologia*, 42, 2000, 149–166. See below, ch. 6.

89  M. Yacob, and S. Swaroop, 'Malaria and Spleen Rate in the Punjab,' *IJM*, 1, 4, Dec. 1947, 469–489.

90  A.T.A. Learmonth, 'Some Contrasts in the Regional Geography of Malaria in India and Pakistan,' *Transactions and Papers (Institute of British Geographers)*, 23, 1957, 37–59, at 48, 38.

91  Macdonald, 'Analysis of Equilibrium in Malaria,' 132; P. Russell, L.S. West, R.D. Manwell, and G. Macdonald, *Practical Malariology* (London: Oxford University Press, 1963), 473.

92  Macdonald's remark appears in discussion of 'constant transmission build[ing] up a firm immunity which prevented epidemic happenings, whereas interrupted transmission permitted a fall of immunity, followed by an epidemic'; 'Analysis of Equilibrium in Malaria,' 132.

93  The one exception was the year 1942 with war-time hyperinflation, poor harvests, and absence of standard relief measures. On this, see Zurbrigg, *Epidemic Malaria and Hunger*, ch. 12.

94  Christophers, for example, was aware of epidemic decline, in his 80s pondering the contribution of flood control; S.R. Christophers, 'Policy in Relation to Malaria Control,' *IJM*, 9, 4, 1955, 297–303, at 301.

95  In hyperendemic areas 'the infective reservoir is almost exclusively in new entrants, either newborn children or immigrants. . . . This type of governing mechanism is susceptible of mathematical analysis . . . but such an analysis is not attempted here'; G. Macdonald, 'Community Aspects of Immunity to Malaria,' in Bruce-Chwatt and Glanville, eds., *Dynamics of Tropical Disease*, at 82.

96  Macdonald, 'Analysis of Equilibrium in Malaria,' 133 [emphasis added].

97  G. Macdonald, 'On the Scientific Basis of Tropical Hygiene,' Presidential address, *Transactions of the Royal Society of Tropical Medicine and Hygiene*, 59, 1965, 622–630, in Bruce-Chwatt and Glanville, eds., *Dynamics of Tropical Disease*, 26. J.A. Nájera remarks that 'the idea that the epidemiology of malaria could be unified in a single theoretical model gave a major impulse to the concept that all malaria situations could be controlled by a single method'; ' "Malaria Control" Achievements, Problems and Strategies,' *Parassitologia*, 43, 2001, 1–89, at 42.

98  W. Byam, and R.G. Archibald, eds., *The Practice of Medicine in the Tropics* (London: Henry Frowde, Hodder, and Stoughton, 1922), vol. 2, 1514. Spleen rates, Christophers once again stressed in 1949, were commonly observed to be much higher among the poor, a pattern attributed not primarily to greater exposure to infection among the poor but to reduced capacity to throw off infection; 'Endemic and Epidemic Prevalence,' 704.

99  Macdonald, 'Analysis of Equilibrium in Malaria,' 135, 145.

100 Wigglesworth, 'Malaria in Ceylon,' 612.

101 Dunn, *Malaria in Ceylon*, 16, 11.

102 See also Meegama, 'Malaria Eradication,' 209.

103 D.L. Doolan, C. Dobaño, and J.K. Baird, 'Acquired Immunity to Malaria,' *Clinical Microbiology Review*, 22, 1, Jan. 2009, 13–36; H. Krisin, et al., 'Malaria in a Cohort of Javanese Migrants to Indonesian Papua,' *Annals of Tropical Medicine and Parasitology*, 97, 6, Sep. 2003, 543–556; J.K. Baird, et al., 'Adult Javanese Migrants to Indonesian Papua at High Risk of Severe Disease Caused by Malaria,' *Epidemiology and Infection*, 131, 1, Aug. 2003, 791–797.

104 With the exception of holo- or hyperendemic conditions where re-inoculation is continuous, the protective effect of a single infective exposure was limited, due to high levels of pleomorphism, multiple 'antigenically distinct races or strains between which [immunological] cross-protection is incomplete'; I.A.

McGregor, and R.J.M. Wilson, 'Specific Immunity: Acquired in Man,' in W.H. Wernsdorfer, and I.A. McGregor, eds., *Malaria: Principles and Practice of Malariology* (Edinburgh: Churchill Livingstone, 1988), 559–619, at 571.

105 S.R. Christophers, J.A. Sinton, and G. Covell, 'How to Do a Malaria Survey,' *Health Bulletin*, No. 14 (Calcutta: GOI, 1931), 110 [emphasis added].

106 Christophers, 'Malaria in the Punjab,' 73; Christophers, 'Endemic and Epidemic Prevalence,' 712. On this, see Zurbrigg, *Epidemic Malaria and Hunger*, 82.

107 Christophers's obituarist described him as a person without rancor, 'impossible to quarrel with,' who 'inspired respect, admiration and affection in all those who worked with him'; M.W. Service, 'Obituary. Sir Rickard Christophers: A Tribute,' *Transactions of the Royal Society of Tropical Medicine and Hygiene,* 72, 1997, 678–680. This degree of collegial respect however could at times leave it difficult to distinguish colleagues' views from his own.

108 Christophers, 'Endemic and Epidemic Prevalence,' 709–710. It has been suggested that with the 1930s' identification of differing anopheline 'sibling' species based on differential feeding habits (animal or human), Christophers came to de-emphasize economic factors in his malaria analysis; H. Evans, 'European Malaria Policy in the 1920s and 1930s: The Epidemiology of Minutiae,' *ISIS,* 80, 1989, 40–59, at 58–59. Yet such a shift is not evident in his later writing: Christophers, 'Endemic and Epidemic Prevalence'; Christophers, 'Measures for the Control of Malaria in India,' *Journal of the Royal Society of Arts,* Apr. 30, 1943, 285–296, at 290.

109 Christophers, 'Endemic and Epidemic Prevalence,' 717–718.

110 Christophers, 'Measures for the Control of Malaria in India,' 289.

111 Christophers, 'Endemic and Epidemic Prevalence,' 715.

112 Great Britain, *Report of the Royal Commission on Agriculture in India* (London: HMSO, 1928), vol. 1, Pt. 1, 145.

113 Macdonald, and Majid, 'Report on an Intensive Malaria Survey,' 466; G. Covell, 'Method of forecasting and mitigating malaria epidemic in India,' LNMC. mimeograph document, C.H./Malaria/257–258, Geneva, Mar. 31, 1938.

114 In his 1957 overview of the Indian malaria literature Learmonth notes earlier discussion of economic factors, but concludes that '[r]ecent work makes one cautious about this nutritional factor,' steering discussion to non-immune young children; 'Some contrasts in the regional geography of malaria,' 48, 38. A recent exception to the sidelining of hunger-induced malaria fulminancy appears in the work of J.A. Nàjera; ' "Malaria control" achievements, problems and strategies,' 23.

115 H.E. Shortt, and P.C.C. Garnham, *Biographical Memoirs of Fellows of the Royal Society,* 25, 1979, 178–207, at 188, doi: 30928. Six years earlier, on the occasion of his birth centenary, Christophers's Punjab study was singled out for praise for 'introduc[ing] the method of mapping the *incidence* of malaria and the possibility of predicting its occurrence on the basis of rainfall records. Control measures by water management were suggested and applied with some success'; L. Bruce-Chwatt, 'Sir Rickard Christophers: The First 100 Years,' *Transactions of the Royal Society of Tropical Medicine and Hygiene,* 67, 5, 1973, 729–730 [emphasis added].

116 P. Russell, 'Some Aspects of Malaria in India,' July 5, 1941, Rockefeller Archive Centre, RG.1.1. S.464 B.11 f.87; as cited in J. Farley, *To Cast Out Disease: A History of the International Health Division of the Rockefeller Foundation (1913–1951)* (Oxford: Oxford University Press, 2004), 123. In another inversion, Russell elsewhere would describe the 'social obstacles' to malaria

control to be 'absence of educated' public opinion, insufficient technical personnel, 'lack of cognizance by public officials as to the cost of malaria' and a 'widespread ineptness in applying . . . the results of research in malariology'; 'Malaria and its Influence on World Health,' *Bulletin of the New York Academy of Medicine*, Sept. 1943, 597–630.

117 Recent research linking increased malaria morbidity and zinc deficiency may be an exception.

# 3

# HUNGER ECLIPSED

## Nutritional science in colonial South Asia

Alongside the dramatic medical science developments in entomology and immunology in the early years of the twentieth century, the 1920s were a period of rapid advances in understanding of the micronutrient constituents of food, a research field initially termed 'chemical hygiene.'[1] In recent years, much scholarship has been directed to the emergence of the 'new science of nutrition,' exploring its powerful influence on Western dietary practices and the rise of commercial food industries.[2] Rather less attention, by comparison, has focused on what was left behind in the process. Within the new medical subdiscipline of nutritional science, earlier concern for quantitative hunger rapidly was overshadowed by that for food quality, seen largely in terms of micronutrient deficiencies. In Western industrialized countries this shift in nutritional focus took place at a time when hunger as a widespread social reality, if not vanquished, was in considerable retreat through a beginning rise in wage levels, and labour and social security legislation. Elsewhere, however, the new dietary science came to compete with, and largely supplant, attention to 'macronutrient' deficiency in societies where both acute and chronic hunger still remained pervasive realities.[3]

The overshadowing of hunger as a medical category and as a central historiographical subject is a question of much broader dimensions and significance for health and demographic history than can be addressed here. In this chapter, we consider simply two aspects of this transformation as it unfolded in colonial India: first, its epistemic impact as one additional strand contributing to the demise in understanding of hunger as a central factor in South Asian malaria mortality history; and second, the principled efforts of a handful of scientists, nascent trade unions, and members of the Indian public who questioned and sought to resist the reductive character and consequences of the new dietary science.

Colonial interest in micronutrient deficiency states in India grew rapidly in the early years of the twentieth century, in no small part propelled by the emergence of the syndrome of beriberi among naval and other institutional populations in eastern and South Asia in the late nineteenth century. One of the early consequences of modern food processing, beriberi in its epidemic form was a paralytic syndrome that notably appeared with the rapid expansion of machine-milling of staple grains, in particular rice. Early on, the disease had been linked to diet, its sudden appearance in the Japanese navy prompting a shift to more varied food rations, a measure that saw the incidence of the syndrome plummet from 30 per cent to nil between 1882 and 1886. By the turn of the century Dutch scientists in Java had concluded that beriberi was a deficiency disease caused by the absence of 'protective' substances in 'polished' rice, minute substances removed in the process of industrial machine-milling. In the Malay peninsula, the syndrome was eliminated following a 1911 government prohibition on highly polished rice supplied to government institutions.[4] The specific seed-coat substance removed in milling would be identified in 1926 as thiamine, termed vitamin $B_1$.[5]

In India, formal nutritional research began in the 1910s, undertaken by Colonel R. McCay, a physiologist at Calcutta Medical College, work that initially focused on protein and its relative content in the region's staple foodgrains.[6] With the identification of specific vitamins through the 1920s, interest rapidly extended to micronutrient deficiencies as well, with a Beri-beri Enquiry initiated in 1921 under Robert McCarrison at the Pasteur Institute at Coonoor in the western hills of the Madras Presidency.[7] Four years later, the institute's mandate broadened to 'Deficiency Diseases' in general, and in 1929, the Nutrition Research Laboratories were formally established also at Coonoor.

As in much of the world, the paradigmatic power of the new science of nutrition was immediate. Where in 1922 the *Indian Medical Gazette* had described insufficient food (hunger) as the overwhelming nutritional problem facing the country and interpreted micronutrient deficiency states as largely problems of poverty (not enough of *any* food), by 1936 a special nutritional issue of the same journal would be devoted exclusively to issues of 'dietary' quality. Frank states of micronutrient deficiency diseases such as beriberi were uncommon, medical advisors acknowledged, but 'milder forms' were now considered a wide-spread form of 'hidden hunger.'[8]

In the early nutritional literature, the term 'malnutrition' was used in its etymological sense of dietary *imbalance* rather than *insufficient* food (undernourishment). McCarrison was at pains to emphasize the distinction, defining malnutrition as 'the impairment of the normal physiological processes of the body consequent on the use of a food which is deficient in quality although it may be abundant in quantity.'[9] Although his interest included specific micronutrient deficiencies such as iodine deficiency in relation to goitre in certain Himalayan hill tracts, a major focus to McCarrison's research was what he considered to be macronutrient *imbalance*: insufficient dietary protein and excess carbohydrate, a problem he considered particularly serious in southern and eastern regions of India where rice was a common staple grain.[10]

The effect of imperfect food in causing a degree of physical inefficiency, which may not be associated with any gross evidence of disease, is exemplified in India as in few other countries in the world. . . . Malnutrition is thus the most far-reaching of the causes of disease in India. It is one of the greatest – if not *the* greatest – problems with which the investigator of disease is faced.[11]

The concern with rice stemmed from what was seen as the grain's low protein content. It was believed that where diets were based primarily on rice, the 'bulk' of such a diet made it difficult to consume quantities sufficient to meet protein requirements. For Western scientists accustomed to meat-based diets, the nature and content of protein in common foods was a long-standing preoccupation.[12] In the early twentieth century adult protein requirement was considered to be above 100 grams per day, almost double the level recognized as adequate in the 1980s.[13]

McCarrison's views on protein deficiency were rapidly embraced in South Asian medical circles. By the 1930s the *Indian Medical Gazette* can be seen correspondingly urging, '[i]n the language of modern dietetics, . . . the ideal should be to provide a 'square meal' . . . well balanced from the point of view of bulk as well as flavour and in the approximately correct proportions of essential constituents.'[14] Here, concern with dietary 'bulk' no longer meant insufficient food (staple grains) but rather its opposite, too much carbohydrate, too much rice in particular. In 1938 a bacteriologist at the recently inaugurated All-India Institute of Hygiene and Public Health was warning that the 'great excess of carbohydrates' was 'directly or indirectly responsible . . . for the most severe ravages of this country by the various tropical diseases, such as malaria, kala-azar, tuberculosis . . . etc.'[15] Thus, in little more than a decade, medical perception of the 'nutrition problem' in India had largely shifted from one of hunger, not enough food, as articulated so clearly in the 1922 pages of the *Indian Medical Gazette*, to instead the *wrong kind* of food – which, in turn, was interpreted as a principal *cause* of economic backwardness and poverty.

These views were rapidly embraced by constituencies well beyond the medical profession. As a prominent witness invited to testify at the 1926–1927 proceedings of the Royal Commission on Agriculture in India (RCAI), McCarrison urged that 'defective' and 'faulty food' was 'the most far-reaching of the causes of disease in India.'[16] 'Cholera, malaria, dysentery, tuberculosis and leprosy kill their thousands every year; but malnutrition maims its millions, and is the means whereby the soil of the human body is made ready for the rank growth of the pathogenic agents of many of those diseases which afflict the Indian people.'[17] In the course of their proceedings, the Commissioners personally toured McCarrison's laboratory at Coonoor, where his experiments comparing growth of laboratory rats fed a wheat- versus rice-based diet garnered intense interest.[18] Commission members came away determined to

dispel the idea that malnutrition and starvation are the same. Actually, a person suffering from malnutrition may be consuming more than his system can utilise. . . . [L]ack of physique and vigour in Bengal was most probably due to a deficiency of protein in the diet . . . owing to the bulkiness of the rice diet.[19]

Deficiency diseases, they emphasized, were not primarily economic in origin. They resulted from 'the absence of some essential element in the diet. Their occurrence is, therefore, no indication of poverty and consequent scarcity of food.'[20] The Commission went on to cite estimates prepared by the 1925 All-India Conference of Medical Research Workers that 'loss of efficiency' due to 'preventable malnutrition and disease was not less than twenty per cent,' and concluded that malnutrition was a major cause of 'physical *inefficiency* and ill-health among the masses of India.'[21]

## 'Nutrient imbalance' questioned

The rapid embrace of dietary quality as the leading nutrition problem in India did not go unopposed. Within the public health administration, officials still attuned to field realities of hunger openly queried the sweeping generalizations of ill-health being offered on the basis of the McCay-McCarrison research. C.A. Bentley was one, whose testimony at the 1927 hearings of the Royal Commission on Agriculture demonstrates the conceptual gulf already at play within the administration. As Director of Public Health for Bengal and leading analyst of agricultural decline in the Presidency, Bentley was a key witness at the Bengal sessions of the Agriculture enquiry. In his written submission to the Commission he had had a great deal to say, not unexpectedly, about the relationship between agriculture, economic prosperity, and health.[22] Many of the questions directed to him in the oral hearings, however, related not to agricultural decline, nor to its relationship with malaria, but rather to nutritional deficiency disease in Bengal.[23]

Following brief enquiries about irrigation, hookworm, and school latrines, the Commission's Chairman turned to querying if Bentley attached 'great importance to the problem of malnutrition in the Presidency,' a question which prompted the following exchange:

BENTLEY: In one sense, yes. There is a very large proportion of the population that at certain times of the year or in certain districts does not get enough nourishment at all.

CHAIR: That is starvation. I want to know whether the diet is badly balanced or whether certain essential food-stuffs are absent? . . . Do they take too much rice?

B: They take too little proteids [sic] The milk-supply is very poor. It is very costly and a large number of people cannot buy milk; they cannot take sufficient quantity of *ghi* also. Most of the people cannot take even fish.[24]

Unsatisfied, the Commission Chairman repeated the question. Was there not an 'excess of rice' in the Bengali diet? 'It is one of those things on which we cannot have too much information,' Bentley replied diplomatically, adding, '[i]t is very difficult to say whether one would place this problem above everything else in importance. But there is no doubt that it is exceedingly important.' Frustrated, a second commissioner reworded the question:

SIR THOMAS MIDDLETON: [I]s it not a most important thing for the public health of the community . . . that steps should be taken to correct the ill-balanced diet?

B: This is a thing in which I myself am very keen; I would like to see it. But I should first like to see them get sufficient food. . . . That is really our problem in Bengal. I have known cultivators when I was investigating malaria in villages . . . who at certain times of the year had practically nothing but the produce of their fruit trees.

M: That would apply only to 10 per cent of the population?

B: No; very much more than that. . . . [I]n certain areas of the Birbhum district, a very large proportion of the population do not have enough to eat, although it has not been considered bad enough to call it a famine. Only a couple of years ago I visited in the Birbhum district in which the bulk of the people had not enough food. I went in connection with cholera, but I found that the people were starving.

M: That is quite likely. But taking the normal position, whereas your statement would refer, one would hope, only to a small percentage. Colonel McCay's conclusion that the general diet is ill-balanced must refer to something like 90 per cent of the population? . . . You are convinced as a medical man that, generally speaking, it is true that the dietary of a Bengali is badly balanced?[25]

To this, Bentley replied with a monosyllabic 'Yes,' a response which prompted, in turn, suggestions for nutritional 'education and propaganda' schemes, as he perhaps had anticipated. '[W]e have not emphasized it so much,' Bentley explained, 'because it is really not so obvious. If we were to start emphasizing the question of diet at the present time, in the beginning we should be looked upon by the bulk of the people as mad men.' Under still more urging, however, he ultimately conceded: 'Yes; we want [dietary] education in our schools; this is a matter which should be taken up.'[26]

What is remarkable in this exchange, aside from the seeming lack of interest in what might be termed 'ordinary' (endemic) starvation, is how thoroughly the idea of qualitative dietary imbalance had already absorbed official attention, notwithstanding the virtual absence of epidemiological evidence as to its significance. Enormous questions remained with respect to the 'great excess of carbohydrates' thesis: among others, how applicable laboratory-based research was to humans; and the degree to which laboratory conditions represented 'native' diets.[27] Nor had any effort been made to examine empirically the 'too much rice' thesis in relation to regional differences in mortality levels, though general death rates were considerably lower in the southern 'rice-eating' Madras Presidency than in the wheat-based northwest.[28]

So compelling was the *idea* of dietary imbalance that the laboratory findings of McCarrison would override direct epidemiological observation, including that coming from Bentley, one of the most experienced colonial Public Health officials in the country. Nor was he alone in questioning the emphasis on dietary quality. In his testimony to the Commission, the Public Health Commissioner with the Government of India, J.D. Graham, also voiced caution in embracing McCarrison's emphasis on protein deficiency. Asked if he thought the 'superior physique of the peoples of northern India' was due to diet, Graham suggested that

> the question is very much *sub judice* at the moment. Colonel McCay went very strongly for the absence of the protein elements in the diet as being the causation; but I showed [in written testimony] how that had been questioned by Dr. Hindhede, a leading Danish dietetic expert, and that is one of the reasons why I say we require more inquiry in India on this particular subject.[29]

Bentley's testimony on the degree and priority of the 'quantitative' nutrition problem however remained unpursued within the RCAI proceedings.[30] Referring back to the work of both McCarrison and McCay, the Commission concluded that 'diet is the all-important factor in determining the degree of physical development and general well-being of the people, and that with a low protein consumption, deficient stamina, mental and physical, must be expected.' Echoing McCarrison, it recommended, in addition to mass dietary education ('propaganda') campaigns, greater production 'of foodstuffs containing the nutrient substances which the staple food lacks.'[31]

As for the protein deficiency thesis itself, it remained just that. By the early 1940s, following analysis of the nutritive value of a range of common Indian foods, it ultimately was recognized that, where staple foodgrain consumption was adequate to meet caloric needs, protein requirement also was generally met. In the case of greater protein requirement among young children, protein content could be made up with very modest levels of traditional pulses (lentils).[32] Staple foodgrain 'bulk' was an issue, but primarily for its quantitative insufficiency: a problem of poverty.[33] But by this point, the concept and terminology of 'malnutrition,' and the thesis of dietary imbalance, had already become broadly entrenched.

Serious micronutrient deficiency states did exist in the Indian subcontinent. These included iodine deficiency in the central sub-Himalayan hills, and keratomalacia caused by severe vitamin A deficiency, a softening and ulceration of the cornea leading to blindness, the latter seen particularly among young children in the end-stages of severe emaciation. It appeared also in relation to famine relief camps along with outbreaks of scurvy (vitamin C deficiency)[34] in situations where access to traditional 'famine foods' (leafy greens, rich in vitamins A and C) was also severely compromised. Non-famine consumption of leafy greens was generally more common amongst the very poor because of their minimal cost as a low status famine food.[35]

Severe thiamine deficiency (beriberi) also was a serious medical condition. But as a phenomenon largely triggered by modern techniques of food processing, its relationship to poverty was somewhat more complex. As we have seen, major beriberi outbreaks had appeared abruptly in the late nineteenth century amongst naval troops, prisons, schools, and large industrial undertakings. These were institutions in which large numbers were fully dependent on centralized provisioning where industrially milled rice was preferred for its greater resistance to spoilage.[36] But 'polished' rice had quickly also assumed a higher social status among the civilian population, in a fashion similar to that for white bread in Europe a century before. By the early twentieth century local outbreaks of clinical thiamine deficiency began to appear as well amongst lower-middle classes in urban centres such as Calcutta for whom machine-polished rice constituted nearly the sole food source.[37]

As for rural prevalence, beriberi was largely localized to the northern deltaic region of the Madras Presidency (now Andhra Pradesh), known as the North Circars. Here the syndrome was overtly a disease of poverty, limited to the agricultural labourer households who produced, and consumed, the rice now highly polished for export markets, and whose intense impoverishment proscribed even minimal consumption of pulses or vegetables. Elsewhere in the southern rice region of the subcontinent, the traditional practice of parboiling harvested paddy ensured that adequate thiamine content remained after milling.[38]

## Micronutrient hunger and the shift of responsibility

What accounts for the ideological power of the new science of dietetics? Historians of nutritional science in recent decades have traced the professional and commercial interests associated with modern nutritional theory in industrialized countries,[39] a critique that has been extended to colonial societies as well in the work of C. Sathyamala, Michael Worboys, V.R. Muraleedharan, and David Arnold, among others.[40] Certainly in South Asia the idea of 'micronutrient hunger' as an invisible menace captured the imaginations of administrators and the educated Indian public as readily as it was doing in other parts of the world. Presented as primarily a 'hidden' hunger, it was, by definition, virtually impossible to assess personal risk. Subclinical degrees of deficiency could, in theory, affect anyone.[41] In his position as the director of the Coonoor Nutrition Research Laboratories, W.R. Aykroyd (1899–1979) in 1935 ominously suggested in his popular writing that '[i]n all probability, there are food deficiency diseases in India which have never been observed or described.'[42] Six years later, the highly respected Indian scientist, Sir P.C. Ray, would warn that with respect to the '[e]lusive chemical substances called vitamins . . . there is a large "no man's land" between frank illness and optimum health, and it is possible to be well without being as healthy as an optimum diet would have permitted.'[43] Like microbial infection, hidden nutrient deficiency states increasingly were perceived as a constant, covert threat.

Interest among medical professionals in South Asia probably was further heightened by the fact that thiamine deficiency presented an epidemiological profile in some ways different from that of most infective diseases in that it was *not* exclusively associated with the rural poor, in Calcutta affecting some urban lower-middle class groups as well. To this extent it offered something of a moral oasis from the litany of 'diseases of poverty' which otherwise surrounded them. But the idea of micronutrient 'health' also offered many positive attractions. For the educated elite it was modern and scientific, promising an open-ended possibility of 'optimum' health. At the same time, for colonial administrations dietary therapy appeared to offer a simple fix for the ill-health and disease of the poor, in theory accessible to everyone. Like mosquito and malaria eradication, it therefore was attractive for its seeming broad democratic appeal.

But the micronutrient diagnosis of ill-health also offered the possibility of shifting responsibility away from the state to the individual. Malnutrition was rapidly being recast as a problem of ignorance regarding choice of qualitatively nutritious foods, the solution to which lay in education. Already, legislation to limit the high degree of rice 'polishing' had been rejected by the government to assuage commercial grain interests.[44] In his October 1926 testimony to the Royal Commission on Agriculture, J.D. Graham, GOI Public Health Commissioner, highlighted the conclusions of a recent British Medical Research Council report pointing to 'maternal [in]efficiency' as key to the nutrition problem in Scotland.[45] By 1931, the Punjab Public Health department was citing 'measures directed against dysgenic habits and customs,' as one of its most important tasks: habits, it stressed, 'that deprive the body of essential food factors (vitamins), and thereby lower resistance to infection or give rise to specific disease.' This, even as the province's annual report continued to be prefaced with data on grain prices, harvest conditions, and wage levels.[46] The influence of the new dietary science in reframing understanding of the nature of the hunger problem in India, in other words, was quite profound.

## Dietetic momentum

Beyond scientific fascination, there was a larger momentum involved, however, similar to that faced by the Government of India in relation to malaria and the related onus to embrace *Anopheles* mosquito eradication.[47] The professional imperative to apply 'scientific' microbiologic knowledge was extremely difficult to resist, even for those with extensive professional experience and administrative authority. In their tenacious grilling of Bentley, members of the Royal Commission on Agriculture were implicitly questioning his professional competence: that '*as a medical man*' he ought to appreciate the importance of ill-balanced dietaries. It was at this point in the proceedings that even Bentley relented, agreeing to the educational priority of balanced dietaries, a view which he clearly saw in the context of rural Bengal as absurd.

As the former chief medical officer to the Empire of India and Ceylon Tea Company, Bentley's concern for hunger could hardly be seen as ideologically driven. As was the case for Christophers and James as well, it was based on extensive field experience and pragmatic common sense. What he was describing to the Inquiry Commissioners was *endemic* acute hunger: recurring, seasonal semi-starvation, superimposed upon general undernourishment ('chronic' hunger).[48] The commissioners clearly did not share either this experience, or apparently his concern. Presumably they would have responded to conditions of frank 'famine' (epidemic starvation), for which by this time there were clear administrative obligations. But *endemic* hunger, acute and chronic, was not a responsibility of medical professionals, unlike nutrient imbalance had now become.

Waning interest in, and indeed comprehension of, 'ordinary' (non-famine) hunger on the part of 1926–1927 Agricultural Inquiry members contrasted starkly with that expressed four decades earlier at the highest levels of the administration in the 1888 Dufferin Inquiry into the condition of the poorer classes. That earlier enquiry sought to assess both aspects of hunger based upon a common understanding of human subsistence precarity, one expressed in terms of prevalence of two, one, or zero meals per day.[49] Undoubtedly, broader administrative interest in 1888 had been prompted by a growing political imperative to avoid famines, and the need to know how close to the edge of starvation the rural poor actually were in the various regions of the subcontinent. Now, in the 1920s, with frank famine largely controlled through major recent changes to the Famine Code,[50] attention to the less politically incriminating form of acute hunger – endemic in form – amongst colonial administrators was fast receding. And so too was its scientific and medical legitimacy as a public health issue.

The problem, of course, lay not in nutritional science itself. Micronutrient deficiency states did exist and in specific cases could hold important epidemiological consequences.[51] Interpretation of their public health significance however was taking place in this period without adequate, indeed often without any, epidemiological investigation. Scientific fascination with the phenomena was outstripping the obligation to place the microbiologic insights in context, and in turn overriding judgement. In the case of thiamine deficiency, the specific menace was connoted to apply to 'diet' *in general*. Little attention was paid in the professional literature to the central role of industrial food processing in its etiology as a public health problem. Nor to ready remedies: simple, minimal additions to staple foods of greens or pulses. The uncritical presumption of scientific expertise left little room for inserting commonplace experience, or for incorporating traditional understanding of 'diet.' As seen above, in many of the southern rice-growing regions, rural understanding of thiamine deficiency historically had been evident in the time- and labour-intensive traditional practice of parboiling rice before milling. Yet one is hard-pressed to find appreciation of such understanding reflected in nutritional tracts of the period. Key insights were thus forfeited, and with them, essential epidemiological perspective. Research into micronutrient disease was not incompatible with concern for macronutrient hunger and its socio-economic dimensions. Nevertheless, as in Britain and other industrial countries, concern for the former largely came to supplant, rather than complement, that for quantitative deficiency.[52]

The academic sidelining of hunger can be seen to reflect a seductive 'logic' inherent to scientific discovery, one where new medical discoveries generally lay in previously 'hidden' microbiologic domains. Any tension between the earlier 'macrobiologic' understanding of hunger and the new microbiologic insights clearly was an artificial one. Nevertheless, the cascading microbial and micronutrient discoveries of the period provided powerful new areas of medical expertise and, as Foucauldians would point out, channels of professional and political control – a reductive momentum that few within the South Asian medical community, or elsewhere, felt able publicly to question. In that process of overshadowing, the visibility and legitimacy of hunger as a medical and public health category was rapidly being undermined.

A further manifestation of this epistemic transformation can be seen in the appropriation of language. The expression 'two square meals a day,' employed in the Dufferin Inquiry, colloquially meaning 'enough to satisfy hunger,' was a quantitative concept from antiquity. In an unwitting sleight of hand, a 1936 *Indian Medical Gazette* editorial on 'dietary and nutritional standards in India' would employ the term instead, however, to convey the new nutritional sense of 'square': 'one which is well balanced from the point of view of bulk as well as flavour and in the approximately correct proportions of essential constituents.'[53] Here, entirely different meanings were being wrapped in an earlier language of hunger in a near-seamless supplanting of quantitative issues by qualitative. Basic concepts were being shed and the very language of hunger itself recast. In the process, the exclusivity of the new 'language of dietetics' was removing access to discussion of hunger from the public domain, and corralling it instead within the sphere of medical specialists. These developments of course were not unique to British India. Added momentum to the new specialty of nutritional science was coming from outside India's borders, in the work of the Health Organisation of the League of Nations (LNHO). And here, also, W.R. Aykroyd played a central role, in work that preceded his 1935 colonial appointment to India.

## The League of Nations and nutrition

By the early 1930s, the mandate of the League of Nations Health Organisation had expanded to include nutrition alongside communicable disease control, a concern heightened by the global effects of the economic Depression.[54] In 1931, a nutrition committee was established under Aykroyd, then a young British nutritionist with epidemiological experience investigating beriberi in the late 1920s among isolated Newfoundland fishing communities dependent on highly refined ('white') wheat flour. In its earliest deliberations, nutrition committee delegates from African colonies and India had stressed the economic dimensions to the nutrition problem: insufficient income and food of any kind.[55] Over time, however, the committee's work veered increasingly to issues of dietary quality, with a particular emphasis on milk protein, a shift evident in Aykroyd's final League of Nations report.[56] Co-authored with Etienne Burnet, the 1935 'Nutrition and Public Health' report set out a rather different tone. 'Thirty years ago,' it began,

> it was generally believed that the dietary requirements of human beings are satisfied so long as they have enough to eat. . . . We now know that the adequacy of a dietary depends on the presence of a considerable number of factors and that *mere* quantitative sufficiency may co-exist with a whole series of qualitative defects.[57]

Thus set out, the remainder of the report was informed largely by concern for 'qualitative defects.' Of its 133 pages, fewer than four dealt with 'nutrition and poverty.' Even where raised, economic aspects generally were qualified. Conclusions from a Czechoslovakian household budgets study at one point were cited, with the comment that 'it was irrational to recommend a higher intake of "protective" foods to people who were only just able to purchase sufficient Calories.'[58] Yet this was followed immediately by the citing of a 1926 British Medical Research Council report[59] that stressed 'maternal inefficiency':

> It is clear that a mere increase in wages or relief would not eliminate all dietary deficiency associated with poverty; education is also necessary. . . . [There was] no reason to doubt that valuable results

can be obtained even among families with very small incomes, by educational means.[60]

Here, once again, the economic dimension was minimized, indeed trivialized, in this case, as 'mere' wages.

But beyond the class-ist and sexist assumptions of maternal 'inefficiency,'[61] the logic of the educational approach was questionable for another reason. Dietary studies undertaken during this period, both colonial and European, consistently showed that household consumption of 'protective' foods declined in tandem with lower levels of income – a predictable consequence in light of their greater cost per calorie. A 1933 Swedish study showed a close relationship, even within the working class, between household income and the price paid per 10,000 calories. In the Netherlands, 'the employed families spent . . . 1.71 [cents] per 100 calories, while the unemployed spent only 1.07 cents.'[62]

What the inter-war nutrition surveys in fact were demonstrating was the fundamental rationality of the poor in maximizing the priority caloric value of the foods chosen in the face of often grossly inadequate income. Ignorance (of dietary principles) and income levels were manifestly *not* of equal importance in explaining the 'nutrition problem.' The overriding barrier was economic.[63]

The larger context for the 1935 Burnet-Aykroyd report, and the League of Nations' engagement in nutrition, was the Depression-aggravated crisis in global agriculture and the broader world economy. The global 'nutrition problem' was clearly linked to international trade structures and the contradictory situation where hunger due to unemployment and lack of purchasing power co-existed with enormous global foodgrain surpluses. Those surpluses had prompted mass destruction of stocks in Western countries as a means of supporting their rural constituencies by increasing foodgrain prices.[64] But by the mid-1930s prevailing economic doctrine that had produced policies to 'restrict production drastically, create scarcity, and wait for prices to rise'[65] was no longer politically tenable. In the words of the Bengali academic and agricultural scientist Nagendranath Gangulee, these policies addressed the dilemma of 'poverty in the midst of plenty by eliminating the plenty instead of the poverty.'[66] Prominent Anglo-Commonwealth figures at this point stepped in, urging, under the rubric of 'a marriage of health and agriculture,' that the problem of global hunger lay in inadequate extension of modern agro-technology, proposals that would soon take shape in the post-war Food and Agricultural Organization (FAO) and 'green revolution'[67] – if without addressing the structural issues of access to food and to productive resources. In the meantime, however, following publication of his 1935 'Nutrition and Public Health,' Aykroyd was appointed to succeed McCarrison as director of the nutrition laboratories at Coonoor in India.

## 'Nutrient imbalance' challenged

Important research on the nutritive value of Indian foods followed under Aykroyd's directorship of the Nutrition Research Laboratories at Coonoor,[68] work that led in 1938 to a re-evaluation of earlier assumptions regarding protein deficiency as a priority nutrition concern in India, as we have seen.[69] Research emphasis now was channelled into defending the protein 'quality' of the native Indian diet and to assessing the relative merits of vegetarian and non-vegetarian diets. This significant work tended also, however, to redirect attention to dietary quality aspects. Already, in the earliest months of his Coonoor appointment, Aykroyd, in his non-academic writing continued to articulate his view of the 'malnutrition problem in India' as one primarily of 'faulty diet.' Policy recommendations, as in many of the major League of Nations reports, were directed to the production of more food of 'superior quality' and mass education to remedy 'ignorance and prejudice' underlying such 'defective diet[s].'[70] For Aykroyd himself, this meant repeated emphasis on the superior quality of milk.[71]

The academic focus on dietary quality however did not go unopposed. From the early 1930s, emerging industrial trade unions in India had been working to re-inject economic dimensions into discussion of the 'nutrition problem' in the country. In their memorandum to the 1931 Royal Commission on Labour, the Bombay Textile Labour Union, for example, submitted a detailed analysis of industrial wages that showed the cost of even a very modest nutritionally balanced diet exceeded prevailing wage rates; indeed, that their caloric purchasing value was lower even than that of prison rations.[72] Subsequent diet surveys of Madras city industrial workers in 1935–1936 showed only 3 per cent of labourer households with food budgets sufficient for a 'well-balanced' diet.[73] For over one-third of households surveyed total food expenditure amounted to barely half the cost of a minimally 'balanced' diet[74] – this, among a group that represented 'a relatively highly paid class.'[75] These data confirmed that the nutrition problem lay overwhelmingly in the economic realm.

By the 1930s the International Labour Organization (ILO) also was urging greater attention to economic dimensions of the nutrition problem, as the human effects of the global Depression continued to deepen. Beyond basic advocacy, the ILO was circulating similar income survey protocols internationally to facilitate such economic studies.[76] Up to this point the nutrition problem in South Asia was assumed to be most severe among the urban labour population.[77] But greater investigation of rural conditions increasingly was being urged, and in 1936 Aykroyd, in collaboration with colleague B.G. Krishnan, initiated a detailed rural household income and dietary survey in the Madras Presidency.[78] What the survey revealed was a pattern similar to that of the European survey results, but much more pronounced: amongst low- and lowest-income households, reliance upon the least expensive food sources, with negligible consumption in the latter case of pulses – though only marginally less 'cheap' than cereals. Even at this, daily food intake averaged less than 2,300 calories per consumption unit in 40 per cent of households.[79] Among poor tenant households (one-quarter of study families), food intake averaged 1,664 calories per consumption unit a day; in 10 per cent of households, less than 1,600 calories.[80] Such levels of severe undernourishment meant that some kind of physiological 'adjustment' occurs, the authors observed: 'basal metabolism is reduced, the body functioning is at a lower level of vitality . . . the under-fed labourer is lethargic and his output of work is small. [It is a] level of food intake which permits only a languid existence.'[81] Such households 'may without exaggeration be described as half-starved,' the report concluded, adding that 'the problem of under- and malnutrition in South India is more serious than has yet been realized.'[82]

Extremely low to nil expenditure on oils, milk, meat, pulses, and vegetables was documented as well in 1941 among Bihar industrial workers, with the single partial exception of the cheapest 'green leafy vegetables.'[83] The consistent nature of the relationship between household income and caloric consumption level highlighted the overriding role of economics underlying low consumption of 'protective' foods. Indeed, in the early 1950s, an estimated 97 per cent of calories obtained by agricultural labourer households in India came from cereals, the cheapest food sources available, and even at this, between one-third and one-half did not meet bare minimum caloric requirement.[84]

The stark economic dimensions to the 'nutrition problem' in India as revealed in these studies would be taken up more comprehensively in 1939 by Nagendranath Gangulee, in a 336-page text, *Health and Nutrition in India*. Gangulee was a soil biologist, not a nutritionist, who as Professor of Agriculture, Animal Husbandry and Rural Economy at the University of Calcutta, had been a member of the 1926–1927 Royal Commission on Agriculture in India. In the years that followed, however, he had directed his investigations increasingly to human nutrition. Concern over the growing tendency for qualitative issues of diet to supplant quantitative in the nutrition literature had in turn prompted him to compile and analyze data from available household income and dietary studies. Among them was a diet survey of Assam tea plantation labourer households that revealed adult consumption levels to be 15 ounces of staple foodgrains a day, amounting to approximately 1,460 calories.[85] Together, such figures made it clear, he concluded, that '[t]he working class suffers from malnutrition, not because it is ignorant but because it is poor.' What was required was not 'palliation,' but 'a profound modification in the economic structure of society.'[86]

Though at times he assumed the nutritionist division of foods into 'energy-producing' and 'protective,' Gangulee did not waver from his insistence on the primacy of the economic diagnosis. In his 1939 text neither the colonial government nor the Indian elite was spared. 'Moneylenders, landlords, traders, priests and hosts of others take away the fruits of the labours [of the poor].' A solution to hunger required structural reforms that addressed the 'enormous disparity in incomes which creates a tiny caste of plutocrats and an immense group of the very poor. . . . [I]n the face of poverty, medical science is rendered impotent.'[87] Structural economic reforms, he urged, started with establishment and enforcement of a legal minimum wage, but extended to land reform and overall taxation policies, quoting the *Report of the Indian Statutory Commission* as describing British India as 'a country in which there are large accumulations of wealth on which the burden of Government rests very lightly.'[88]

His most scathing critique was directed to the 'backward state of agriculture' as the root of the rural hunger problem, pointing out that the 'land could yield at least twice or three times as much human food as it does at present,' and outlining in the final chapters fundamental reforms required to remedy agricultural impoverishment, low productivity, and endemic undernourishment.[89] Here he was also sceptical of purely technological solutions to agriculture productivity such as chemical fertilizers, arguing instead for green and farmyard manuring, composting, crop rotation, and seed selection, practices that had produced far higher yields in eastern Asia, but which required far greater re-investment of agricultural profits into production. Above all, he urged effective credit extension to small producers. In his critique of 'the combined forces of feudalism and capitalism,' Gangulee at times could lapse into somewhat idealized notions of Indian rural society and possibilities for voluntary self-help.[90] Hunger, and its causes, nevertheless were starkly articulated as the overriding 'nutrition problem,' both unnecessary and illegitimate.

## Allure of the scientific

The key questions raised by the trade unions and figures like Gangulee in the 1930s however would remain largely unaddressed within the nutritional science discipline. Emphasis on the economic roots of 'malnutrition' was unsustained in British India, a pattern common well beyond South Asia. At one level, attraction to the narrow framework was a function, in part, of the sweeping euphoria of the time for science and technology. In the context of the immense failures faced by Western industrial societies – the demonstrated bankruptcy of economic orthodoxy; the catastrophic consequences of internecine warfare that enveloped their imperial domains; and imperial decline itself – science offered a ready antidote to ebbing confidence and optimism. Overarching faith in science could transcend political boundaries, however, as seen in Soviet Russia as well.

In the medical arena, the career of Aykroyd serves as an example of the professional search for progress through science, though there can be little doubt that he understood poverty to be the 'basic cause of malnutrition.' In 1940, for example, he signed his name as co-author to an astute analysis of the economic 'rationality' of south Indian villagers in their rapid adoption of power milling of rice. The study took into account the time and energy burden required of women in the hand-milling of rice and the added constraints this work posed for their children's nourishment, and their own.[91] The 84-page monograph once again acknowledged that concerns over protein insufficiency had been 'exaggerated by certain workers' and questioned the 'myth' of the supposed 'indigestibility' of 'bulky' rice diets.[92]

Yet in his popular writing and in his advisory roles, Aykroyd would continue to articulate a technical view of the 'malnutrition problem' in India. Citing prospects for vitamin tablets, alongside education and 'development of agriculture,' he insisted that 'if the resources of science are brought to bear on the problem, progress can be made, however formidable the obstacles of poverty.' Acknowledging that the 'idea of giving malnourished school children in India a daily capsule, at present seems rather outlandish,' he nevertheless urged that 'science . . . usually has a few aces up her abundant sleeve. Even in existing economic circumstances . . . much can be done.'[93] Technology, in other words, could circumvent constraints of poverty and its messy underlying socio-political determinants. In one of his last formal publications in India, he continued to urge the 'spread of knowledge,' school feeding programs, and agricultural policies aimed at correcting 'the deficiencies in the diet of the population . . . [and] the diseases to which faulty feeding gives rise.'[94]

C. Sathyamala highlights this deeply contradictory stance, noting that '[e]ven where brief reference was given to poverty or lack of income,' Aykroyd 'would often minimise their importance by adding additional factors such as ignorance of food values etc as reasons for undernutrition.'[95] In this, however, he was hardly alone. A parallel shift from insufficient food to micronutrient deficiencies was taking place as well in the Colonial Office. Michael Worboys has documented the rewriting ('emasculat[ion]') of a draft report submitted in 1936 to an enquiry on malnutrition in Africa which similarly shifted focus from economics to ignorance in the final published version.[96]

As expert advisor, Aykroyd consistently gave in to the professional expectation to come up with 'interventions' in the technical realm. It was, after all, the mandate of the nutritional scientist to offer optimism that something could be done[97] – though the option remained of speaking, *as a scientist*, to both the economic and the biomedical, as Gangulee continued to do. Instead, circumvention of the economic and political had become a recurring pattern. Insufficient food, he suggested at one point, was an issue separate from nutritional science, the former already being addressed by the appropriate authorities: 'These are questions of special interest to those concerned with labour problems and they are at present being actively studied by the International Labour Office.'[98] Nutritional scientists could quite legitimately focus on qualitative issues, he was suggesting, which, after all, was their area of competence.

This compartmentalization of professional responsibilities was mirrored in a new concept of food itself. Human sustenance had now been categorized into two groups: 'protective' foods containing essential vitamins, minerals, and 'first-class protein' of animal origin, on the one hand, and 'energy' foods, on the other.[99] By this definition, the diets of most of the world's population based on staple foodgrains were automatically 'unbalanced,' inherently so. Ignored in this formulation was the fact that most staple foodgrains supplied a broad range of micronutrients, as well as protein, in addition to complex carbohydrates. Nutritional science, in effect, was casting blanket disparagement on a fundamental aspect of colonized societies, and in doing so, positing yet another realm of 'native' culture as requiring Western enlightenment. In the process also, this binary conceptualization misconstrued the very nature of food, with 'protective' foods, rather than staple foodgrains, now those 'most necessary for good health.'[100] It was a powerful recharacterization. Despite deep reservations for many of McCarrison's conclusions, even M.K. Gandhi would come to refer to polished rice as 'pure starch.'[101] And it was one that would leave a legacy of misunderstanding of basic food needs long into the future. Only in the 1970s did nutritionists distance themselves from what was the general thesis of protein deficiency in the low-income world.[102] In the meantime however, the new nutritional science would come to inform two major reports in the dying days of British rule.

## Nutritionist expertise and the Bengal famine

Administrative concern over hunger would reappear starkly in the early 1940s with the Bengal famine bringing to a head the longstanding crisis in food production in British India. Of any official document of this period, the report by the Bengal Famine Commission tabled in 1945 might have been expected to address hunger unequivocally and its relationship to mortality from infective disease. This would hardly be the case however, as we will consider below. First, by way of context, a brief overview is offered of the famine itself.

Much has been written recently about the wartime famine in Bengal in which over 2 million Bengalis perished in 1943–1944.[103] In 1981, Amartya Sen reclaimed key insights into its causes: most prominent among them was the fact that starvation was triggered not by harvest failure (food availability decline) but primarily by hyperinflation: the soaring cost of foodgrains.[104] Numerous disastrous errors in foodgrain administration in the province followed the 1942 Japanese occupation of Burma (Myanmar). Wartime hyperinflation and the British administration's preoccupation with ensuring rice supplies to the war-related industrial workforce in Calcutta, culminated in

1943 in a 500 per cent increase in grain prices throughout Bengal. Despite desperate pleas from district-levels officials, the government blocked implementation of the Famine Code, relief measures otherwise routinely applied from the 1920s on when grain prices rose over 40 per cent above normal levels.[105] For a large portion of the landless poor, purchasing power was reduced to a tiny fraction of its already bare-subsistence level, and epidemic starvation ensued.

Sen's study highlighted as well that the 'gigantic' rise in mortality across the famine period mirrored the normal seasonal pattern of deaths in non-famine years, 'just linearly displaced severely upwards' (Figure 3.1).[106] Paramount among the excess deaths was post-monsoon malaria mortality, though rainfall and environmental conditions were unchanged. In earlier work, I have explored the central role of starvation underlying the dramatic rise in malaria lethality in Bengal in 1943,[107] and argued that the extremely

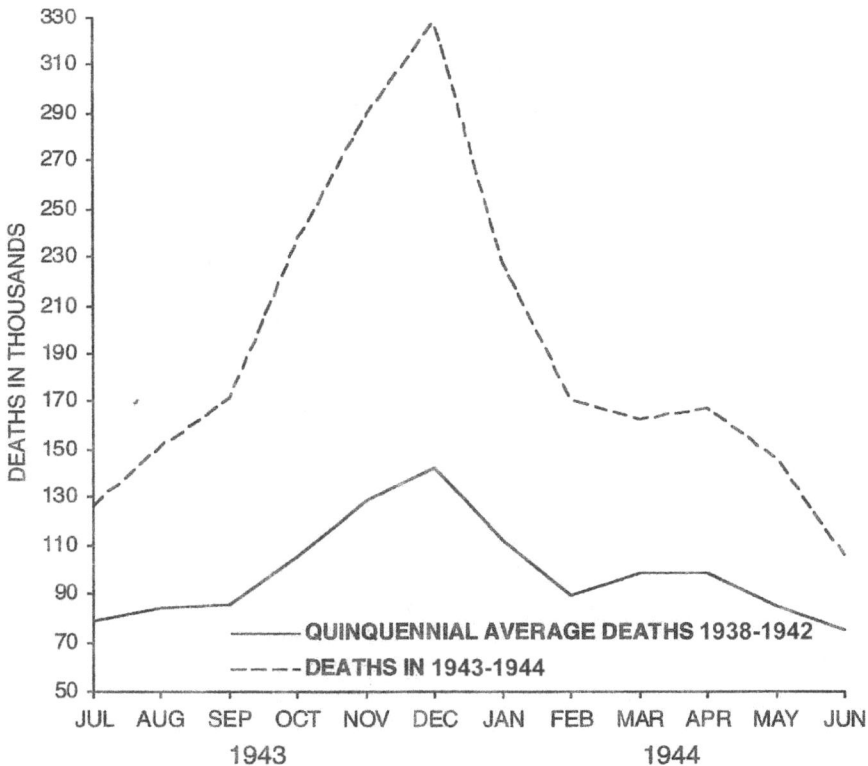

*Figure 3.1* Mortality, by month, Bengal province, July 1943–June 1944

Source: Based on Famine Inquiry Commission, India. *Report on Bengal*, 1945, p. 113.

close seasonal timing of mortality in 1943 relative to non-famine years strongly suggests magnified lethality of endemic diseases rather than substantial change in exposure to microbes and malaria vectors. In this sense, the Bengal famine is a particularly stark example of the power of hunger to shift infection lethality.

If the Bengal famine is also an abject example of the consequences of 'scarcity' in the absence of the Famine Code, it is a demonstration as well of how close to the edge of destitution much of the population in the final years of British rule remained. At the close of the colonial period, calorie consumption for the bottom 10 per cent of households in India was estimated at bare basal metabolic requirement, levels suggesting endemic borderline semi-starvation, with little capacity for regular work.[108] In the absence of fundamental structural reforms in agriculture, per capita foodgrain availability had declined steadily after 1920 with the control of famine (epidemic starvation).[109] Colonial land tenure and lack of affordable credit for the vast majority of smallholders and tenant cultivators continued to block increased foodgrain production that otherwise ought to have accompanied modest growth in population after 1920.[110]

It is notable, then, that the medical portion of 1945 Bengal Famine Commission report[111] largely failed to address the underlying context to the famine: prevailing endemic hunger. The final report of the Famine Inquiry Commission did acknowledge that

> a well-balanced and satisfactory diet is beyond the means of a large section of the population. The poor man is forced, in order to satisfy hunger, to depend largely on the cheaper kinds of food. The lack of purchasing power is thus a most important, perhaps the most important cause of malnutrition.[112]

Yet even here, equivocation remains. It is conceivable that by 'satisfactory diet' and 'malnutrition' the intended meaning was a quantitative one: enough to eat. But with the terms employed there is no way really to know. Clarity on the issue of hunger, in other words, even in a famine report, was elusive with the use of the term 'well-balanced.'

Moreover, the remark appears to imply that poverty (lack of purchasing power) was a problem primarily in terms of food *quality*.[113] But was this actually the case? Did the cheaper staple foods of the poor necessarily place them at risk of micronutrient deficiencies? The staple grains consumed by much of the rural population were millets such as ragi (finger millet), jowar (sorghum), or bajra (pearl millet), grains somewhat richer in micronutrients and protein content typically than the more expensive grains such as rice. Leafy greens were cheapest of all – food of the poor, as 'famine foods' – and were an abundant source of vitamins and minerals.[114] What does seem clear is that with the lay language of hunger dispensed with, or in the case of 'square' meals per day appropriated, the imprecision of the new dietary discourse made the shift from macro- to micronutrient deficiency that much easier.

In the immediate aftermath of the 1943–1944 Bengal famine, far-reaching measures of food rationing and price control measures were instituted, such that by October 1946 over half the population of British India, more than 150 million people, were included in these policies.[115] Accompanied by a brief post-war economic boom, the modest, but real, shift in food security through these distribution programs was associated with a pronounced decline in mortality levels. In Punjab province, for example, the crude death rate fell from 27.8 in 1944 to 19.8 in 1946.[116] With the acute war-time food crisis under relative control, however, perception of the nature of the food problem rapidly narrowed once again to one of food *availability* rather than food *access*. Addressing hunger was becoming primarily a macro-managerial task directed to increasing overall production.

The question of food availability was not, of course, an unimportant one. Food production in India in 1957 was still estimated at only 2,200 calories per adult.[117] But in the post-war era, technological methods became a pre-eminent focus, to the relative neglect of structural barriers to increased productivity (land reform, tenancy, assured credit access for small producers). Issues of *access* to food – 'underfeeding,' wages, conditions of work for women, and maldistribution of all resources – raised with such clarity in the 1930s – would once again recede into the background, and with it, medical engagement with that vast domain of undernourishment and endemic starvation: 'normal' hunger.'[118]

With rapid expansion of Western technical assistance in the immediate post-war and post-Independence periods, academic interpretation of the nutrition problem in India reverted increasingly to the domain of nutritional science and its overriding framework of dietary quality. In the place of wage legislation and fundamental land reform, nutritional policy was directed to production of the right *kinds* of foods and nutritional education.[119] Administratively, this retreat from quantitative hunger would be formally reflected in 1946 in the pages of the *Report of the Health Survey and Development Committee*, chaired by Sir Joseph Bhore.

## Hunger and the Bhore report

Commissioned in the final days of the colonial administration as a thorough overhaul of the medical and public health care systems in India, the Bhore report has been applauded, justly, for its emphasis on extension of primary and preventive health care beyond the urban medical enclaves. In addressing the underlying 'nutritional' determinants of ill-health in India, however, the Committee largely adopted the narrow framework and language of the new nutritional science. 'Faulty nutrition,' the introductory paragraph to chapter 5 ('The Nutrition of the People') read, 'is directly and indirectly responsible for a large amount of ill-health in the community.' Based upon a report by the Nutrition Advisory Committee, the Bhore Committee's nutrition assessment and recommendations closely reflected those of Aykroyd who headed the special committee. 'Defective nutrition,' it offered, 'may take two forms resulting either from an ill-balanced diet, which fails to provide the required constituents of food in their proper proportions, or from the energy value of the food being insufficient to provide for all the activities of the individual concerned.'[120] Here, the quantitative dimensions of the problem – not enough food – is mentioned, but in such terms that one might be forgiven for failing to recognize the phrasing to mean hunger.

A single reference is made to Aykroyd's earlier assessment that an estimated 30 per cent of the population did not get enough to eat. But the admission was followed in the same sentence by a description of Indian diets as 'almost invariably ill-balanced . . . in terms of food factors, a deficiency in fats, vitamins, and proteins of high biological value.'[121] Further on, 'the main defects of the average Indian diet' are described as, first, 'an insufficiency of proteins' particularly 'first class protein' of animal origin; then, of mineral salts and vitamins.[122]

It is puzzling why Aykroyd continued to stress protein deficiency in his role as advisor to the Bhore committee when his earlier research indicated otherwise.[123] But equally so, why the central issue of 'insufficient energy value' was not followed up with specific policy recommendations, aside from education, in the 19 pages that detailed the nature of defective nutrition. In all, only one example of the 'Economic Aspect of the Problem' appears in the 25-page nutrition section of the Bhore report, injected abruptly, as if the ghost of Nagendranath Gangulee were wafting by the committee room door: passing reference to the Rs 15 per month wage of peons in the Government Secretariat, a wage level well below the cost of even a very modest 'balanced' diet for a family, estimated to be Rs 16–24. 'These figures,' the text read, 'give a striking illustration of the gulf that existed between the expenditure necessary on food and that which large numbers of workers could afford.'[124]

Yet with the exception of expanded training of nutrition specialists and school feeding programs, policy measures aimed at addressing the economic dimensions of the nutrition problem were absent. In their place were recommendations for fortification of foods (iodized salt), future distribution of synthetic vitamin tablets, and 'local nutrition committees . . . to teach the people satisfactory dietary habits and spread knowledge of nutrition.' As for poverty, '[a]n increase in the prosperity of the country, associated with a rise in agricultural production,' it was argued, 'will . . . automatically produce a general improvement in nutrition.'[125] Curiously, the report 'refrained from making any reference to the activities of the Food Department of the GOI . . . confining our review . . . to the period ending with the year 1941.'[126] Thus the monumental food ration distribution system enacted across the country in the aftermath of the Bengal famine was left invisible, and also any discussion of its continuation or its impact on the public's health.

Elsewhere, in a chapter on occupational health, the Bhore report did recommend wage levels to permit 3,000 calories per day for manual workers in industrial work; also, limiting hours of work for women, and a statutory obligation of industries employing more than 50 women to provide crèches and free milk to children.[127] These brief recommendations however were largely lost within the 724 pages of the overall report. Moreover, to the extent that poverty, hunger, and the conditions of work that underlay endemic hunger remained the domain of public health, they no longer belonged within the ambit of 'nutrition' discussion. Hunger was no longer the mandate of nutritional science, as Aykroyd had signalled earlier, but belonged to the domain of economists or labour organizations. Indeed, the very word by this point had slipped from view.[128]

How then did the sidelining of hunger in nutritional science analysis affect understanding of malaria? We return to Paul Russell's assertion in 1941 that 'better food' failed to offer protection from malaria and the academic circumstances that may have bolstered this claim, as an important example.[129]

## Nutritional science and malaria

In 1940, researchers at the Nutrition Research laboratories at Coonoor published the results of a study on the effect of diet on the course of malaria infection.[130] The study involved monkeys experimentally infected with malaria and subsequently assessed for intensity of infection in terms of ensuing blood parasite levels. Two groups of laboratory animals were tested: one fed a wheat-based diet with ample milk, pulses, ghee, and vegetables; the second group, an 'ill-balanced' diet limited largely to parboiled milled rice, and 'particularly deficient in vitamins C and A and calcium.' The dietary framework employed for assessing 'malnutrition' impact was based, in other words, on qualitative dietary factors rather than quantitative levels of hunger. Average maximum parasite prevalence was found to be similar in both groups, and the authors concluded that '[t]he course and severity of primary attacks of malaria were unaffected by the difference in the state of nutrition of the monkeys previous to infection.'[131]

In discussing their results, Passmore and Sommerville cited at some length Christophers's 1911 report, *Malaria in the Punjab*. In doing so, however, they questioned his 'scarcity' conclusions, offering simply that the scarcity-epidemic link could instead be explained on the basis of entomological factors alone: drought-induced waning acquired immunity and vector deviation (increased cattle mortality resulting in enhanced mosquito vector feeding on humans). Suggesting that their own experimental findings put to question the earlier Punjab study conclusions, they went on to advise that '[t]he mere association of malnutrition and a high malaria mortality in such circumstances cannot be taken as proof that malnutrition *per se* is an important or essential factor in the causation of malaria epidemics.'[132]

It is difficult to see the paper as ideologically influenced, for Passmore was not disinterested in the issue of hunger. A decade later, for example, he appealed, in the pages of the *Lancet*, for less punitive conditions of famine relief and a 'thorough overhaul' of policies, arguing that the Famine Codes 'have neglected the basic physiology of work.'[133] All the more so, then, the Passmore-Sommerville article reflects the profound conceptual shifts in disease and nutritional thought that had taken place in the intervening three decades since publication of Christophers's 1911 epidemic malaria report. Their conclusion – that severity of malaria was 'unaffected by the state of nutrition' – rested upon a micronutrient definition of 'nutrition' (qualitative malnutrition), and additionally, upon a microbiologic measure of 'severity' (blood parasite levels).[134] It thus addressed questions bearing little resemblance to the questions Christophers had explored in the earlier Punjab study – enhanced malaria lethality in relation to acute hunger – nor those that Sri Lankan observers had sought to raise regarding the 1934–1935 malaria epidemic. Remarkably enough, such basic distinctions by 1940 had become so blurred as to be now unrecognizable.[135]

Despite such interpretative problems, and the manifest methodological difficulties with the study itself,[136] the Passmore-Sommerville conclusions would figure prominently in subsequent malaria literature. Russell's 1941 definitive claim that '[w]ell fed soldiers in perfect physical condition go down with malaria as rapidly and as seriously, with as high a death rate as average villagers'[137] appears in an article he published in the *Indian Medical Gazette* that same year.[138] It was a claim repeated in his 1946 text, *Practical Malariology*, and again in the text's third edition in 1963.[139] In each case the single reference given was the 1940 Passmore-Sommerville paper, although by the mid-1940s, more comprehensive experimental research on diet, both quantitative and qualitative aspects, was suggesting quite different results.[140]

The influence of the Passmore-Sommerville article, however, extended well beyond Russell's writing. The 1940 paper would centrally inform a brief discussion of the question of 'nutritional status and malaria' in Boyd's prominent 1949 compendium of malaria research.[141] Epidemiological studies such as *Malaria in the Punjab* and *Malaria in the Duars*, in contrast, were missing from the brief review. Possibly they were alluded to in the acknowledgement that '[m]any writers have suggested that [malaria] infection is of more severe character in ill-nourished populations.' If so, they appear to have been dismissed as unscientific with the follow-up comment that '[u]ntil recently no experimental data on this subject were available.'[142] To qualify as scientific, a role for hunger now required experimental (microbiologic) validation (and indeed, appears in this case to have rested upon its impact on the malaria parasite) though immunological hypotheses, however uncorroborated by epidemiological experience, as seen in the preceding two chapters, did not.[143]

## Conclusion

In his overview of the emergence of nutritional science in India, Arnold has observed that '[m]etropolitian [nutritional] science was reworked and remoulded to meet local needs.' And indeed, as he points out, the food production crisis, which assumed acute form with the Bengal famine, was used as a 'critique of colonial neglect.'[144] But it is less clear that this 'reworking' did in fact better address 'local needs.' Certainly, it held the potential of such a critique. Yet in veering to dietary quality, it offered instead a reprieve, arguably a diversion, from the reality of widespread undernourishment and subsistence insecurity. Moreover, the focus on qualitative aspects of Indian agriculture would serve in the post-colonial period to draw attention further away from fundamental structural reforms and the underlying problems of servitude and class.

Thus if the new science of nutrition was being remolded, it is unclear to what extent those needs encompassed the priorities of the endemically hungry. The 'dietary critique' which non-nutritionist voices had succeeded momentarily in transforming into a critique of colonial agricultural policies was in fact already being edged off the stage. That critique did exist. But it lay largely outside the professional domain of nutritional science. Instead, hunger as a medical reality was quickly fading from public health view. In its place was left a term, 'malnutrition,' which in its original use was never intended to encompass hunger.[145] McCarrison in all his writing had insisted on the distinction between qualitative 'malnutrition' and quantitative 'underfeeding' – in modern terminology, 'undernutrition' – in order to stress what he saw as the overriding public health importance of the former. Like McCarrison, Nagendranath Gangulee also was scrupulous in distinguishing the two, though for very different reasons. Recognizing the growing confusion, he urged that the term 'malnutrition' 'be avoided as often as under feeding will do the work': urging, in effect, 'say what you mean.'[146]

It was not to be. Increasing use of the term 'malnutrition' brought further blurring of the two very different nutritional issues. In the process, both the concept and the very term 'hunger' was being lost, and with it, other basic language and concepts as well: scarcity, destitution, physiological poverty. The consequences were profound. Margaret Pelling describes the 'scientising of diet in the twentieth century,' pointing to Shryock's 1936 *Development of Modern Medicine*,

> in which the index entry for 'diet' . . . directs the reader first to 'malnutrition' and secondly to 'vitamins', while an entry for 'nutrition'

refers simply to medical criticism of the feeding of babies, and to nineteenth-century physiological chemistry. This is one reflection of the scale of the physician's abandonment of the broader interpretative aspects of nutrition.[147]

Pelling's 'broader nutrition,' it would seem, encompasses daily subsistence. Even where 'malnutrition' was employed to refer to hunger, the meaning conveyed had become something rather different. Malnutrition was now a medical syndrome, a clinical state, rather than a social and political concern. As a medical diagnosis rather than the product of structural economic conditions, the narrowed diagnostic framework lent itself in turn to equally narrow solutions, those appropriate for the acute care health worker but not for framing preventive policy. With underfeeding as both the condition (diagnosis) and now also the cause (etiology), the solution (treatment) was more feeding, thus less ignorance (on the part of poor women), a condition considered amenable to educational interventions: 'spread of knowledge' about correct diet. Shorn of their economic and social dimensions, the factors which brought about 'undernutrition' – wage levels, conditions of women's productive and reproductive work, and so on – were also being allowed to fade from view. In this sense, the 'discovery of colonial malnutrition' in 1920s South Asia is better understood as a *supplanting* of an earlier understanding of hunger as quantitative insufficiency of food and precarity of access, with qualitative issues of diet, maternal behaviour, and in the 1950s the term 'protein-energy malnutrition' (PEM) in turn. In the process, a central reality that has shaped so much of human history had also come to be set aside.

That consideration of the 'Human Factor' in malaria epidemicity could be sidelined so casually from medical and intellectual discourse speaks to the epistemological power of modern biomedical science, narrowly applied. In this sense, the reshaping of the 'Human Factor' in South Asian malaria history is a dual transformation: from non-specific to acquired immunity, and from hunger to micronutrient imbalance, in an arena of conceptual and linguistic abstraction and conflation that made the 'uncoupling' of disease and destitution much more likely. It is a legacy that continues to bedevil historical enquiry to the present day. Almost a half-century after the Passmore-Sommerville article's publication, a major review of the role of 'nutrition' in malaria would also conclude, that

[w]hile there is some evidence that malaria can adversely influence the nutritional status of humans, there is little which supports a concept that malnutrition enhances the severity of malarial infections in man. Indeed, the balance of available evidence indicates that malnutrition in humans is more commonly antagonistic to malaria.[148]

The role of acute hunger in malaria lethality, as documented in the South Asian colonial malaria literature, was never refuted. In the preoccupation with immunological and micronutrient developments in the final decades of the colonial period, it simply came to be set aside.[149] In a sense, the subdiscipline of 'malariology' could no longer 'see' what was missing because basic concepts and indeed the very language with which to do so were gone as well. But as recent historiography of Western public health suggests, the loss of language and concepts of human hunger did not begin with the twentieth-century disciplines of immunology and nutritional science. Set in larger historical context, the demise of the 'Human Factor' in malaria understanding was an expression of a much broader transformation in the conceptualization of health and disease in Western medical thought, one that can be seen more than a century earlier within the sanitary movements of western Europe.

Moreover, among local public health officials in India, the sidelining of economic conditions from epidemic understanding did not go unopposed. And here the voluminous pages of the colonial sanitary records offer, in addition to their important vital registration data, a fascinating window on the struggle by individual public health figures who questioned the reductionist tide set in train by the sanitationist and biomedical revolution, a chapter of the region's health history to which we now turn.

# Notes

1 By 1934 there were over 2,700 members of the American Dietetic Association, most 'actually earning their living by nutrition work'; E. Burnet, and W.R. Aykroyd, 'Nutrition and Public Health,' *Quarterly Bulletin of the Health Organisation of the League of Nations*, 4, 2, June 1935, 323–474, at 389 [hereafter, *QBHO*].

2 For an overview of nutritional science development, see H. Kamminga, and A. Cunningham, 'Introduction,' in H. Kamminga, and A. Cunningham, eds., *The Science and Culture of Nutrition, 1840–1940* (Amsterdam: Rodopi, 1995), 1–14.

3 M. Worboys, 'The Discovery of Colonial Malnutrition Between the Wars,' in D. Arnold, ed., *Imperial Medicine and Indigenous Societies* (Manchester: Manchester University Press, 1988), 208–225.

4 W.R. Aykroyd, *Conquest of Deficiency Diseases* (Geneva: World Health Organization, 1970), 20; F. Dunn, 'Beriberi,' in K.F. Kiple, and K.C. Ornelas, eds., *Cambridge World History of Food* (Cambridge: Cambridge University Press, 2008), 914–919.

5 Aykroyd, *The Conquest of Deficiency Diseases*, 20–21.

6 D. McCay, *Investigations on Bengal Jail Dietaries: With Some Observations on the Influence of Dietary on the Physical Development and Well-Being of the People of Bengal* (Calcutta: Superintendent Govt. Print., 1910).

7 R. McCarrison, *Studies in Deficiency Diseases* (London: Henry Frowde, Hodder & Stoughton, 1921); J.A. Shorten, 'The Role of Vitamins in Tropical Diseases,' *Indian Medical Gazette*, May 1922, 164–169 [hereafter, *IMG*].

8 Editorial, 'The Economic Factor in Tropical Disease,' *Indian Medical Gazette*, 57, Sept. 1922, 341–343 [hereafter *IMG*]; Editorial, 'Dietary and Nutritional Standards in India,' *IMG*, July 1936, 405–406.

9 R. McCarrison, 'Memorandum on Malnutrition as a Cause of Physical Ineffi-ciency and Ill-Health Among the Masses in India,' in Great Britain, *Report of the Royal Commission on Agriculture in India* (London: HMSO, 1928), vol. 1, Pt. II, 100 [hereafter *RCAI*], republished in H.M. Sinclair, *The Work of Sir Robert McCarrison* (London: Faber and Faber, 1953), 261–283.

10 R. McCarrison, 'Problems of Nutrition in India,' *Nutrition Abstracts and Reviews*, 2, 1932, 1–2, as cited in *The Work of Sir Robert McCarrison*, 268–269.

11 McCarrison, 'Memorandum on Malnutrition,' 96–97.

12 K.J. Carpenter, *Protein and Energy: A Study of Changing Ideas in Nutrition* (Cambridge: Cambridge University Press, 1994).

13 H.N. Munro, 'Historical Perspective on Protein Requirement: Objectives for the Future,' in K. Blaxter, and J.C. Waterlow, eds., *Nutritional Adaptation in Man* (London: John Libby, 1985), 155–168.

14 Editorial, 'Dietary and Nutritional Standards in India.'

15 S.C. Seal, 'Diet and the Incidence of Disease in India,' *IMG*, May 1938, 291–301, at 297, 300, 296.

16 McCarrison, 'Memorandum on Malnutrition,' 96–97.

17 Ibid., 95.

18 *RCAI*, vol. 1, Pt. I, 494.

19 Ibid., 493, 494.

20 Ibid., 495.

21 Ibid., 481–482, 494; Resolution of the All-India Conference of Medical Research Workers held at Calcutta on 27th to 29th October 1924 and on 15th to 17th December 1925; reproduced in *RCAI*, vol. I, Pt. I, 1928, Appendix III, 155.

22 *RCAI*, vol. IV, Bengal Evidence, 240–247.

23 Ibid., 248–271.

24 Ibid., 253.

25 Ibid., 259. [emphasis added]

26 Ibid., 260. Bentley's frustration at one point prompted overt critique of imperial fiscal policies: he argued that the Presidency was 'treated so badly by the finan-cial settlement . . . [that] of every 6 or 8 rupees of revenue raised in Bengal only 2 rupees remain in the Province, and it does not give us a fair chance'; ibid., 259.

27 For a comprehensive account of the absorbing focus on protein requirement and its overestimation among European scientists, see Carpenter, *Protein and Energy*; K.J. Carpenter, 'A Short History of Nutritional Science: Part 4 (1945–1985),' *Journal of Nutrition*, 133, 2003, 3331–3342. C. Sathyamala points to the remarkable absence of empirical investigation in human communities to support the 'too much rice' thesis; 'Nutrition as a Public Health Problem (1900–1947),' International Institute of Social Studies, Working Paper No. 510, Dec. 2010.

28 Mean 1931–39 crude death rate figures: Punjab, 23.9; Bombay, 24.8; Central Provinces and Berar, 32.8; Madras, 22.7; Bengal, 22.7; *Stat. Abst.*

29 *RCAI*, vol. I, 143, 163.

30 This, despite reference by Graham to '[t]he economic side of the labour wage in so far as it affects malaria,' a subject that 'has been worked out in a very interest-ing way in regard to the tea gardens in the Duars by Christophers and Bentley in a report now fifteen years old'; *RCAI*, vol. I, 145.

31 *RCAI*, vol. IV, 493.

32 W.R. Aykroyd, *Nutrition*, Oxford Pamphlets on Indian Affairs, No. 21 (Bom-bay: Humphrey Milford, Oxford University Press, 1944), 17.

33 Poverty and livelihood precarity also meant overriding time constraints for women in feeding young children sufficiently frequently through the day, as well as negligible access to more costly, energy-dense cooking oils.

34 W.R. Aykroyd, and B.G. Krishnan, 'Diets Surveys in South Indian villages,' *Indian Journal of Medical Research*, 24, 3, Jan. 1937, 667–688, at 685 [hereafter, *IJMR*]; J.D. Graham, Public Health Commissioner with the GOI, 'Replies to the Questionnaire,' *RCAI*, vol. I, 140–148, at 145.

35 Among Jamshedpur (Bihar) industrial labourers, for example, daily consumption of leafy greens was observed to be higher among the poorest income group than among the highest (1.2 ozs. compared to 0.1 oz); W.R. Aykroyd, 'Economic Aspects of the Problem of Nutrition in India, *Indian Journal of Social Work*, 2, 3, Dec. 1941, 269–282, at 278; W.R. Aykroyd, *Diet Surveys in India* (Cawnpore: The Job Press, 1948), 3. A sense of stigma associated with leafy greens as a famine food perhaps explains a substantial prevalence of subclinical vitamin A insufficiency in the general population.

36 Beriberi afflicted the Brazilian navy and workers engaged in constructing the Panama Canal, and also British soldiers in 1916 subsisting on bread made from refined wheat flour during the siege of Kut in Mesopotamia (Iraq); Aykroyd, *Conquest of Deficiency Diseases*, 18.

37 *RCAI*, vol. IV, 253; Editorial, 'The Economic Factor in Tropical Disease, *IMG*, Sept. 1922, 341.

38 Referring to beriberi in the North Circars as 'a poor man's disease,' McCarrison noted that it commonly appeared 'following attacks of some debilitating illness (diarrhoea, dysentery) or in sufferers from some chronic debilitating malady' and typically during or shortly following the winter monsoon rains, the season of peak agricultural stress; R. McCarrison, and R.V. Norris, 'The Relation of Rice to Beri-beri in India,' *Indian Medical Research Memoir*, No. 2 (Calcutta: Thacker, Spink & Co, 1924), in Sinclair, *Work of Sir Robert McCarrison*, 238.

39 Among the substantial literature: S.M. Horrocks, 'The Business of Vitamins: Nutrition Science and the Food Industry in Inter-war Britain,' in Kamminga and Cunningham, eds., *Science and Culture of Nutrition*, 235–258; D.F. Smith, ed., *Nutrition in Britain: Science, Scientists and Politics in the Twentieth Century* (London: Routledge, 1997), 219; H. Levenstein, *Paradox of Plenty: A Social History of Eating in Modern America* (New York: Oxford University Press, 1993); J. Vernon, *Hunger: A Modern History* (Cambridge, MA: Belknap Press of Harvard University Press, 2007); M. Nestle, *Food Politics: How the Food Industry Influences Nutrition, and Health* (Berkeley: University of California Press, 2007); I. Mosby, *Food Will Win the War: The Politics, Culture, and Science of Food on Canada's Home Front* (Vancouver: University of British Columbia Press, 2014).

40 Sathyamala, 'Nutrition as a Public Health Problem'; Worboys, 'The Discovery of Colonial Malnutrition'; V.R. Muraleedharan, 'Diet, Disease and Death in Colonial South India,' *Economic and Political Weekly*, Jan. 1–8 1994, 55–63; D. Arnold, 'The "Discovery" of Malnutrition and Diet in Colonial India,' *Indian Economic and Social History Review*, 31, 1, 1994, 1–26; D. Arnold, 'British India and the "Beriberi Problem", 1798–1942,' *Medical History*, 54, 2010, 295–314.

41 In 1941 the American Medical Association warned that 'hidden hunger' struck those who 'satiate[d] themselves with vast quantities of food' but did not eat enough essential nutrients; 'National Nutrition,' *Journal of the American Medical Association*, 116, Jun. 28, 1941, 2854, cited in Levenstein, *Paradox of Plenty*, 23.

42 W.R. Aykroyd, 'The Problem of Malnutrition in India,' *Current Science*, 4, 2, Aug. 1935, 75–77.

43 Sir P.C. Ray, 'The Problem of Nutrition in India,' *The Indian Review*, 42, Apr. 1941, 209–212.

44 N. Gangulee, *Health and Nutrition in India* (London: Faber and Faber, 1939), 136.

45 *RCAI*, vol. I, 149; D.N. Paton, and L. Findlay, *Child Life Investigations. Poverty, Nutrition and Growth. Studies of Child Life in Cities and Rural Districts in Scotland*, Medical Research Council Special Report Series, no. 101 (1926); as cited in D. Smith, and M. Nicolson, 'Nutrition, Education, Ignorance and Income: A Twentieth-Century Debate,' in Kamminga and Cunningham, eds., *Science and Culture of Nutrition*, 288–318 at 294, note 2.

46 *Report on the Public Health Administration of the Punjab*, 1931, 8.

47 On this, see S. Zurbrigg, *Epidemic Malaria and Hunger in Colonial Punjab: 'Weakened by Want'* (London and New Delhi: Routledge, 2019), ch. 7, 264–266.

48 For discussion of categories of hunger in physical and epidemiological terms, see Appendix II.

49 For references to meals-per-day, excerpted from the provincial reports submitted to the confidential 1888 Dufferin Inquiry, see Government of Punjab, *Report on the Famine in the Punjab in 1896–97* (Lahore: Civil and Military Gazette Press, 1898), Appendix II. 'Normal condition of the poorer classes,' No. 263 S., dated Simla, June 23, 1888, xxxvii–xlii at xlii, cited in Zurbrigg, *Epidemic Malaria and Hunger*, 110. See also W. Digby, *'Prosperous' British India: A Revelation from Official Records* (London: T. Fisher Unwin, 1901), 472, 511; B.M. Bhatia, *Famines in India* (Delhi: Asia Publishing House, 1963), 147–149.

50 Zurbrigg, *Epidemic Malaria and Hunger*, chs. 10–11.

51 Incidence of the infantile form of beriberi, for example, rose markedly in the 1950s in Burma and the Philippines with expansion of power-mills to rural areas; M.S. Meade, 'Beriberi,' in F. Kiple, ed., *Cambridge World History of Human Disease* (Cambridge: Cambridge University Press, 1993), 606–611, at 608.

52 Worboys, 'The Discovery of Colonial Malnutrition,' 221–222, 209. See also, Smith and Nicolson, 'Nutrition, Education, Ignorance'; C. Petty, 'Food, Poverty and Growth: The Application of Nutrition Science, 1918–1939,' *Bulletin of the Society for the Social History of Medicine*, 1987, 37–40.

53 Editorial, 'Dietary and Nutritional Standards in India.'

54 League of Nations, 'The Problem of Nutrition,' vol. I, *Interim Report of the Mixed Committee on the Problem of Nutrition* (Geneva: LNHO, 1936).

55 Medical representatives from both African colonies and India, for example, urged that '[i]n an under-nourished population, especially if it is subjected to periods of famine or semi-famine, the mere treatment of disease . . . will achieve but negligible results. . . . [T]he first task before the administrations of predominantly native territories is the raising of the economic status of the population'; 'Report on an International Conference of representatives of health services of African Territories and British India,' *QBHO*, II, 1933, 104, cited in Worboys, 'Discovery of Colonial Malnutrition,' 215.

56 Burnet and Aykroyd, 'Nutrition and Public Health.' 'For practical public health work, a standard of from 70 to 100 grams of protein may well be employed, and the desirability that a reasonable proportion should be of animal origin may be emphasized'; ibid., 347. This, despite serious questioning of the protein insufficiency thesis from within the League of Nations itself, as seen in the work of E.F. Terroine; 'Report on the Protein Component of the Human Diet,' *QBHO*, 4, 1935. See also Gangulee, *Health and Nutrition in India*, 44.

57 Burnet and Aykroyd, 'Nutrition and Public Health,' 327 [emphasis added].
58 Ibid., 385.
59 Paton and Findlay, 'Poverty, Nutrition and Growth,' 294.
60 Burnet and Aykroyd, 'Nutrition and Public Health,' 386.
61 W. Hannington, secretary of the Unemployed Workers Movement (UK) responded: 'I think the workers are entitled to be indignant at the patronising insults of those who suggest that the ill-health of their families is due to the ignorance of the harassed housewife'; *The Problem of the Distressed Areas*, as cited in Smith and Nicolson, 'Nutrition, Education, Ignorance,' 302.
62 League of Nations, *Final Report of the Mixed Committee of the League of Nations on The Relation of Nutrition to Health, Agriculture and Economic Policy* (Geneva: LNHO, 1937), 248–274, at 251, 274.
63 Micronutrient deficiencies, rather than macro-, were singled out as 'paving the way' for infectious disease and physical inefficiency, and remedial emphasis was on education; Burnet and Aykroyd, 'Nutrition and Public Health,' 327.
64 A.L.S. Staples, *The Birth of Development: How the World Bank, Food and Agriculture Organization, and World Health Organization Changed the World, 1945–1965* (Kent, OH: Kent State University Press, 2006), 71–76; T. Boon, 'Agreement and Disagreement in the Making of *World of Plenty*,' in Smith, *Nutrition in Britain*, ch. 8.
65 W.R. Aykroyd, 'International Health – A Retrospective Memoir,' *Perspectives in Biology and Medicine*, 11, 2, 1968, 273–285, at 279.
66 Gangulee, *Health and Nutrition in India*, 21.
67 J.H. Perkins, *Geopolitics and the Green Revolution: Wheat, Genes, and the Cold War* (Oxford: Oxford University Press, 1999); Staples, *Birth of Development*, 74.
68 Aykroyd, *The Nutritive Value of Indian Foods*.
69 Aykroyd in 1948 again observed that 'intake of total protein is usually sufficient when cereals form the bulk of the diet and calorie yield is adequate,' and repeated his 1937 observation that up to one-third of the rural population 'does not get enough to eat'; *Diet Surveys in India*, 4–5, 3. See also, Aykroyd, *Nutrition*, Oxford Pamphlets, 3, 17.
70 See, e.g., Aykroyd, 'The Problem of Malnutrition in India.'
71 W.R. Aykroyd, and B.G. Krishnan, 'The Effect of Skimmed Milk, Soya Bean, and Other Foods in Supplementing Typical Indian Diets,' *IJMR*, 24, 1937, 1093–1115.
72 GOI, *Report of the Royal Commission on Labour in India* (Calcutta: GOI Central Publication Branch, 1931), vol. I, Pt. I, 316–317. Here too, however, the notion that cereal-based diets were 'too bulky' and unbalanced is evident; ibid., 28.
73 N.K. Adyanthaya, *Report on the Enquiry into the Family Budgets of Industrial Workers in Madras City, 1935–1936* (Madras: Superintendent, Govt. Press, 1940), as estimated by Aykroyd in 'Economic Aspects,' 276, 275.
74 'The cost of a "well-balanced" diet was estimated at between Rs 4 to 6 per adult monthly'; Aykroyd, 'Economic Aspects,' 271.
75 Ibid., 273. A detailed overview of the results of nutritional surveys is given in Muraleedharan, 'Diet, Disease and Death.'
76 P. Weindling, 'The Role of International Organizations in Setting Nutritional Standards in the 1920s and 1930s,' in Kamminga and Cunningham, eds., *Science and Culture of Nutrition*, 319–332, at 327–329.
77 Gangulee, *Health and Nutrition in India*, 27.
78 Aykroyd and Krishnan, 'Diet Surveys in South Indian Villages.'

79 The measure 'calories per consumption unit per day' takes into account differing requirements by age and gender, thus making comparison between households possible.

80 Aykroyd and Krishnan, 'Diet Surveys in South Indian Villages,' 674–675, Table II, 688.

81 Half of the poorest households consumed regular, if small, amounts of green leafy vegetables, a larger proportion than among the highest-income group; and for all, hand-pounded parboiled rice and millets formed the staple grain. All households were found to consume tamarind, a good source of thiamine and limited amounts of vitamins C and A; ibid., 684.

82 Ibid., 687.

83 Aykroyd, 'Economic Aspects,' Table 3, 278.

84 India, Directorate of the National Malaria Eradication Programme. *Agricultural Labour in India, Intensive Family Survey* (Delhi: Ministry of Labour, GOI, 1955), vol. I, 150–151, cited in R.P. Sinha, *Food in India: An Analysis of the Prospects for Self-sufficiency by 1975–76* (Bombay: Oxford University Press, 1961), 20. Corresponding percentages arrived at by the ICMR were 83.4 for agriculturalists and 75.2 for industrial wage-earners; ibid.

85 Dr. Margaret Balfour, 'Maternity conditions and anaemia in the Assam Tea-gardens, *Journal of the Association of Medical Women in India*, vol. 24, 1936, cited in Gangulee, *Health and Nutrition in India*, 230.

86 Ibid., 228, 234, 74, 112. In his research Gangulee may well have come across Christophers's *Malaria in the Punjab,* noting that 'it has been demonstrated that a direct relationship exists between the price of essential foodstuffs and the epidemic malaria'; ibid., 78.

87 Ibid., 81, 111, 212.

88 Ibid., 25–26, 225–226, 306.

89 Ibid., 225, 269, 277, 306.

90 Ibid., 277, 302.

91 W.R. Aykroyd, B.G. Krishnan, R. Passmore, and A.R. Sundarajan, 'The Rice Problem in India,' *The Indian Medical Research Memoirs*, No. 32, Jan. 1940, 1–84, at 65, 61–71.

92 Ibid., 18, 13. See also, W.R. Aykroyd, 'Nutrition, International and National,' *Current Science*, Mar. 1936, 639–642, at 639. Earlier, Aykroyd had also acknowledged that nutritional education 'propaganda may easily become insulting if it is directed at a population struggling to feed itself on a totally inadequate wage or allowance'; W.R. Aykroyd, 'Diet in Relation to Small Incomes,' *QBHO*, 2, 1933, 130–153, at 150.

93 Aykroyd, 'Economic Aspects,' 280–282.

94 Aykroyd, *Nutrition*, Oxford Pamphlets, 32, 29, 15.

95 Sathyamala, 'Nutrition as a public health problem,' 19. In a small monograph published in Britain in 1937, Aykroyd acknowledged that 'to ascribe the ill-feeding of the children of poor mothers to "maternal inefficiency" is heartless and on the whole unjustifiable'; yet in the next sentence he urged that 'the education of young mothers on dietetics might produce useful results'; W.R. Aykroyd, *Human Nutrition and Diet* (London: Thorton Butterworth, 1937), 224. In 1948, poverty and ignorance would be conflated overtly: 'Everybody knows that the basic cause of malnutrition is poverty, and the illiteracy and ignorance which accompany poverty'; W.R Aykroyd, Director, Nutrition Division, FAO, *Proceedings of the Fourth International Congress on Tropical Medicine and Malaria*, Washington, D.C., May 10–18, 1948, 1178.

96 By the early 1940s, Worboys observes, malnutrition was reinterpreted as a technical problem: 'ignorance as to what to grow, how to grow it, what to eat and how to cook it'; with the 'growing tendency to "scientise" or "medicalise" social problems,' the nutrition problem became 'depoliticised . . . chang[ing] from one of inappropriate structures to one of inadequate knowledge,' with remedies increasingly 'sought, not through structural changes, but by "technical fixes": dietary supplements and nutritional education'; 'The Discovery of Colonial Malnutrition,' 221–222, 209.

97 Aykroyd, *Nutrition*, Oxford Pamphlet, 27. 'An incidental and no doubt intended consequence of this change of emphasis,' Worboys observes, 'was to shift the tone of the [Colonial Office] Report from one of pessimism to one of optimism'; 'Discovery of Colonial Malnutrition,' 220.

98 Aykroyd, 'Nutrition, International and National,' 641.

99 This division had been formalized earlier at LNHO meetings held at the LSHTM in November 1935 where two separate subcommittees were formed on ' "energy-bearing" substances and protective foods'; Sathyamala, 'Nutrition as a Public Health Problem,' 14.

100 United Nations Conference, 'Final Act of the United Nations Conference on Food and Agriculture, Hot Springs, Virginia, United States of America, 18th May–3rd June 1943,' reproduced in 'United Nations Conference on Food and Agriculture: Text of the Final Act,' *The American Journal of International Law*, 37, 4, Supplement: Official Documents (Oct. 1943), 159–192.

101 M.K. Gandhi, *Diet and Diet Reform* (Ahmedabad: Navajivan Publishing House, 1949), 33–34.

102 See, e.g., J.C. Waterlow, and P.R. Payne, 'The Protein Gap,' *Nature*, 258, 113–115; D. McLaren 'The Great Protein Fiasco,' *Lancet*, Jul. 13, 1974, 93–96. For an overview of changing estimates of protein requirement, see H.N. Munro, 'Historical Perspective on Protein Requirement: Objectives for the Future,' in K. Blaxter, and J.C. Waterlow, eds., *Nutritional Adaption in Man* (London: John Libby, 1985), 155–168; also, Carpenter, *Protein and Energy*, 180–203.

103 T. Dyson, and A. Maharatna, 'Excess Mortality During the Bengal Famine: A Re-Evaluation,' *Indian Economic and Social History Review*, 28, 3, 1991, 281–297.

104 A. Sen, *Poverty and Famines: An Essay on Entitlement and Deprivation* (Oxford: Oxford University Press, 1981).

105 For an overview of early twentieth-century reforms in famine relief policy, see Zurbrigg, *Epidemic Malaria and Hunger*, ch. 11.

106 Sen, *Poverty and Famines*, 216. As the Commission subsequently suggested, 'the presence of famine accentuated the lethal effect of disease present in lesser degrees in normal times'; Famine Inquiry Commission, *Report on Bengal* (New Delhi: GOI, 1945), 112–113.

107 S. Zurbrigg, 'Did Starvation Protect from Malaria? Distinguishing Between Severity and Lethality of Infectious Disease in Colonial India,' *Social Science History*, 21, 1, 1997, 27–58.

108 GOI. Ministry of Labour, *Agricultural Labour: How They Work and Live* (New Delhi: All-India Agricultural Labour Enquiry, 1952), cited in D. Narain, *Distribution of the Marketed Surplus of Agricultural Produce by Size-Level of Holding in India* (Bombay: Asia Publishers House, 1961), 36–37. An early 1940s rural Bengal survey found 10.7 per cent of 'households living on Rs 100 a year or less, equivalent to daily grain consumption of 11 ounces per capita (312.5 grams), amounting to 1,150 calories.' Though encompassing both child

and adult consumption levels, this figure nevertheless indicated severe caloric insufficiency; R.B. Lal, and S.C. Seal, *General Rural Health Survey, Singur Health Centre, 1944* (Calcutta: GOI Press, 1949), 95. A similar finding has been estimated for the bottom 10 per cent of the population in pre-Revolutionary France; R. Fogel, 'Second Thoughts on the European Escape from Hunger: Famines, Chronic Malnutrition, and Mortality Rates,' in S.R. Osmani, ed., *Nutrition and Poverty* (Oxford: Clarendon Press, 1992), 243–280.

109 For an account of WW2-related famine conditions in southeastern Punjab in 1942, see Zurbrigg, *Epidemic Malaria and Hunger*, 371–372.

110 P. Mohapatra, 'Coolies and Colliers: A Study of the Agrarian Context of Labour Migration from Chotanagpur, 1880–1920,' *Studies in History*, 1, 2, n.s., 1985, 297–299; E. Boserup, *The Conditions of Agricultural Growth* (Chicago: Aldine, 1965), 98–100; G. Omvedt, *The Political Economy of Starvation: Imperialism and the World Food Crisis* (Bombay: Leela Bhosale, 1975), 27–35.

111 *Report on Bengal*, ch. II, 'Causes of Disease and Mortality,' 116–123.

112 *Famine Inquiry Commission: Final Report* (Delhi: Govt Press, 1945), 112.

113 Although the Famine Inquiry report did acknowledge that an estimated 30 per cent of the population 'does not get enough to eat,' most of its eight-page chapter on 'The Problem of Nutrition' was directed to insufficient production and consumption of 'protective' foods; ibid., 105–112.

114 Interestingly, Aykroyd in 1970 would attribute the decline of beriberi 'to far-reaching changes in economic circumstances and conditions of employment' as well as 'scientific understanding of its cause'; Aykroyd, *Conquest of Deficiency Diseases*, 25. Long before, however, the idea of beriberi had already established a micronutrient prominence in nutritional science.

115 H.F. Knight, *Food Administration in India, 1939–47* (Stanford: Stanford University Press, 1954), 189, 215, 307–8; Zurbrigg, *Epidemic Malaria and Hunger*, ch. 12.

116 Zurbrigg, *Epidemic Malaria and Hunger*, ch. 12.

117 Ministry of Food and Agriculture. Department of Food, *Report of the Foodgrains Enquiry Committee* (New Delhi: GOI, 1957), 40.

118 'As in Britain,' Worboys observes, 'the technical dimensions of the problem allowed for this radicalism to be lost as the definition of the problem changed from one of inappropriate structures to one of inadequate knowledge'; 'Discovery of Colonial Malnutrition,' 222.

119 For a succinct account of the protein insufficiency thesis as informing the work of FAO and broader UN agencies in the 1950s and 1960s, see Carpenter, 'A Short History of Nutritional Science,' 3331–3342.

120 Famine Inquiry Commission, India, *Report of the Health Survey and Development Committee* (New Delhi: GOI, 1946), vol. 1, 12, 54. For background to the appointment of the Health Survey, see S. Amrith, *Decolonizing International Health: India and Southeast Asia, 1930–65* (Basingstoke: Palgrave Macmillan, 2006), 57–63.

121 Famine Inquiry Commission, India, *Health Survey and Development Committee*, vol. 1, 57.

122 Ibid., vol. 2, 70.

123 See note 68.

124 Ibid., vol. 1, 56.

125 Ibid., vol. 2, 71.

126 Ibid., vol. 1, 58.

127 Ibid., vol. 2, 130.

128 C. Sathyamala points to an alternative report by a health subcommittee headed by Col. S.S. Sohkey, appointed in 1938 by the National Planning Committee of the Indian National Congress [*National Health*. National Planning Committee Series (Bombay: Vora & Co. Publishers, 1948)] that addressed the 'root cause of disease' as 'found in the poverty – almost destitution – of the people' where per capita income for many is 'barely sufficient to provide one meal per day'; 'Nutrition as a Public Health Problem,' 23–24.

129 P. Russell, 'Some Aspects of Malaria in India,' Jul. 5, 1941, Rockefeller Archive Centre, RG.1.1. S.464 B.11 f.87; cited in J. Farley. *To Cast Out Disease: A History of the International Health Division of the Rockefeller Foundation (1913–1951)* (Oxford: Oxford University Press, 2004), 123.

130 R. Passmore, and T. Sommerville, 'An Investigation of the Effect of Diet on the Course of Experimental Malaria in Monkeys,' *Journal of the Malaria Institute of India*, 3, 4, Dec. 1940, 447–455.

131 Ibid., 455.

132 Ibid.

133 Ibid., 448.

134 Ibid., 455.

135 'By increasing metabolic demands, the code lowers the effectiveness of the relief. . . . Clearly relief would be more effective if the large camps and works could be abolished and the people helped in their own villages'; R. Passmore, 'Famine in India,' *Lancet*, Aug. 1951, 303–307.

136 Information on only 15 malaria-symptomatic animals is given: eight in the 'ill-balanced' rice diet group, and seven in the 'well-balanced' diet group, making the possibility of statistically significant conclusions unlikely. Moreover, half of the animals in the 'ill-balanced' diet group lost weight during the pre-inoculation period, two deaths occurring among those with greatest weight loss, compared to one death among the 'well-balanced' diet group. Thus, though the study's intent was to look at qualitative *mal*nutrition rather than acute hunger, the monotonous 'malnourished' (rice) diet appears to have led to moderate quantitative deficiency in some animals as well, further confounding results; Passmore and Sommerville, 'An investigation of the effect of diet.'

137 See ch. 2, above.

138 P.F. Russell, 'Some Social Obstacles to Malaria Control,' *IMG*, Nov. 1941, 681–690.

139 P. Russell, L.S. West, and R.D. Manwell, *Practical Malariology* (Philadelphia: W.B. Saunders, 1946), 540–541. 'The results clearly added weight to the view that one may not hope to control malaria simply by combating malnutrition'; Russell, West, Manwell, and Macdonald, *Practical Malariology*, 3rd ed., 1963, 625.

140 M.M. Brooke, 'Effect of Dietary Changes upon Avian Malaria,' *American Journal of Hygiene*, 41, 1945, 81–108.

141 J.D. Fulton, and B.G. Maegraith, ch. 38, 'The Physiologic Pathology of Malaria,' in M.F. Boyd, ed., *Malariology: A Comprehensive Survey of All Aspects of This Group of Diseases from a Global Standpoint* (Philadelphia: W.B. Saunders, 1949), 904–934, at 915–916. Results of two other studies also were cited that suggested thiamine and biotin deficiency states increased malaria severity; however, in both cases the extreme diets required to ensure absence of the specific micronutrient appear to have confounded results; ibid.

142 Ibid.

111

143  For discussion of experimental research on quantitative hunger and malaria carried out by S.P. Ramakrishnan in the early 1950s, see S. Zurbrigg, 'Did Starvation Protect from Malaria?: Distinguishing Between Severity and Lethality of Infectious Disease in Colonial India,' *Social Science History*, 21, 1, 1997, 27–58.

144  Arnold, 'The "Discovery" of Malnutrition and Diet,' 26.

145  See above, at note 9.

146  Gangulee, '*Health and Nutrition in India*,' 81.

147  M. Pelling, *The Common Lot: Sickness, Medical Occupations and the Urban Poor in Early Modern England* (London: Longman, 1998), 61.

148  I.A. McGregor, 'Malaria and Nutrition,' in W.H. Wernsdorfer, and I.A. McGregor, eds., *Malaria: Principles and Practice of Malariology* (London: Churchill Livingstone, 1988), 754–777, at 763. It is unclear the meaning of 'malnutrition' intended by McGregor here, but undernourishment seems implied. Curiously, only 14 years earlier McGregor, after several decades of malaria work in the Gambia, rued that '[w]e have tended to forget what the very distinguished Italian school of malariologists taught us many years ago, namely, that the real bulwarks against malaria lie in the progressive "bonification" of a country, that is to say, in progressive improvement in the economic, the educational, the agricultural, and . . . the health standards of a country'; 'Darling Foundation Award,' *WHO Chronicle*, 1974, 28, 356–358.

149  Hamlin similarly observes that '[t]he role of predisposition was not something that could be disproved' by Chadwick in his 1842 *Sanitary Report*, 'but it could be ignored'; C. Hamlin 'Predisposing Causes and Public Health in Early Nineteenth-Century Medical Thought,' *Society for the Social History of Medicine*, 5, 1, Apr. 1992, 43–70, at 70.

# 4

# THE LARGER SANITATIONIST
# CONTEXT

[U]nless some better support both in Quantity and Quality of
provisions can be procured . . . some putrid epidemic disease
must be the Consequence.
—— Henry Legge to John King 13 May 1800;
cited in Douglas Hay, 'War, Dearth and
Theft in the Eighteenth Century: The Record
of the English Courts,' *Past and Present*,
95, 117–160, 129

The demise within medical discourse of hunger's role in malaria mortality across the final years of the colonial period reflected a much broader
transformation taking place in concepts of infective disease and epidemic
causation in Western medical thought, a reductive trajectory apparent from
the early nineteenth century. Historians of public health in recent years have
extended analysis beyond narrowly framed institutional accounts of the
early modern sanitary movement in industrializing Europe to investigate
the far-reaching transformation in understanding of health and disease that
movement represented, and its consequences.[1] Christopher Hamlin in particular has explored the 'uncoupling of disease and destitution'[2] in medical
theory that took shape in mid-nineteenth-century Britain under the mantle
of Edwin Chadwick's 1842 Sanitary Report: how an earlier 'predispositionist' understanding of epidemic causation that encompassed conditions of
hunger and physical debility in the human 'host' was set aside, leaving the
recurring 'fever' epidemics in the burgeoning industrial urban slums narrowly attributed to atmospheric vapours emanating from 'filth' in the external environment.[3]

A similar conceptual narrowing, if less complete, can be seen within the
Indian Medical Service in the later nineteenth century with the transfer
of the sanitationist epidemic paradigm – and soon laboratory and 'tropical' (primarily vector-based) medicine – to British India. In the case of
malaria, by the final years of colonial rule this epistemic shift had led to a

113

fundamental redefinition of the nature of the 'malaria problem' in South Asia, and in turn to a rapid reshaping of theoretical approaches to its control. It was to the earlier, pre-Chadwickian understanding of 'predisposing' factors in epidemic causation that Christophers was turning, in his 1911 epidemic malaria enquiry report, and attempting to reclaim. In tracking, then, the ultimate demise of the 'Human Factor' in malaria epistemology in the Indian subcontinent, this earlier experience in the British metropole provides essential context.

This chapter briefly traces the sanitationist transformation in epidemic thought in nineteenth-century Britain. It goes on to explore, in the pages of the colonial sanitary records, how the narrowed doctrine of 'miasmic filth', transported to South Asia, was perceived in Punjab by district-level sanitary officers, and contested. In the process, it highlights the larger economic content implicit in earlier 'climatist' theories of epidemic disease: dimensions that encompassed harvest and land drainage conditions, aspects often unrecognized in modern critiques of pre-bacteriological epidemic thought. In doing so, it reinterprets the 'clash' of epidemic paradigms encountered at the professional level within the Indian Medical Service to be, at the local administrative level, instead a reasoned accommodation of both the so-called climatist and new microbial understandings of epidemic disease – an accommodation that would be increasingly challenged by the paradigmatic power of the rapidly emerging subspecialisms of modern laboratory-based medicine.

## Context to the nineteenth-century sanitationist epidemic model

The singular environmental focus of Edwin Chadwick's 1842 Sanitary Report in its etiological assessment of epidemic 'fever', primarily typhus,[4] in industrializing Britain had its roots, in part at least, in earlier climatist (often referred to as 'anticontagionist') theories of epidemic disease causation. Atmospheric conditions had long been considered conducive to noxious vapours responsible for a range of fevers. Climatist theories however were not generally exclusivist, but to varying extents took into account additional co-existing factors underlying disease causation. Constitutionist theory, for example, considered various disease diatheses, hereditary or induced, which rendered an individual more vulnerable to a morbid or mortal disease outcome. Related, but broader still, was a 'predispositionist' understanding of disease, where physical exhaustion ('physiologic poverty') resulting from hunger, mental anxieties, and debilitating conditions of work and living was seen as a central underlying determinant of human vulnerability to disease and to epidemic occurrence. The common endemic fevers such as typhus, relapsing fever, and malaria, where direct human-to-human 'contagion' was only irregularly evident, were thought to be triggered by miasmas (in the latter case, 'mal-aria' or bad air) emanating from rotting organic waste or waterlogged soils and thus affected by climatic conditions. These miasmas, however, in many cases were considered 'exciting' or proximate causes, understood to require physical debility ('predisposition') among the afflicted for their morbid expression to take form in epidemic mortality.[5]

The importance of predisposition was expressed most transparently perhaps in the writing of Johann Frank in his late eighteenth-century text, *The People's Misery: Mother of Diseases*:[6]

> The weaker the organism and the more exhausted from troubles the human machine is, the sooner *miasmas and contagions* penetrate it like a dry sponge. . . . Even a light infection, localized in a small spot, soon develops into a deadly disease similar to jail or hospital fever and spreads among relatives and friends who are exhausted by misery and predisposed for it.

Recognition of a key role for human destitution underlying epidemic disease also underlay Rudolf Virchow's famed assessment of the cause of the major typhus epidemic in the impoverished rural tracts of Upper Silesia in the late 1840s.[7] 'Physiological misery' was recognized also as endemically at play in recurring typhus epidemics in Britain and documented in the writing of prominent medical figures such as William Pulteney Alison of Edinburgh, as well as in the testimony of local Poor Law medical officers to the 1839 Sanitary Inquiry chaired by Chadwick.[8] What distinguished the nineteenth-century sanitationist view of epidemic causation articulated in the 1842 Sanitary Report was the singular focus on external filth to the exclusion of conditions of the human host.

The neologism 'sanitary,' derived from the French term *cordon sanitaire*, appears to have been first used as an English term in the mid-1820s, Margaret Pelling has suggested, initially in a pejorative sense in referring to quarantine laws.[9] By the early 1830s, however, the term had been given a 'positive, environmental connotation' by the Benthamite sanitarians, associating it with water provision, waste removal (conservancy), and sewer infrastructure. Simply through use, it quickly came to commandeer an authority which pre-empted awkward definitional questions, Hamlin suggests, making the exclusion of issues such as poverty and hunger possible.[10]

The reception accorded the narrowed Chadwickian-sanitationist model of epidemic fever in Britain at one level can be understood in the context of scientific developments of the period. From the early nineteenth century, physico-chemical investigation of fermentation had led to greater specification within miasma theory where diseases were considered to be caused by specific poisons (ferments or 'zymes'). William Farr employed the term 'zymotic' in his initial vital registration classification system in the late 1830s to refer to fevers considered to be caused by broad atmospheric conditions conducive to organic decay of environmental filth, thus diseases associated with particular regions or localities.[11] With ongoing developments in pathology that identified discreet anatomical lesions, medical attention turned increasingly to specific miasmic agents and the differentiation of individual disease entities (nosology). During these years, Hamlin observes, 'an older *physiological* conception of disease was giving way to an *ontological* one'; in the process, as Michael Worboys also notes, making 'diseases "things" or entities that were separate from the patient.'[12]

At another level, the emergence of a narrowed miasmic theory of epidemic disease in Britain took place in the context of extremely rapid urbanization, in a society unprepared infrastructurally and philosophically, with the ascent of *laissez-faire*, to deal with the human consequences. Between the late eighteenth century and 1900, the proportion of the population living in urban areas in Britain grew from 15 to 85 per cent, with recurring waves of Irish famine refugees adding fuel to the urban fires of epidemic typhus. Municipal provision of minimal water supply and sewage disposal was a reactive response to a profound crisis of unmet basic human needs, but also to the fears and panic of the non-poor.[13]

Yet there was a larger context involved as well. As secretary to the Poor Law Commission preceding his appointment to head the 1839 Sanitary Inquiry, Chadwick was at the centre of 1832 reforms to the Elizabethan Poor Laws, changes that reduced poor relief expenditure by half by restricting relief only to those willing to reside within the repellent (and often pestiferous) confines of workhouses.[14] Thus, though the promise of water and sewers, achieved in the final decades of the nineteenth century, was unquestionably a 'public good,' it came at the expense of the earlier system of parish relief, itself meagre, and with an undermining of notions of social obligation. Epistemically, it came also with a redefinition of epidemic fever causation. Environmental miasma, Chadwick now argued, was the principal *cause* of destitution ('pauperism') in industrializing Britain through the debility and illness it triggered, rather than underlying hunger and conditions of work. A number of leading medical observers disagreed.[15] But their testimony to the 1839 Sanitary Inquiry was largely omitted from the pages of the 1842 Sanitary Report.[16]

Identification of specific microbes in the final decades of the nineteenth century would further amplify the reductive trajectory. Much of the new laboratory research was channelled into bacteriology's twin discipline of immunology: techniques to induce or bolster 'acquired' immunity to specific microbes (vaccines and anti-toxins), spurred by the compelling, if somewhat unrepresentative, example of smallpox (*vaccinia*) vaccination, and initial successes in animal husbandry in the case of an anthrax vaccine. In the process, attention slipped further away from those conditions of the human host that undermined general immune *capacity*, conditions that underlay epidemics of typhus[17] and as well the lethality of very many other endemic infections such as tuberculosis, and common respiratory and diarrheal infections.[18] Disease increasingly was equated to *infection* and microbial transmission *per se* ('invading germs'), with little attention to the response of the human host to this infection, a response mediated by the immune capacity of the individual. This conflation was expressed linguistically in the growing prominence of the term 'infectious disease.' By the late nineteenth century, the earlier 'seed and soil' under-standing of disease saw 'soil' increasingly viewed principally in terms of 'acquired' immunity, and a central goal of public health now that of inducing specific immunity through vaccines[19] – an approach that further reinforced a focus on germ (infection) transmission and a movement away from conditions of the human host conducing to morbid disease. Though such an approach would prove invaluable for infections of major inher-ent virulence such as tetanus, diphtheria, and whooping cough, 'public health' by the early twentieth century, Galdston would observe, was

> no longer humanist – but rather microbist . . . no longer concerned with working conditions, hours, wages, literacy, child labor, in a word, with man's total environment. It is interested in germs, in vaccines, in serums, in fumigation, sterilization, and quarantine.[20]

### The sanitary paradigm transported to India

The epistemic shift taking place in disease theory in Europe was transported to British India in the later decades of the nineteenth century, in this case as 'tropical hygiene.' Hamlin does not attempt to explore the broader impact of the sanitationist paradigm transferred to the colonial context. Yet his work sets the stage for such analysis by identifying the conceptual and lin-guistic levers in Britain that first effected the demise of hunger as a public health category there: among them, the removal of starvation as a medi-cal cause of death from the mortality registers of mid-nineteenth-century England.[21] Such was the power of the sanitary paradigm in both concept and terminology that hunger would be formally invisible in colonial Indian vital registration ledgers as well – in a land where destitution as an engine underlying epidemic disease was that much more manifest even than in the proliferating slums of mid-nineteenth-century Britain.

South Asian public health historiography has yet to fully integrate the conceptual implications of the nineteenth-century sanitarian movement into the study of the colonial sanitary regime established in India. Recent critiques of British Indian public health policy, including malaria control policy, have been directed to its 'enclavist' character and reluctance on the part of mid-nineteenth-century sanitary officials to immediately embrace the new laboratory medicine.[22] Much less attention has been directed to the model itself. The story of public health policy under the British Raj, how-ever, is considerably more complex. There were, for example, compelling epidemiological reasons for colonial sanitary officers' reluctance to set aside earlier pre-germ-theory understanding of epidemic disease causation. As in Britain, there were those who questioned, and resisted, the view of epidemic disease mortality as primarily 'filth' mediated.[23] A major element to pre-Chadwickian hygiene policy, in British India as in pre-industrial Europe, was the prevention of a broad spectrum of diseases through 'environmental' changes relating to land drainage, if in the case of the former only rarely applied.[24] The deleterious effects of waterlogged soils on the health of an agricultural population was explained in terms of miasmic vapours associated with moisture-induced organic fermentation. But an underlying concern and purpose to land drainage was clearly understood as economic, centred on productivity of the soil. In the case of the Jumna Canal inquiry in 1840s eastern Punjab, for example, agricultural impoverishment due to waterlogging was recognized as a key factor in predisposing to 'intense' malarial fever in the waterlogged tracts,[25] and led ultimately to a realignment of the Jumna and Lower Bari canals.

Such an understanding is apparent as well in the 1863 *Report of the Royal Commission of Inquiry into the Sanitary State of the Army in India.* Epidemics in the Indian subcontinent, the report noted, 'appear, disappear and reappear in different periods and at different degrees of intensity but always occur among populations exposed to certain unhealthy conditions.' Of the 'unhealthy' conditions listed, the first one cited by the Commission related to agricultural drainage.

> [I]ntermittent [malarial] fever disappeared from places which it formerly ravaged after drainage of the soil and improved cultivation. . . . It is evident that when men are exposed to the operation of very unhealthy places, many of the weak are cut off at once . . . and others . . . so enfeebled that they rapidly succumb.[26]

Implicit in the concern with drainage, in other words, lay agricultural prosperity: an understanding that economic hardship underpinned the virulent (epidemic) form of fevers.[27]

Within the British Indian army itself, there was of course less concern for frank destitution, with troops insulated from the vicissitudes of harvests and foodgrain markets. The physical debility that did exist in the army came by virtue of class recruitment, indifferent attention to ration adequacy and palatability, and above all the physical exhaustion of military campaigns. In the wake of the 1857 Rebellion, the administration had been forced to acknowledge, and better attend to, such physical exhaustion among both British and Indian troops.[28] The 1866 edition of the hygiene manual of Edmund Parkes, the basic text for sanitation work in British India, devoted several chapters to the effects of heat and physical debility associated with campaigns, particularly among new recruits, and the need for rest, protected water supply, and improved quality of food. With regard to malaria specifically, the manual read,

> it is well known in many diseases that two sets of causes are in operation – one external, and one internal to the body (exciting, and pre-disposing). . . . The internal disposition [to 'the paroxysmal fevers'] is greatly heightened by poor feeding, anaemia, and probably by scurvy. To remove the internal causes, our only means at present are the administration of antiperiodics, especially quinine; and good and generous living, . . . [with] warm clothing, warm coffee, and a good meal before the time of exposure to the malaria.[29]

Radhika Ramasubban notes that after 1863, troop 'vitality' and efficiency began to be remedied through greater attention to the palatability of food rations and the physical demands made on troops. Morale, she suggests, was managed less through unlimited supplies of liquor[30] than through better food and minimally humane conditions of military work and life.

## Vital registration's window

After 1863, greater attention of course was also directed to controlling the environment in and around military populations through a system of rural cantonments, and periodic stationing of British troops and administrative staff in cooler hill stations.[31] Still, the military could not be fully insulated from the health conditions of the general population. This understanding underlay establishment of a civilian vital registration system in the wake of the 1863 report. In addition to mortality figures, information on harvest conditions and prevailing foodgrain prices would be routinely recorded in the annual provincial Sanitary Commission reports, data considered key to anticipating epidemic patterns among the civilian population.

The significance of vital registration for imperial rule, however, very quickly extended beyond that of an early warning system for the colonial army. Lower-level (district) officials were soon confronting the magnitude of fever mortality, pre-eminently malarial, as the leading non-enclave 'public health' issue, and coming to appreciate the power of economic conditions underlying its highly lethal form.[32] The 1880 second edition of the *Madras Manual of Hygiene*, for example, included as an Appendix, an exacting analysis of epidemic mortality in relation to foodgrain price levels and starvation across the 1876–1877 South Indian famine prepared by the Madras Sanitary Commission, W.R. Cornish.[33] Thus within only a few years of its establishment, a registration system set up to track the epidemic diseases of priority to the government and imperial trade (cholera and smallpox) was revealing malaria, and the destitution underlying its epidemic form, as the leading 'sanitary' problem facing much of the subcontinent. In effect, the provincial sanitary ledgers were pulling back the miasmic curtain on price starvation, and the human cost of the *laissez-faire* doctrines upon which the imperial project rested.[34] In Punjab, the same reports were also shedding light on the locally disastrous economic consequences of interruption in surface drainage, conditions often greatly exacerbated by extensive road and rail infrastructure construction. Alongside climatist notions of the debilitating effects of heat and humidity on imperial forces, the overriding power of economic hardship in determining epidemic mortality among the general population was a reality rapidly permeating sanitary consciousness.

It was in this same period, of course, that the influence of sanitationist and germ-based laboratory medicine was taking medical attention in another direction. By the late nineteenth century, for example, the 1894 edition of the 433-page *Indian (Madras) Manual of Hygiene* no longer included the Cornish appendix detailing epidemic mortality patterns in the 1876–1877 Madras famine.[35] Attention to broader economic dimensions in epidemic analysis was rapidly ebbing at the academic level with identification of specific disease microbes in the final two decades of the nineteenth century, if 'on the ground' the vital registration ledgers continued to throw into sharp relief the impact of harvest and price conditions on death rates. The development of immunological 'interventions' (vaccines, antitoxins) and understanding of newly identified vectors was further shifting attention to microbe transmission,[36] giving imperial medicine much finer tools for protecting the colonial administrative populations in what quickly took conceptual shape as 'tropical medicine' – although in practice most of the rural population continued to be excluded.[37] Pushing policies further to a narrowed germ-transmission focus was the outbreak of plague in 1896, with sanitary practice absorbed by the demands of anti-plague immunization and, from 1907, vector (rat) extirpation, even if both measures in practice were largely ineffective.[38] Together, imperial economics, international trade obligations, and the new laboratory medicine were pushing sanitary attention at the administrative level in India to focus ever more narrowly on specific disease interventions and to a wholly 'contagionist' (germ-transmission) interpretation of epidemic causation.

## Reinterpreting the 'Clash' of paradigms

In recent critiques of the colonial public health service in British India, historians have highlighted the largely enclave framework to nineteenth-century sanitary efforts that excluded most of the general population,[39] as well as the reluctance of many within the colonial sanitary service to abandon 'anti-contagionist' (climatist, miasmic) views of disease causation following the identification of specific microbes and their modes of transmission. Undoubtedly, a climatist theory of cholera epidemics, as Mark Harrison suggests, was convenient for the British colonial regime, 'a powerful tool against advocates of quarantine and those who pressed government to intervene more directly in public health.'[40] Yet while clearly congruent with imperial trade interests, avoidance of quarantine measures was not the only reason underlying the regime's reluctance to embrace a 'contagionist' view of epidemic disease. Miasmic theory in fact fit well with epidemiological observation in much of the Indian subcontinent. In a region where fevers (pre-eminently malarial) were manifestly associated with moisture, monsoon rainfall, and, in pernicious form, with waterlogged soils and human destitution, a focus on broader determinants beyond simply contagion was understandable. There were compelling empirical reasons, in other words, to view the leading epidemic diseases, malaria and cholera, as climate related, if the economic dimensions to climate fluctuations often went unarticulated. Empirically, germ transmission (contagion theory) could not explain epidemiological patterns of epidemic mortality on its own, even for cholera. John Snow's 1854 waterborne theory of cholera[41] was considered dangerous by many Indian Medical Service (IMS) officials not because it was wrong but because it was insufficient to explain epidemic mortality patterns observed. Contagion could explain local transmission in an outbreak, but neither the timing nor the often vast extent of the major recurring epidemics.

Nonetheless, from the mid-1880s with the development of diphtheria antitoxin, there was growing absorption with the specifics of microbe transmission, enthusiasm further heightened with confirmation of mosquitoes as vectors of diseases such as filariasis and malaria and the rapid emergence of an institutional 'tropical medicine' at the turn of the century. These were laboratory advances that appeared to hold out the promise of technical solutions to modify specific diseases, or to interrupt their transmission altogether, what Paul Ehrlich (1854–1915), who developed the first effective medicinal treatment (Salvarsan) for syphilis, would in 1906 term 'magic bullets.'[42] Inevitably perhaps, the doctrinal collision between earlier climatist theories of disease causation and a narrowly-applied germ-theory model of disease triggered increasing policy debate within the senior ranks of the Indian Medical Service.

These intra-professional tensions have been a major focus of recent South Asian public health historiographic analysis. J.C. Hume importantly points out that there were other sources of intra-professional conflict as well, with the transformation to laboratory-based medicine. Among them were deepening professional tensions arising from the Punjab administration's proposal to employ 'traditional' *hakims* as sanitary inspectors.[43] Thus the advent of scientific medicine was bringing into sharp relief an entire range of questions as to *who* provided *how much* of *what* services (preventive or curative) and for *whom* (enclave or public). The ensuing debate and dissension so prompted, Harrison has suggested, may well have allowed room for continuing equivocation on the part of the Government of India, serving to further postpone systematic public health policy.[44]

These questions were, and remain, central to analysis of South Asian colonial public health policy and practice. But the concerns they raise involve largely intra-professional issues. They fail to convey how the paradigmatic collision between pre-germ theory views and laboratory medicine played out in sanitary practice at the local level. In terms of their practical application, there was general accommodation between climatist ('anticontagionist') theories that urged drainage, and contagionist views that focused on 'germ' transmission, though the underlying etiological theory differed.[45] In the practical policy domain of water supply, for example, little contradiction existed between contagionists and climatists: a clear understanding existed of water contamination, and the need for testing water supplies for organic matter. For the miasmatist, the precise nature of the contamination (fermentative 'poisons') differed from that identified by the later microbiologists. But the actual preventive measure or *practice* was similar. This was the case as well for 'conservancy,' sewerage methods and policy. In practice, both approaches were employed in India as well, certainly in the urban context where some effort was made at improving and protecting water supply beginning from the 1880s. At the level of practice, in other words, there was less conflict than within academic halls of theoretical debate.[46]

Characterization of medical theory divisions of this period as a contest between miasmatist 'versus' germ-theory views is problematic also, however, because it overlooks the deeper 'tension' faced by the British Raj in regard to public health policy: the overarching economic (predispositionist) dimensions to epidemic patterns. Deficiencies in the effectiveness of the civilian sanitary service under the British Raj entailed more than grossly inadequate funding, differences in theoretical underpinnings, or choices of personnel 'delivering' sanitary interventions. A more fundamental problem lay in the insufficiency of both the 'contagionist' and 'climatist' disease models where the latter was increasingly reduced in the later nineteenth century to 'sanitationist' (filth) dimensions: that is, to factors external to the human host. Neither offered the measures required for a civilian population presenting a very different 'soil' than that of imperial military and administrative populations, one of widespread undernourishment and recurring famine conditions, to a large extent unmitigated.[47] In this sense, historiographic focus on coverage or funding failures of the colonial public health service arguably has left the limitations of the nineteenth-century sanitary model itself unexamined. And with it, a dominant dimension to sanitary deliberations of the period.

## 'General Sanitation': not a mere footnote

The 1911 All-India Sanitary Conference marked the moment of epistemic truce in the epidemic causality debate, historians have noted. 'No longer was there thought to be any fundamental contradiction between the aims of research scientists and those who struggled on a day-to-day basis with practical sanitation.'[48] At the level of public optics, this indeed appears to have been the case. Yet the differences resolved at the Sanitary conference in November 1911 did not lie primarily between contagionist (germ-theory) and narrowly defined miasmatist views. What was being acknowledged in the meeting's Presidential address, and to a limited degree resolved, was a broader economic content to the term 'practical sanitation.'[49] Only weeks before, Christophers's report, 'Malaria in the Punjab,' had finally been tabled.[50] In the wake of its official release, the accommodation arrived at in Bombay involved a re-insertion of the 'Human Factor' (destitution) into the epidemic equation. Tucked within the conference president's linguistic envelope of 'practical sanitation' was acknowledgement of the central importance of agricultural productivity and prosperity. In the case of Punjab this was pre-eminently a matter of adequate surface drainage, as in the case of the Jumna canal realignment; elsewhere, such as deltaic Bengal, restoration of inundation irrigation flows. But nor was surface or inundation 'drainage' the only economic action authorities had in mind at this point in relation to agricultural improvement. 'Practical sanitation' also encompassed fundamental changes in famine relief and foodgrain price policy, changes in economic policy that would pre-empt mass destitution ('famine') and associated fulminant malaria conditions and begin to stem the recurring loss of human and agricultural capital out of the rural economy triggered by recurring famines.[51]

What the 1911 epistemic compromise represented in effect was a reinsertion of a broader 'climatist' perspective into epidemic causality, one where climate was understood in terms of its specific subsistence consequences: harvests, livelihood, and staple foodgrain access (prices). Christophers's spatial mapping of 1908 malaria epidemic mortality had confirmed what already was suggested by the clinical and class profile of epidemic malaria mortality: such patterns could not be understood merely on the basis of malaria transmission. The broad geographic pattern to malaria epidemicity distinguished the phenomenon from contagion alone, calling to mind instead earlier 'zymotic' dimensions of fever epidemics, the nineteenth-century European term employed to convey posited atmospheric conditions conducive to fermentation as the causal agency at play. Christophers in subsequent writing would alter the term to emphasize the specific economic dimensions to the spatial mortality pattern, coining the neologism 'zymonic' for the purpose.

> The word epidemic, applied as it is to outbreaks of disease on a small scale, does not sufficiently characterise such vast exhibitions of the power of zymotic disease, and I propose to call such phenomena *zymonic* from their likeness in distribution to cyclonic disturbances in the atmosphere.'[52]

As in his earlier 'Malaria in the Punjab' analysis, Christophers would refer to the economic nature of that different causal agent with concerted delicacy: in this instance, adding a single key sentence: 'Almost coming under the phase of zymones, were the famines that once decimated tracts in India'; then adding that '[f]ortunately these no longer figure on our list as direct causes of mortality.'[53] Significantly, he also went on to suggest that 'epidemics of this magnitude . . . [were] by no means confined to malaria.'

> Immense cholera epidemics have been of frequent occurrence. They are ascribed to infection carried by pilgrims returning from the pilgrim *melas* . . . but there must be something more at the back of them than the *mere fact of such dissemination*, some condition peculiarly favourable to the spread of cholera in such years.[54]

Here Christophers was bringing the microbiologic (contagionist) and predispositionist understandings together, under the rubric of 'general sanitation,' the term he had used in his 1909 'Human Factor' paper to refer to measures that addressed human destitution.[55]

Part of the historiographical difficulty in interpreting theoretical debate and policy developments taking place in British India in this period, one can suggest, lies with the level of abstraction in colonial officials' use of the term 'general sanitation.' Hidden within the term could be almost any economic measure. As with the nineteenth-century Jumna canal realignment, it included drainage (waterlogging remediation) in which the paramount effect was understood as economic. After 1908, 'sanitary' measures also extended to flood-, drought-, and price-relief, and in time more systematic 'bonification' measures in Punjab in the form of surface water drainage.[56] In his 1917 report on malaria in Amritsar, C.A. Gill explicitly employed the term 'General Sanitation' in referring to measures directed to ameliorating those conditions that tend 'to bring about repeated relapses . . . [such as] poor and insufficient food, bad housing, excessive exposure to climatic conditions.' 'All measures,' he continued, 'which promote the well-being of the people and their powers of resistance to disease come indirectly within the scope of anti-malarial measures.'[57]

Certainly for Christophers, his use of the term was as code for alleviating destitution. Repeatedly in his published writing he employed the term 'general sanitary reforms' in circumstances where the sole meaning could only be economic. Thus he concluded the 1911 Punjab inquiry urging that 'the immediate removal or prevention of flood water, *should be the first step in the sanitation of a rural tract*,'[58] where the economic consequences of flood conditions had been vividly articulated at the Simla malaria conference two years earlier.[59] To subsequent analysts, however, this larger content to the term could easily be missed.[60]

In other words, the 'compromise' reached among top officials in the Indian Medical Service in December 1911 was not a mere footnote to the competing medical theory debates and professional discord of the period. Instead it involved acknowledgement of the primacy of hunger in the public health burden of malaria in India, an issue that lay at the core of the epistemic contest within the sanitary administration at this point, and which was the pivot around which subsequent colonial public health policy, and arguably the region's health history, revolved. Yet if the 'fundamental contradiction' between public health figures seemingly was resolved in formal declarations in 1911, deep dissension remained among individual members of the Indian Medical Service regarding disease theory and policy approaches,[61] and views of the sanitarian's task, as will be considered in chapter five. But first we consider how the late nineteenth-century 'collision' of disease theories played out in the practical experience of sanitary officers working 'in the field,' a rather different story from that taking place at the level of academic debate.

## Epidemic causation: view from the field

All three perspectives on epidemic causality – contagion, climate, and predisposition (destitution) – are evident in the early sanitary records of Punjab province, as are tensions arising in relation to them as succeeding provincial sanitary commissioners responded to recurring epidemics and the dramatic microbiologic developments of the later nineteenth century. Thus in addition to their important quantitative data, the annual sanitary reports offer a vivid portrait of the response at the local level to the epistemological shifts in health understanding taking place with the emergence of a germ-theory-based medicine and sanitary practice, and correspondingly the vicissitudes of predisposition as a concept within public health thought.

Debate over epidemic causation was most acute in relation to cholera, the disease of paramount concern to the British Raj in much of the nineteenth century for its effects on imperial trade and the ever-present threat of international quarantines. By virtue of geography, cholera was of additional concern for the Punjab administration, the eastern portion of the province having been the site where cholera had, for a period, compromised British efforts to regain military control during the 1857–1858 Indian Rebellion. But as well, major Indian army cantonments were located in the province which bordered the northwest frontier region where military campaigns in Afghanistan continued through the remainder of the nineteenth century. Thus cholera statistics and theoretical discussion of cholera causation loom large in the provincial records, far overshadowing those for fever (primarily malaria). In this context, it is hardly surprising that the first provincial sanitary commissioner for Punjab would be an IMS officer ardently committed to developing protected water supply systems.

Over the course of his 1867–1875 tenure, A.C.C. DeRenzy would become increasingly adamant in urging modern water-supply infrastructure for the province, arguing that even 'covered wells were a hazard.'[62] At the central level, in contrast, the post of Sanitary Commissioner to the Government of India was filled by a 'climatist,' J.M. Cuningham, whose reluctance to embrace a contagionist view of cholera would trigger increasing criticism from more junior members of the sanitary service. Most prominent among them was DeRenzy, whose ridicule of Cuningham's 'anti-contagionist' views in the pages of the *Lancet* ultimately led in 1875 to the former's transfer to a less prestigious posting in Assam.[63]

Emphasis on cholera continued, however, under DeRenzy's successor, H.W. Bellew. Fifty-one pages of the 1879 Punjab sanitary report, a year of famine in the province, were devoted not to fever mortality, which was enormous, but to cholera. Unlike DeRenzy however, Bellew's views of cholera etiology were distinctly climatist, directed more to 'conditions of the climate' and of the soil in explaining patterns of the disease.[64] Moreover, Bellew's attention would increasingly turn to the very much greater mortality burden being recorded under the category of fever deaths, in his 1882 report describing fever as 'the most deadly and most baneful disease which we have to contend against in this Province.' Here, too, his perspective was climatist, noting that severe epidemics occurred 'when seasons of unusual drought are followed by copious rainfall,' a view that broadened in time to encompass 'defect[s] in food supply' and 'unusual exposure to fatigue [and] privations.'[65] In this, Bellew had the support of leading medical figures such as Joseph Fayrer, Surgeon-General and President of the India Office Medical Board, who continued to advocate a broader epidemiological and 'natural history' approach to understanding epidemic behaviour in the subcontinent.[66] As to remedial measures, however, Bellew's recommendations took an increasingly moralistic tone, urging villagers to adopt domestic cleanliness, to wear clothing 'appropriate to the climate' and to heat their homes through the night to avoid chills and sickness, admonishments that revealed a level of behaviouralist naïveté that in time became difficult even for his superiors to ignore.[67]

It was in the middle of Bellew's 1875–1885 tenure that the malaria plasmodium was identified by Alphonse Laveran. Two years later in 1882, Robert Koch identified the tuberculosis bacillus, and the following year, the cholera vibrio. Already, however, the colonial government was itself beginning to shift its 'climatist' views to accommodate the new microbiologic research, inaugurating in 1880 the first scientific medical journal, *Scientific Memoirs by Medical Officers of the Army of India*. Five years later Cuningham was replaced as Sanitary Commissioner with the Government of India by Surgeon-General B. Simpson, an ardent proponent of the new laboratory medicine. That same year in Punjab, Bellew would be succeeded by A. Stephen as provincial sanitary commissioner.

Stephen brought a much more rigorous analytic approach to his observations of epidemic mortality, in the case of cholera initiating a detailed system of mapping outbreaks and mortality across the province. Like his predecessor, he also drew attention to the inordinately greater mortality recorded under the category of fever, calculating fever deaths in 1887 to be 51 times greater than cholera mortality; in 1889, 54 times greater than smallpox deaths and 151 times greater than cholera.[68] Like Bellew, Stephen saw climatic conditions of rainfall and waterlogging as prime determinants of local health conditions. But in his concern with locality and soils, Stephen gave greater emphasis to the economic consequences of waterlogging on autumnal fever mortality, pointing increasingly to rail, road, and canal embankments as directly contributing to the problem.[69]

Under the more sympathetic vice-regency of Lord Dufferin (1884–1888), Sanitary Boards were established in 1888 in each province and Stephen enthusiastically oversaw beginning efforts at improving rural drainage, supervising district-level surveys of areas where surface drainage was blocked by infrastructure embankments. At the March 1891 Sanitary Board meeting, he urged that '[e]fficient drainage [was] the only effectual means of preventing outbreaks of malarial fevers and their sequellae.'[70] Deputy Commissioners were instructed to

> report on all areas . . . in which drainage has been intercepted by railways, canals or other works carried out by Government. . . . Projects for the drainage of water-logged areas should be undertaken, and sufficient water-way should always be provided when embankments are raised in constructing railways, canals, and roads.[71]

At the same time, he took direct aim at the administration of the canal irrigation system, highlighting the 'evil effect on health of excessive irrigation by canal water.'

> [U]nless special precautions are undertaken canals are not an unmixed good. When canal water is allowed to flow over an almost level country, unless arrangements are made to get rid of the surplus, the subsoil gradually becomes water-logged, and malarial fevers with enlargement of spleen become very prevalent.[72]

But along with drainage operations, Stephen also stressed the need for immediate relief for flood-paralyzed villages:

> [W]hile the country remains liable to such floods . . . sickness and mortality will be excessive, and . . . the inhabitants will certainly undergo physical deterioration *unless they are speedily relieved.* . . . Were those suffering from malarial fevers among the general population as carefully treated, fed and nursed as fever patients in Jails and in the Native Army, the mortality from these causes would be very much smaller than it is.[73]

Though no doubt aware at this point of the malaria plasmodium, he continued to advance the 'classical' hygienic measures of surface drainage works, and to articulate the pre-sanitationist distinction between triggering factors in malaria epidemics and underlying factors. In his 1887 report he quoted affirmatively a district-level Civil Surgeon's assessment of the severe epidemic conditions that autumn who had described 'the predisposing cause [of the 1887 epidemic] as debility produced by scarcity of food and the exciting cause as waterlogging of sub-soil from excessive rainfall and floods.'[74]

By the mid-1890s, however, drainage efforts by the provincial Irrigation Department appear to have stalled over financing disputes between central and local levels of government,[75] an impasse perhaps reflecting a change in viceregal leadership. In the meantime, major famines in the final years of the nineteenth century and the outbreak of plague in 1897 further diverted attention and funds from surface drainage. Few accounts of major flood control projects appear in the annual sanitary reports after 1895, until the 1920s.

Nonetheless, while Stephen was the first provincial sanitary official to openly question the unalloyed benefits of canal irrigation, his annual reports were surprisingly silent regarding the effects of soaring grain exports out of the province – export earnings upon which the fiscal foundation of the British Raj rested. It would be Land Revenue administration officials, rather than members of the Sanitary Department, who in published form warned of the effects of the booming export trade on public health. Certainly, Stephen was aware of the severity of these epidemics, pointing to 1890 as the first year on record that deaths in the province exceeded births, in that year by 11.3 per mille, and acknowledging the effect of the high prices in 'reducing the physical powers' of the population. But elsewhere he would downplay the recurring grain-price crises that marked his tenure, giving little hint of the extraordinary shifts in food security taking place.[76] '[N]o *real* scarcity,' existed in 1890, he reported, 'and the health of the people was probably not appreciably affected by the slight [price] rise.'[77] Blocked surface drainage was considered to be remediable, but price behaviour apparently was not. To the extent that he addressed the social distribution of mortality in the province, attention was directed not to class differentials which were large, but to politically safer differences among the major religious groups and increasingly to sex differentials in infant mortality.[78]

It was under the 1894–1897 tenure of Stephen's successor, W.A. Roe, a microbiologist, that public health analysis would veer sharply to a reductive framework. With 1895 rainfall 'considerably below the average,' Roe concluded that 'meteorological conditions were more favourable to health.' The offending cause of fever mortality was now reduced to 'moisture,' and its absence equated to 'health.'[79] Roe's tenure as Punjab Sanitary Commissioner predated Ross's confirmation of the role of mosquitoes in malaria transmission, yet already understanding of 'health' had come to be reduced to the 'exciting' or triggering factor in fulminant malaria: monsoon rainfall levels.

The narrowness of Roe's logic was too much, it seems, even for the British Raj to ignore. A GOI directive in early 1896 prodded provincial sanitary officials to be 'considering, as far as may be possible, the influence of weather and food prices on the death rate.'[80] Yet conditions following a second year of drought in 1896 would again be described by Roe as 'remarkably dry and very healthy.'[81] Absent was any hint of the economic livelihood effects of two consecutive years of drought. Indeed, the famine year of 1897 would be described as 'on the whole a healthy one,' on the basis it seems that though the monsoon rains had returned, they were slightly below average levels.[82] Yet 1897 mortality rates in the province had risen by 50 per cent against the previous decade average, itself a level already elevated by a series of major price-related epidemics in the late 1880s and early 1890s.[83] In his annual report for that year Roe limited his narrative remarks to one-third of a page, with no reference to the autumn malaria epidemic in the southeastern region of the province.

The equating of 'health' in the province to below-normal rainfall continued under Roe's successor, C. J. Bamber, the latter perhaps concerned lest he court ridicule by adhering to 'old school' miasmatist theories of epidemic disease in the wake of Ronald Ross's confirmation in 1897 of the vector role of mosquitoes in malaria transmission. Though monsoon rainfall in 1899 stood at record low levels, Bamber's annual sanitary report for the year contained no hint of the broader consequences of extreme drought once again afflicting the countryside. Indeed, for the first time since initiation of vital registration reporting in the province in 1867, no foodgrain price data were included in the annual report, though the province was plunging headlong into 'the great famine' of the century. In its aftermath Bamber acknowledged that the province had suffered severely, but even here his admission was remarkably sanguine. '[G]eneral scarcity and dearness of food,' he concluded, 'does not appear to have affected the health of the population to any material extent, except in Hissár and Karnal districts, where insufficient and unwholesome food helped to raise the death-rate by decreasing the power of the people to resist disease.' In fact, crude death rates had risen to over double non-famine levels in the majority of the province's 24 plains districts, much of the mortality occurring at the close of the famine with return of normal monsoon rains and malaria transmission in their wake. In three districts, 1900 mortality rates had tripled, with one-tenth of the entire population succumbing. 'With the exception of a few districts,' Bamber observed in a seemingly reassuring tone, 'the dearness of food did not lead to a demand for higher wages. On the other hand, . . . labourers and artisans . . . [were] found willing to work for lower wages owing to increased competition from famine.'[84]

One is tempted to interpret the reluctance of sanitary officials to discuss the health implications of harvest failure as stemming from official pressures to avoid the politically sensitive issue of starvation deaths. Certainly, the highest echelons of the administration a decade earlier had concertedly discouraged criticism of grain exports and their impact on price levels.[85] Yet by the late 1890s the Government of India itself was urging provincial sanitary officials to consider economic conditions in their annual reporting. In the wake of the 1900 famine, the GOI issued another directive, this time insisting on more details than casual rote data on harvests, foodgrain prices, and wage levels.[86] Mention of meteorological, crop, and foodgrain price conditions would re-appear in the Punjab sanitary report in 1903. But the subsequent year's report contained no information on harvests, though rainfall and humidity conditions received several pages' commentary. 'Fortunately,' the sanitary commissioner again concluded, 'the rainfall in 1904 was below the normal and this accounts for the moderate death rate recorded from fevers.'[87]

A similar reading of drought as good fortune due to reduced malaria transmission would appear in somewhat different form that same year with the decision to eliminate all irrigation channels at the rural military cantonment at Mian Mir (Lahore) and environs in pursuit of anopheles extirpation, a policy that reduced the area to its former near-desert state.[88] In the meantime, initial trials of mosquito destruction had been initiated in municipal areas of several Punjab districts in 1903.[89]

## Reductionism respite

Marked reluctance on the part of Punjab sanitary officials to address economic conditions at the turn of the twentieth century would be broken three years later by Bamber's successor. Despite preoccupation with plague mortality that continued to soar in the province, Major E. Wilkinson in his 1907 provincial sanitary report pointed with alarm also to poor monsoon rains, 'short crops,' and rising prices.[90] A year later in the aftermath of the disastrous 1908 fever epidemic, malaria lethality would be linked explicitly to prevailing scarcity and harvest failure along with widespread destruction and economic paralysis triggered by flooding.[91] The 1908 sanitary report went further, pointing to the epidemics of 1892 and 1900 as similar examples of the association of malaria mortality with conditions of 'scarcity' (famine-level prices). Three years later in 1911 the centrality of food security to mortality in the province would formally be acknowledged with official publication of Christophers's 'Malaria in the Punjab' report. Much, of course, had transpired in the preceding two-decade interval – including publication of the 1901 Famine Commission Report in which starvation unambiguously was named as the key agent transforming endemic malaria in the country into its disastrously lethal epidemic form.[92] Deputed to conduct an enquiry into the 1908 Punjab malaria epidemic, Christophers had begun by seeking out the experience of earlier provincial sanitary commissioners. From the annual reports of Bellew and Stephen he would have come across their graphs of annual fever mortality and rainfall data painstakingly and cumulatively charted year by year. Impressed, it seems, by Stephen's mapping of cholera mortality during his tenure, Christophers employed similar techniques to delineate 1908 autumn malaria mortality across the province, using what appears to be the same district- and *thana*-level maps.[93] He then went on to devise statistical techniques to quantify the relationship between rainfall and prices on malaria mortality, stimulated perhaps by this earlier work.

Beginning in 1908, the annual provincial sanitary reports would include more detailed reviews of monsoon and harvests conditions, in addition to price and wage trends, as economic preamble. And for the remainder of the colonial period two voices, one microbiologic, the other overtly economic, would frame analysis contained in the annual reports.[94] The 1927 provincial report, for example, highlighted 'the profound influence upon the state of the public health [of] . . . meteorological conditions, and more particularly abnormal seasons . . . where health and to a large extent prosperity, is a gamble in rain.'[95] The following year the Public Health Commissioner with the Government of India prefaced his own annual report with seven pages detailing all-India rainfall, agricultural, and economic conditions.[96] And in the early days of the global Depression, the Punjab Director of Public Health (formerly provincial 'Sanitary Commissioner') described infant mortality rates as 'a delicate test of economic stress.'[97] Six years later the 1937 annual report for the GOI advised that 'public health cannot be regarded as an entity distinct from the general, social and economic life of the community,' and called for

> further legislation which will undoubtedly have far-reaching effects on the economic life and general well-being of the people. Agricultural indebtedness, land tenure and industrial problems, to cite a few examples, are all receiving serious attention and . . . mention is made of these wider aspects of community life in order to emphasise the necessity of viewing health problems from the widest possible angle.[98]

It was of course this 'widest possible angle' that had been sought in the enquiry into the 1908 Punjab malaria epidemic almost three decades earlier, and cogently argued in the 1922 pages of the *Indian Medical Gazette*.[99] In other words, whatever theoretical disagreement had existed at the academic level at the turn of the twentieth century regarding epidemic disease causation, little gulf remained in the 1910s and early 1920s at the level of the public health administration between the microbiological dimensions of disease transmission and economic determinants of disease lethality. If public health officials could do little in the way of directly addressing these key economic conditions, their advocacy in this regard nonetheless had become prominent and unambiguous.

131

## A different kind of tension

Yet despite the seeming accommodation of the two perspectives – economic and microbiological – a tension of another kind permeated the pages of the Punjab public health reports through the final decades of colonial rule. From the mid-1920s on, one can trace a sense of growing professional frustration with the limited level of funding made available, in practice, for surface drainage and flood control, and the limits to then-standard public health technical interventions.[100] Quinine distribution efforts were 'merely palliative,' W.H.C. Forster lamented in his 1923 public health report, urging that 'schemes for land drainage must be regarded as the most effective method of mitigating or preventing the occurrence of these disastrous epidemics.'[101] Further fiscal retrenchment in the early 1920s prompted Gill, appointed the following year as officiating Punjab Public Health director, to utter the ultimate sanitationist blasphemy: that rural surface drainage schemes were a far greater priority than conservancy work (sewage disposal) and drainage inside rural villages.

> [T]he execution of water supply and drainage projects in small villages is not a sound proposition from the economic point of view, nor . . . [of] urgent importance from the view of public health. Here land drainage schemes designated to prevent floods . . . are peculiarly calculated to benefit the rural population.[102]

Such questioning of prevailing 'germ-intervention' orthodoxy would be voiced even more openly a decade later, the Public Health Commissioner for the GOI openly contesting exclusive attention to many standard public health measures:

> Abundant supplies of quinine, and the multiplication of tuberculosis hospitals, sanatoria, leprosy colonies, and maternity and child welfare centres are no doubt desirable, if not essential, but none of these go to the root of the matter. The first essentials for the prevention of disease are a higher standard of health, a better physique, and a greater power of resistance to infection.[103]

This hardly amounted to a rejection of specific public health 'interventions,' but rather acknowledgement of their deep insufficiency.

As additional context to this growing frustration within the public health service was the ever-expanding number of preventive techniques becoming available, and corresponding work demands placed on staff. Through the final years of the nineteenth century, the new laboratory-based medicine presented ever more avenues for micro-'intervention' measures: techniques for containment of disease transmission, or in the case of cholera and plague, vaccines for inducing specific immunity. Most were poorly tested and many would later be considered to be of questionable efficacy.[104] Even before the outbreak of plague in 1896, the demands on provincial public health staff already were enormous. Provincial sanitary commissioners were expected to be constantly on tour (until the 1930s, still largely non-motorized) across a province of over 100,000 square miles of territory, in 50,000 scattered villages, inspecting the sanitary condition of the country and investigating both village and urban outbreaks of cholera, fever (malaria), and a growing number of diseases identified as important such as typhus and relapsing fever in the hill regions, in addition to plague from the final years of the nineteenth century. Touring was in addition to statistical reporting responsibilities. These duties – identifying plague and cholera cases, 'extirpating' rats, then mosquitoes and intestinal hookworms – Forster would describe in 1924 as 'exceptionally onerous.'[105] In the face of continuing outbreaks of plague in the province through the 1910s and 1920s, it is hardly surprising that sanitary officials 'on the front lines' were desperate for certitude, and simultaneously lured to, and frustrated by, promises of simple fixes. In the deluge, the central historical question of what turned endemic 'common' infections into highly lethal pestilential epidemics would quietly recede into the background.

For others, the mounting preventive and containment duties were seen increasingly as obscuring and pre-empting attention to the economic issues underlying epidemic conditions. In his 1924 public health report, Gill would quote a recent statement by Sir George Newman, Chief Medical Officer of the British Ministry of Health, that 'summarised the relationship of preventive medicine to the body politic':

> Public Health is purchasable, but only in the long run, and only on a true understanding of scientific facts. Merely to send post-haste a Medical Inspector to visit on a preventive mission an area suffering from an acute and exceptional prevalence of disease is to shut the stable door when the horse has escaped, . . . It is neither State-craft nor science. . . . In public health work this means *sanitation*, nutrition, the establishment of immunity, and what Dr John Simon called 'the necessaries of health. . . . [I]t must be said quite plainly that the prompt attack . . . to chlorinate the water, disinfect the drains, boil the milk, provide a temporary hospital, or get vaccinated . . . has become so insistent, central and locally, that its tendency has been to absorb attention. . . . What is needed for the health of a community is that which is needed for the health of an individual, a wholesome and resistent [sic] constitution.[106]

Perhaps the greatest frustration for public health officials in British India of this period stemmed from being professionally sidelined from such broader economic policies. As late as 1927, Gill ruefully recorded that '[t]he Public Health Department is not directly in touch with the Water-logging Committee' regarding the several land drainage schemes undertaken during the year.[107] In Punjab few details of either drought or flood relief measures, military food lifts, or surface drainage operations appear in the annual public health records.[108] That information, as in the 1890s, was published primarily in the Land Revenue Administration records because it was land revenue officials who were responsible for most relief activities at district level. Clearly, this jurisdictional separation of economic measures from public health duties was a source of intense personal frustration on the part of provincial public health officials like Gill and Forster, seen as reinforcing the reductive trajectory of public health as a discipline.

But there was yet another source for disquiet on the part of public health officials in the immediate post-war period, one that came from within the medical professional itself. Despite concerted efforts at reconciliation at the 1911 Sanitary conference in Bombay, the dispute that had erupted at the Medical Congress in the same city two years earlier between malaria 'eradicationists' (vector sanitation) and 'ameliorationists' ('quininists') had not in fact receded. The 1914 *Indian Sanitary Policy* Resolution[109] had given formal recognition to anti-mosquito strategies in malaria control policy. But vector extirpation programs had not been pursued beyond trial projects in urban settings such as Saharanpur. Aspirations for anti-mosquito programs on the part of proponents of 'vector sanitation' thus had not been satiated. As we will consider in chapter five, advocates of mosquito extirpation were increasingly turning to more inflated arguments for action on malaria transmission control, the disease now framed as a primary 'block' to economic development in the subcontinent,[110] what in contemporary public health analysis has come to be referred to as the malaria-blocks-development (MBD) thesis.[111] And in this they would be joined by prominent medical luminaries such as William Osler who had recently come to describe malaria as 'the greatest single destroyer of the human race.'[112]

Such was the force of this advocacy that Forster as Punjab Sanitary (Public Health) Commissioner felt compelled in 1921 to dispute publicly in the pages of his annual report the surging rhetoric that attributed the subcontinent's economic stagnation to malaria. 'I am not one of those,' he wrote, referring evidently to W.H.S. Jones's recent text, *Malaria: A Neglected Factor in the History of Greece and Rome*,[113]

> who believes that malaria, *qua* malaria, is capable of extinguishing an Empire. Remove the stimulus of gain, then malaria might quite well do what is claimed of it, but the stimulus must first be removed. . . . [Regarding] the unhealthiness of Gurgaon [district], the fundamental cause . . . is loss of the economic stimulus. The soil

is poor, the water saline, and the agricultural conditions generally unfavourable. . . . the "Bunds" [have] ceased to function.[114]

Four years later, Forster would even more pointedly 'repudiate the doctrine that malaria *per se* is capable of destroying empires.'[115]

But the impetus for a narrowed and unidirectional reading of malaria as the cause of the subcontinent's poverty was now coming from a different direction, one even more powerful perhaps than the personal advocacy of Ross: that of fiscal retrenchment. Deep budgetary cutbacks were fanning aspirations among public health workers for sources of alternate funding from beyond India's shores, creating an opening for the involvement of private philanthropic institutions where momentum was fast growing for the inverted doctrine of malaria as a cause of global underdevelopment.

## Notes

1 Foucauldian analysis has explored consequences of late- and post-eighteenth-century state engagement with health, disease, and medical care in relation to institutional and political powers of social control; M. Foucault, and C. Gordon, *Power/Knowledge: Selected Interviews and Other Writings, 1972–1977* (Brighton: Harvester Press, 1980). A further dimension to public 'control' related to food and hunger, and societal norms and obligations regarding human destitution, though less directly addressed in analysis of shifts in socio-political power resulting from the sanitationist redefinition of illness and disease. On this, see D. Smith, and M. Nicolson, 'Nutrition, Education, Ignorance and Income: A Twentieth-Century Debate,' in H. Kamminga, and A. Cunningham, eds., *The Science and Culture of Nutrition, 1840–1940* (Amsterdam: Rodopi, 1995), 288–318.

2 D. Brunton, Review of C. Hamlin, 'Public Health and Social Justice,' *Journal of the Society of the Social History of Medicine*, 13, 1, Apr. 2000, 173–174.

3 C. Hamlin, *Public Health and Social Justice in the Age of Chadwick* (Cambridge: Cambridge University Press, 1998); C. Hamlin, 'William Pulteney Alison, the Scottish Philosophy, and the Making of a Political Medicine,' *Journal of the History of Medicine and Allied Sciences*, 62, 2, 2006, 144–186. See also D. Porter, *Health, Civilization and the State: A History of Public Health from Ancient to Modern Times* (London: Routledge, 1999), 86; M.W. Flinn, 'Introduction,' *Report on the Sanitary Condition of the Labouring Population of Gt. Britain* (Edinburgh: Edinburgh University Press, 1965), at 63–64.

4 Typhus is caused by a rickettsial bacterium (*R. prowazekii*) transmitted inadvertently by the human louse, and endemically present historically in temperate region populations, characteristically taking epidemic form under conditions of destitution, related crowding, and incapacity for elemental hygiene, variously termed famine fever, goal distemper (neurological symptoms), ship or camp fever. Following initial infection, latent organisms can reactivate years later under conditions of physical stress and immune suppression. In 1934 Zinsser correctly hypothesized that Brill's disease was a recrudescent form of typhus, a view confirmed in the 1950s, the disease renamed Brill-Zinsser disease; V.A. Harden, 'Typhus, Epidemic,' in K.F. Kiple, ed., *Cambridge World History of Disease* (Cambridge: Cambridge University Press, 1993), 1080–1084.

5 For an insightful overview of 'pre-germ theory' predispositionist understanding of 'infectious' and epidemic disease, and its demise under nineteenth-century 'sanitationism,' see C. Hamlin, 'Predisposing Causes and Public Health in Early Nineteenth-Century Medical Thought,' *Society for the Social History of Medicine*, 5, 1, Apr. 1992, 43–70; J.V. Pickstone, 'Death, Dirt and Fever Epidemics: Rewriting the History of British "Public Health", 1780–1850,' in T. Ranger, and P. Slack, eds., *Epidemics and Ideas: Essays on the Historical Perception of Pestilence* (Cambridge: Cambridge University Press, 1992), 125–148.

6 Johann Peter Frank, *Academic Address on The People's Misery: Mother of Diseases,* An Address, delivered May 5, 1790 at the University of Pavia. Translated from the Latin, with an Introduction by H.E. Sigerist, *Bulletin of the History of Medicine*, 9, 1941, 81–100, at 98.

7 For an overview of Virchow's analysis, see R. Taylor, and A. Rieger, 'Rudolf Virchow on the Typhus Epidemic in Upper Silesia: An Introduction and Translation,' *Sociology of Health and Illness*, 6, 2, 1984, 201–217; G. Rosen, 'What is Social Medicine?,' *Bulletin of the History of Medicine*, 21, 1947, 674–685.

8 W.P. Alison, *Observations on the Management of the Poor in Scotland, and Its Effects on the Health of Great Towns*, 2nd ed. (Edinburgh: Blackwood, 1840), 10–11; R.B. Howard, 'On the Prevalence of Diseases Arising from Contagion, Malaria, and Certain Other Physical Causes amongst the Labouring Classes in Manchester,' in *Sanitary Condition of the Labouring Population of Great Britain. Local Reports for England and Wales, Parliamentary Papers* (House of Lords, 1842), 317, as cited in Hamlin, *Public Health and Social Justice*, 197. See also Hamlin, '*Public Health and Social Justice*, 54–61, 188–201; Hamlin, 'Predisposing Causes and Public Health,' 43–70.

9 M. Pelling, *Cholera, Fever and English Medicine 1825–1865* (Oxford: Oxford University Press, 1978), 30–31.

10 Hamlin, *Public Health and Social Justice*, 101–102.

11 M. Worboys, *Spreading Germs: Disease Theories and Medical Practice in Britain* (Cambridge: Cambridge University Press, 2000), 39–42; Hamlin, 'Predisposing Causes'; M. Harrison, *Public Health in British India: Anglo-Indian Preventive Medicine 1859–1914* (Cambridge: Cambridge University Press, 1994), 52.

12 C. Hamlin, 'Could You Starve to Death in England in 1839? The Chadwick-Farr Controversy and the Loss of the "Social" in Public Health,' *American Journal of Public Health*, 85, 6, Jun.1995, 856–66 at 859; Worboys, *Spreading Germs*, 5.

13 A. Hardy, *The Epidemic Streets: Infectious Disease and the Rise of Preventive Medicine, 1856–1900* (Oxford: Clarendon Press, 1993), 1. John Duffy suggests that in the urban United States the germ theory 'awakened the upper classes to the realization that bacteria were no respecters of economic or social position,' giving impetus to both public health and antipoverty programs; 'Social Impact of Disease in the Late Nineteenth Century,' *Bulletin of the New York Academy of Medicine*, 47, 1971, 797–811, at 809.

14 S. Szreter, 'Rapid Economic Growth and "the Four Ds" of Disruption, Deprivation, Disease and Death,' *Tropical Medicine and International Health*, 4, 2, Feb. 1999, 146–152, at 148. Hamlin traces shifting notions of social obligation through the eighteenth and early nineteenth century; 'State Medicine in Great Britain,' in D. Arnold, ed., *Warm Climates in Western Medicine: The Emergence of Tropical Medicine, 1500–1900* (Amsterdam: Rodopi, 1996), 132–164. Douglas Hay describes the British State's judicial abandonment of prohibitions on 'engrossing and forestalling' at the turn of the nineteenth century and thus any normative role in food security; 'The State and the Market: Lord Kenyon and Mr Waddington,' *Past and Present*, 162, Feb. 1999, 101–162.

15 Alison, *Observations on the Management of the Poor*, 10–11; W.P. Alison, *Observations on the Famine of 1846–7 in the Highlands of Scotland or Ireland* (Edinburgh: Blackwood & Sons, 1847). For a detailed account of Alison's work, see Hamlin, 'William Pulteney Alison.'

16 Hamlin, *Public Health and Social Justice*, 153–154. None of the testimony by the Manchester Poor Law medical officer, R.B. Howard, on the powerful role of poverty and destitution in typhus epidemicity appeared in the 1842 *Sanitary Report*; 'On the Prevalence of Diseases Arising from Contagion,' 317, as cited in Hamlin, *Public Health and Social Justice*,197.

17 See above, note 4.

18 The HIV-AIDS virus is anomalous historically speaking in targeting directly the immune system itself; and in turn, exceptional in its potential to undermine economies directly, in particular low-income populations where there are as yet limited social support and public health networks.

19 Worboys, *Spreading Germs*, 6, 278–289.

20 I. Galdston, 'Humanism and Public Health,' *Bulletin of the History of Medicine*, 8, Jan. 1940, 1032–1039.

21 Hamlin, 'Could You Starve to Death in England?'

22 J.C. Hume, 'Colonialism and Sanitary Medicine: The Development of Preventive Health Policy in the Punjab, 1860 to 1900,' *Modern Asian Studies*, 20, 4, 1986, 703–724; S. Watts, 'British Development Policies and Malaria in India 1897-c.1929,' *Past and Present*, 165, 1999, 141–181.

23 M. Harrison, *Climates and Constitutions: Health, Race, Environment and British Imperialism in India, 1600–1850* (New Delhi: Oxford University Press, 1999), 170–177.

24 M. Worboys, 'Germs, Malaria and the Invention of Mansonian Tropical Medicine: From "Diseases in the Tropics" to "Tropical Disease",' in David Arnold, ed., *Warm Climates in Western Medicine*, 196.

25 W.E. Baker, T.E. Dempster, and H. Yule, *The Prevalence of Organic Disease of the Spleen as a Test for Detecting Malarious Locality in Hot Climates* (Calcutta: Govt. Printing, 1848), reprinted in *Records of the Malaria Survey of India*, 1, 2, Mar. 1930, 69–85 [hereafter, *RMSI*]; W.E. Baker, T.E. Dempster, and H. Yule, 'Report of a committee assembled to report on the causes of the unhealthiness which has existed at Kurnaul, and other portions of the country along the lane of the Delhie canal, with Appendices on Malaria by Surgeon T.E. Dempster,' 1847; reprinted in *RMSI*, 1, 2, Mar. 1930, 1–68. On this, see S. Zurbrigg, *Epidemic Malaria and Hunger in Colonial Punjab: 'Weakened by Want'* (London and New Delhi: Routledge, 2019), ch. 7.

26 *Report of the Commissioners Appointed to Inquire into the Sanitary State of the Army in India, Parliamentary Papers* (London: HMSO, 1863), vol. I, 58 [emphasis added]. See also, E.A. Parkes, *A Manual of Practical Hygiene, Prepared Especially for Use in the Medical Service of the Army* (London: John Churchill, 1866), as cited in Harrison, *Public Health in British India*, 52. In her overview of the development of imperial sanitary policy in British India, Ramasubban notes it was 'well-known' early on that 'intensity and frequency of disease' in the army depended upon the health of surrounding populations; 'Imperial Health British India, 1857–1900,' in R. MacLeod, and M. Lewis, *Disease, Medicine and Empire* (London: Routledge, 1988), 38–60, at 40.

27 Parkes, *Manual of Practical Hygiene, 52.*

28 In the latter case, debility also was addressed simply through discharge from the army.

29 Parkes, *Manual of Practical Hygiene, 444–45* [emphasis added].

30  Ramasubban, 'Imperial Health British India, 1857–1900,' 41. Arnold notes that annual death rates among both British and Indian troops in the 1860s were cut in half by the late 1880s, to approximately 15 per 1,000, and reduced further to 4.4 deaths per 1,000 by 1914; *Colonizing the Body: State Medicine and Epidemic Disease in Nineteenth-Century India* (Berkeley: University of California Press, 1993), 75.

31  R. Ramasubban, *Public Health and Medical Research in India: Their Origins under the Impact of British Colonial Policy* (Stockholm: SIDA, 1982), 15; Harrison, *Public Health in British India*, 101.

32  W.R. Cornish, *Report of the Sanitary Commissioner for Madras for 1877* (Madras: Govt Press, 1878), 11, 142, xxviii. See Zurbrigg, *Epidemic Malaria and Hunger*, 187.

33  Surgeon-Major H. King, *The Madras Manual of Hygiene*, 2nd ed. (Madras: E. Keys, Govt Press, 1880), Appendix I, 371–383.

34  For details, see Zurbrigg, *Epidemic Malaria and Hunger*, ch. 5.

35  Surgeon-Captain H.E. Grant, *The Indian Manual of Hygiene being King's Madras Manual*, rev. ed. (Madras: Higginbotham & Co., 1894), 326. For discussion of early nineteenth-century colonial miasma theories, see K.T. Silva, 'Malaria Eradication as a Legacy of Colonial Discourse: The Case of Sri Lanka,' *Parassitologia*, 36, 1994, 149–163, at 154.

36  The first paragraphs of Patrick Manson's classic 1898 tropical medicine text read, 'The malaria parasite . . . is by far the most important disease agency in tropical pathology. . . . it undermines the health of millions; predisposing them to other disease . . . impairing their powers of resistance and repair; and otherwise unfitting them for the active business and enjoyment of life. Directly and indirectly it is the principal cause of morbidity and death in the tropics and sub-tropics'; *Tropical Diseases: A Manual of the Diseases of Warm Climates* (London: Cassell and Co., 1898), 1.

37  'Tropical medicine was given marching orders – to secure the safety and improve the productivity of the British Empire,' MacLeod colourfully articulates. 'The French, Belgians, and Germans soon joined the fray. From the 1880s, the practice of medicine in the empire became a history of techniques and policies – of education, epidemiology, and quarantine – the discovery of pathogens and vectors and the segregation of races. Simultaneously, tropical medicine became a history of *mentalités*, shaped by the Pasteurian revolution, which lent a conceptual strategy to complement Europe's political mission'; 'Introduction,' in R. MacLeod, and M. Lewis, eds., *Disease, Medicine and Empire*, 1–18, at 7. It was a sanitary model, he observes, that increasingly 'obscure[d] the relationship of disease to social structure.'

38  R. Chandavarkar, 'Plague Panic and Epidemic Politics in India, 1896–1914,' in T. Ranger, and P. Slack, eds., *Epidemics and Ideas* (Cambridge: Cambridge University Press, 1992), 203–240; I. Catanach, 'Plague and the Tensions of Empire: India, 1896–1918,' in D. Arnold, ed., *Imperial Medicine and Indigenous Societies* (Manchester: Manchester University Press, 1988), 149–171; F. Norman White, *Twenty Years of Plague in India with Special Reference to the Outbreak of 1917–1918* (Simla: Government Central Branch Press, 1929).

39  R. Ramasubban, 'Imperial Health British India, 1857–1900,' 38–60; J.C. Hume, 'Colonialism and Sanitary Medicine,' 721–722; Harrison, *Public Health in British India*, 57; Harrison, *Climates and Constitutions*; D. Arnold, 'Crisis and Contradictions in India's Public Health,' in D. Porter, ed., *The History of Public Health and the Modern State* (Amsterdam: Rodopi, 1994), 335–355.

40  Harrison, *Public Health in British India*, 102.

41  Snow, considered one of the founders of modern epidemiology, famously identified the Broad Street pump in Soho as the common domestic water source for a cholera epidemic in London.

42  In 1908, Ehrlich received the Nobel Prize in Physiology or Medicine for his contributions to immunology.

43  *Hakims* were practitioners of *yunN-I-tibb*, or Greek medicine, the medical system associated with Indian Muslims; Hume, 'Colonialism and Sanitary Medicine.'

44  Harrison, *Public Health in British India*, 116; D. Arnold, "Introduction: Disease, Medicine and Empire,' in Arnold, ed., *Imperial Medicine and Indigenous Societies*, 1–26, at 20.

45  For articulation of the contagionist-anticontagionist framework, see E. Ackerknecht, 'Anticontagionism Between 1821 and 1867,' *Bulletin of the History of Medicine*, 22, 1948, 562–593. For critique of the framework, see C. Hamlin, 'Commentary: Ackerknecht and Anticontagionism: A Tale of Two Dichotomies,' *International Journal of Epidemiology*, 38, 1, 2009, 22–27; Pelling, *Cholera, Fever and English Medicine*, 109. On the mid- to late nineteenth-century evolution of medical concepts of malaria etiology, see M. Worboys, 'From Miasmas to Germs: Malaria 1850–1879,' *Parassitologia*, 36, Aug. 1994, 61–68.

46  Worboys argues this was often the case in European experience as well; *Spreading Germs*.

47  Zurbrigg, *Epidemic Malaria and Hunger*, chs. 5, 10.

48  Harrison, *Public Health in British India*, 115.

49  Despite laudatory words offered to Ronald Ross (in absentia) and IMS Dir-Gen Lukis, the conference president in his opening address reaffirmed, in words quintessentially those of Christophers, that 'the forefront of a sanitary programme [in India] must be a reasoned account of the conditions and circumstances which affect *mortality* and the increase and decrease of populations,' requiring 'the study of the relative effects of . . . social and economic conditions'; *Progs. All-India Sanitary Conference, held at Bombay on 13th and 14th November 1911* (Calcutta: Superintendent Govt. Print., 1912), 1–2.

50  S.R. Christophers, 'Malaria in the Punjab,' *Scientific Memoirs by Officers of the Medical and Sanitary Departments of the Government of India* (New Series), No. 46 (Calcutta: Superintendent Govt Printing, GOI, 1911), 107 [hereafter, *Sci. Mem. Off. Med. San. Dep.*]

51  For analysis of early twentieth-century changes in famine relief policies, see Zurbrigg, *Epidemic Malaria and Hunger*, chs. 11–12.

52  S.R. Christophers, 'What disease costs India: A statement of the problem before medical research in India,' *Indian Medical Gazette*, Apr. 1924, 196–200; Christophers, 'Malaria in the Punjab,' 24, 26. On this, see also Zurbrigg, *Epidemic Malaria and Hunger*, 69–74.

53  Christophers, 'What Disease Costs India,' 199. Writing in 1924, Christophers at this point, it seems, felt some confidence in the famine *prevention* measures being enacted in the wake of the 1908 epidemic, allowing him to finally utter the term 'famine' in his published writing.

54  Ibid., 197 [emphasis added]. It perhaps is this understanding that helps explain the marked decline in cholera research in twentieth-century colonial India that Pratik Chakrabarti notes; in *Bacteriology in British India: Laboratory Medicine and the Tropics* (Rochester: University of Rochester Press, 2012), 190–192.

55  S.R. Christophers and C.A. Bentley, 'The Human Factor,' in W.E. Jennings, ed., *Transactions of the Bombay Medical Congress, 1909* (Bombay: Bennett, Coleman & Co., 1910), 78–83, at 83.

56  Zurbrigg, *Epidemic Malaria and Hunger*, 344–45.

57  C.A. Gill, *Report on Malaria in Amritsar, Together with a Study of Endemic and Epidemic Malaria and an Account of the Measures Necessary to their Control* (Lahore: Miscellaneous Official Publications [Punjab], 1917), 90–91.

58  Christophers, 'Malaria in the Punjab,' 132 [emphasis in original]. Perhaps the most overt use of the term 'sanitary' in relation to acute hunger appears in a 1878 account of Burdwan fever in lower Bengal. 'The most dreadful fever we have ever had in India,' Sir Arthur Cotton recounted, 'is that which has desolated the country around Calcutta, solely from want of water. This is entirely unirrigated and undrained. When the Engineer, and the Medical Officer were ordered to enquire into this, they both reported that the first cause of this fatal fever was the shocking state of the people in respect of even food, that they were so dreadfully underfed that they had no stamina, but succumbed at once to fever, that they might have otherwise thrown off with ease. . . . Nothing can be more certain than that for one death caused by fever from Irrigation, a hundred are prevented by all the *sanitary* effects of regulated water. And what shall we say to the deaths caused by Famine?'; Sir Arthur Cotton, letter to Editor of the *Illustrated News*, June 29, 1877, in anon., *The Great Lesson of the Indian Famine; with Appendix; Containing Letters from Sir A. Cotton* (London, 1877) [emphasis added].

59  GOI, *Proceedings of the Imperial Malaria Conference held at Simla in October 1909* (Simla: Government Central Branch Press, 1910), 5 [hereafter, Simla Conf.].

60  Already in 1904, Christophers's recommendation for 'well-directed sanitary reforms' as an alternate approach to malaria mortality control in light of the 'extreme difficulties' of eradicating mosquito breeding at the Mian Mir cantonment would be derisively interpreted by Ronald Ross as provision of 'night soil buckets'; S.R. Christophers, 'Second Report of the Anti-malarial Operations in Mian Mir, 1901–1903,' *Sci. Mem. Off. Med. San. Dep.*, No. 9, 1904; R. Ross, 'The Anti-malarial Experiment at Mian Mir,' Annual Meeting of the British Medical Association, July 1904: Proceedings of Section of Tropical Diseases, *British Medical Journal*, Sep. 17, 1904, 632–635.

61  On this, see Zurbrigg, *Epidemic Malaria and Hunger*, ch. 8.

62  Hume, 'Colonialism and Sanitary Medicine,' 716–717.

63  *Lancet*, Jan. 14, 1871, 52; cited in Harrison, *Public Health in British India*, 110.

64  *Report on the Sanitary Administration of the Punjab*, 1882, 12 [hereafter, PSCR].

65  *PSCR* 1882, 12, 18; *PSCR* 1878, 29.

66  Sir Joseph Fayrer, *On the Climate and Fevers of India*, Croonian Lecture, Mar. 1882, (London: J&A Churchill, 1882).

67  *PSCR* 1885, 15. See also Hume, 'Colonialism and Sanitary Medicine,' 720.

68  *PSCR* 1887, 33; PLGP, in *PSCR* 1889, 5.

69  *PSCR* 1887, 37; *PSCR* 1891, 17.

70  *PSCR* 1892, 18; 'When this extensive flooding occurs while the temperature is high, it is invariably followed in the Punjab by a severe outbreak of malarial fever'; *PSCR* 1892, 18.

71  *PSCR* 1890, 17.

72  Ibid.

73  *PSCR* 1887, 36 [emphasis added]; *PSCR* 1890, 16.

74  *PSCR* 1887, 36.

75  Hume, 'Colonialism and Sanitary Medicine,' 723.

76  For details, see Zurbrigg, *Epidemic Malaria and Hunger*, 167–174.

77  *PSCR* 1891, 5 [emphasis added]; also, *PSCR* 1892, 5, 16.

78 Zurbrigg, *Epidemic Malaria and Hunger*, 189–190.
79 *PSCR* 1895, 3.
80 PLGP, in *PSCR* 1895, 2. In its review of the 1895 *PSCR*, the provincial government would upbraid the Sanitary Commissioner for rote parroting of price and rain data with no discussion of their implications upon the health of the population, suggesting that '[a]n undigested statement of weather conditions and a table of prices does not help us . . . [in the absence of analysis] pointing out what particular effect the climatic conditions . . . had on the health of the people'; ibid.
81 *PSCR* 1896, 14.
82 PLGP, in *PSCR* 1897, 1. The provincial CDR rose to 45 per mille against a previous 10-year average of 30 per 1,000.
83 Zurbrigg, *Epidemic Malaria and Hunger*, ch. 5.
84 *PSCR* 1900, 3.
85 Zurbrigg, *Epidemic Malaria and Hunger*, ch. 5.
86 PLGP, in *PSCR* 1901, 1.
87 *PSCR* 1904, 12.
88 Zurbrigg, *Epidemic Malaria and Hunger*, ch. 7.
89 *PSCR* 1903, 13.
90 *PSCR* 1907, 1.
91 Simla Conf., 5.
92 *Report of the Indian Famine Commission 1901* (London: HMSO, 1901), 61–62.
93 *PSCR* 1893, opp. page 14.
94 In 1921, the title of the sanitary service was changed to 'public health': at the central level, Public Health Commissioner with the GOI; at the provincial level, 'Directors of Public Health.' The corresponding reports became: *Annual Report of the Public Health Commissioner with the Government of India* (GOI-PHC), and *Report of the Public Health Administration of the Punjab* (PPHA).
95 *PPHA* 1927, 1.
96 *GOI-PHC* 1928, Section I: 'On the State of the Public Health in British India,' The 'key principle' of public health work was the 'study of the character and incidence of disease, its causes and predisposing conditions, its mode of spread, its social factors which increase or reduce it'; ibid., 2.
97 *PPHA* 1931, 3.
98 *GOI-PHC* 1937, 2.
99 Editorial, 'The Economic Factor in Tropical Disease,' *Indian Medical Gazette*, 57, Sept. 1922, 341–343.
100 Zurbrigg, *Epidemic Malaria and Hunger*, ch. 9.
101 *PPHA* 1923, 18.
102 *PPHA* 1924, 20–21.
103 *GOI-PHC* 1935, 2–3.
104 See David Arnold's discussion of the limited effectiveness of cholera vaccines in the late colonial period; 'Cholera Mortality in British India, 1817–1947,' in T. Dyson, ed., *India's Historical Demography: Studies in Famine, Disease and Society* (London: Curzon, 1989), 261–284, at 276); also C. Hamlin, *Cholera: The Biography* (Oxford: Oxford University Press, 2009), 284–285.
105 *PPHA*, 1924, 24.
106 Ibid., 25.
107 *PPHA* 1927, 21. For a similar separation of poverty and public health policy in Edwardian Britain and the existential dilemma it posed for public health professionals, see J. Lewis, 'The Origins and Development of Public Health in

the UK,' in R. Daetels, et al., eds., *Third Oxford Text Book of Public Health* (Oxford: Oxford University Press, 1997), vol. 2, 27. As 'the issue of poverty shifted to social welfare – national insurance and old-age pensions,' Lewis observes, 'their role became increasingly one of technicians, applying the specific interventions that germ research threw up . . . which were to earn the MOH [Medical Officer of Health] the derogatory title of "drains doctor", and subsequently, "mother-craft" educators'; ibid.

108 A partial exception is famine relief activities during the 1939–1940 Hissar district famine.

109 *Indian Sanitary Policy. Being a Resolution issued by the Governor General in Council on the 23rd May 1914* (Calcutta: Office of the Superintendent, Govt Printing, 1914).

110 A. Balfour, and H. Scott, *Health Problems of the Empire* (London: W. Collins Sons & Co., 1924).

111 P.J. Brown, 'Malaria, Miseria, and Underpopulation in Sardinia: The "Malaria Blocks Development" Cultural Model,' *Medical Anthropology*, 17, 3, May 1997, 239–254.

112 W. Osler, *The Evolution of Modern Medicine: A Series of lectures delivered at Yale University on the Silliman Foundation in April 1913* (New Haven: Yale University Press, 1921), 223.

113 W.H.S. Jones, *Malaria: A Neglected Factor in the History of Greece and Rome* (London: Macmillan, 1907).

114 *PPHA* 1921, 3.

115 *PPHA* 1925, 12.

# 5

# COLONIAL RETRENCHMENT
# AND 'SELLING' VECTOR
# CONTROL

## Forster's unease: 'Malaria as Block to Development'

What explains Forster's 'repudiation' of the doctrine of malaria as 'destroyer of empires'? What worried him in 1925? One immediate concern no doubt was a practical one: advocacy for mosquito extirpation in colonial India was now seen to be in direct competition for increasingly scarce public health funds, a concern heightened in 1923 by the Inchcape Commission's prescription for yet further fiscal retrenchment. That consternation could only have intensified with the 1924 publication of Balfour and Scott's *Health Problems of Empire*, where 'everyday malaria' would be described as 'the truly "Imperial" disease, the chronic relapsing malaria which saps life and energy, alters mentality and leads to invalidism and poverty.'[1] As director of the newly expanded London School of Hygiene and Tropical Medicine, and fresh from his Gorgas-esque vector-extirpation anti-malaria triumph in Khartoum, Andrew Balfour's prominence no doubt would have seemed virtually unchallengeable. In the climate of extreme financial stringency, it was perhaps inevitable that those public health officials in India who continually struggled for enhanced quinine supplies and funding for agricultural 'bonification' measures would see advocacy for expanded anti-larval control programs as a dangerous distraction. Yet from the ardency of Forster's words, one senses a deeper concern as well: it suggests a more general alarm over an impending demise in understanding of the broader socio-economic conditions underlying human health. For by the mid-1920s, disease as the primary cause of India's poverty had emerged as rhetorical argument at the highest levels of the public health administration. Despite his later skepticism regarding the protein deficiency thesis, J.D. Graham had argued in his 1924 report as GOI Public Health Commissioner that the prevention of malaria's 'almost incalculable and disastrous results . . . [was] fundamental in the growth of India into a strong nation.'[2]

Forster was hardly alone in his consternation over the hegemonic power of the germ-centred model of health, if perhaps one of the earlier public health workers in colonial South Asia to express such reservations in official documents. The reductive direction in modern disease theory was also by this time becoming a central concern for a handful of Euro-U.S. public health analysts, evident in the writing of Galdston and Ackerknecht[3] and the emergence of the concept of 'social medicine.' But it seems that the concern for Forster was particularly acute in the case of malaria. Beyond the immediate funding contest, it appears he had begun to gauge the full ideological force of the microbiological model of (ill-)health rapidly re-shaping colonial public health debate: sensing the myriad conveniences, professional and political, that were nourishing a narrowed view of the malaria problem in India, and their potential consequences.

Here in this chapter, the inter-war exclusionary trajectory is explored as it played out in colonial South Asia over the final decades of colonial rule. This period offers a key portal for tracking the intersection of medical subspecialisms, Western corporate philanthropy, professional interests, and imperial exigencies that allowed malaria to become a key vehicle post-WW2 through which socio-economic understanding of the global infective disease burden would be shed.

## The 1925 Conference of Medical Research Workers

The disease-as-cause-of-poverty thesis would be articulated formally in 1925 in the proceedings of the All-India Conference of Medical Research Workers at Calcutta: 'the greatest cause of poverty and financial stringency in India is loss of efficiency resulting from preventable disease.'[4] In a manner presaging present-day 'disability-adjusted life year' (DALY) calculations,[5] 'loss of efficiency . . . from preventable malnutrition and disease' was estimated as 'not less than twenty per cent' of the country's economic output, costing India 'several hundreds of crores of rupees each year.' Deemed 'a grave emergency,' the Conference called for a 'thorough enquiry into the wastage of life and the economic depression in India.'[6]

Admirable in its acknowledgement of the *extent* of ill-health in the country, the Conference's causal framework nevertheless turned upside down the view of 'the economic factor in tropical disease' articulated so frankly in the *Indian Medical Gazette* scarcely three years earlier.[7] Proceedings from the 1925 conference, unfortunately, do not appear to have been circulated: unlike for the earlier pre-war Sanitary Congresses, transactions from the annual Medical Research Workers conferences, initiated in 1923, were not made public. However, brief accounts of resolutions adopted at the conference appear episodically in subsequent publications: in particular, in the October 1927 issue of the *Indian Medical Gazette*.[8] The journal's eight-page conference commentary suggests the proceedings may have been framed around a 1924 paper by W.G. King in which the cost to India exacted by malaria was estimated to reach £20 million annually in lost lives and labour.[9] Long-retired from posts as provincial sanitary commissioner, King had been greatly frustrated with Christophers's analysis of epidemic malaria in Punjab at the Simla malaria conference 15 years earlier, conclusions that laid the basis for subsequent policy to be directed to the control of malaria's mortality burden rather than its vector-transmission.[10] Through his 1924 paper it appears King was channelling that disaffection into deliberations at the Medical Research Workers conference planned for the following year.

The unidirectional 'disease-as-cause-of-poverty' argument was not, of course, a new one. The doctrine was already central to the tropical medicine subspecialism of 'malariology' that emerged at the turn of the twentieth century and held a key place in the writing of Ronald Ross.[11] Continents away, the general thesis had reached perhaps its most frank expression within the Rockefeller Foundation's Sanitary Commission, established in 1913, and its global mission of public health training and education, epitomized in the Foundation's reputed creed that saw 'disease . . . [as] the main source of almost all other human ills – poverty, crime, ignorance, vice, inefficiency, hereditary taint, and many other evils.'[12] But the thesis had an earlier pedigree in the nineteenth-century sanitationist reformulation of epidemic theory, with filth-engendered disease deemed the primary cause of urban industrial pauperism.

Such theses, of course, contain an element of truth. In the case of malaria as a 'block to development,' the view undoubtedly derived from European imperial experience with malaria in West Africa where conditions of extremely intense (holoendemic) transmission had long delayed extensive European settlement and economic exploitation along 'the gold coast.'[13] Malaria affected imperial balance-sheets in South Asia as well. Hyperendemic malarial conditions had rendered rail construction in specific hill tracts difficult and particularly costly.[14] Malaria also raised the labour recruitment costs of the plantation industry on the northeastern tea estates. In the latter case, however, it did so largely in the context of broader factors – conditions of human destitution associated with specific indentured labour practices. Indeed, in their 1909 *Malaria in the Duars* report, Christophers and Bentley had openly challenged the thesis.

> In a warm country like India there is perhaps every *a priori* reason to expect malaria to be both prevalent and intense; but if by such intensity we mean the condition so characteristic of the African coast we shall have to modify our conception. . . . [L]arge tracts of India are not particularly malarious in the sense that many tropical countries are. . . . [T]his disease does not prevent the prosperity and natural increase of the population.[15]

The characterization of malaria in much of India as 'prevalent' but 'not particularly malarious' was a pointed rejection of the argument articulated by W.H.S. Jones two years earlier in his *Malaria: A Neglected Factor in the History of Greece and Rome*, a work for which Ross had contributed the introductory chapter.[16] Yet the thesis of malaria as a central cause of poverty prevailed. Extrapolated to malaria *in general*, it increasingly coloured malaria and general public health debate in India, notwithstanding the *Indian Medical Gazette*'s explicit 1922 editorial statement to the contrary.[17]

## 'What malaria costs India': the Sinton monograph

Not surprisingly perhaps, the view of malaria as the cause of India's underdevelopment found a receptive audience within the broader colonial administration. 'Malaria,' the 1928 Royal Commission on Agriculture in India (RCAI) report asserted, 'slays its thousands and lowers the economic efficiency of hundreds of thousands.' Extending the argument further to hookworm disease and kala-azar as well,[18] the RCAI commissioners urged authorities to '[r]elease from the strangle-hold of disease . . . large areas of the country,' action that promised to 'enormously enhance its general prosperity.'[19] A decade later the thesis was argued much more prominently by J.A. Sinton in a monograph entitled 'What Malaria Costs India.'[20] At the end of his tenure as Director of the Malaria Survey of India, Sinton was determined to see malaria control efforts extended beyond the isolated economic enclaves of tea estates, military cantonments, and railway establishments, and openly rued the fact that malaria 'in ordinary times, excites comparatively little comment among the lay public . . . [or] in the Indian Legislature.'[21] But in a fiscal climate of retrenchment, malaria transmission control programs required raising taxes, and that meant convincing those footing the bill that the cost of doing nothing was even greater. Government and local provincial authorities, in other words, were unlikely to be persuaded unless economic productivity, and tax (land) revenues in particular, were considered in jeopardy. In this vein, Sinton cited a 1919 U.S. Public Health service editorial describing malaria as leaving a population 'generally subnormal physically, mentally and economically.'[22]

What was the case for malaria undermining the colonial economy, most of which was based on rural agriculture? For advocates of general anti-mosquito measures it was difficult to point to examples of land going out of production *because of* malaria. Certainly, there were localized tracts where agricultural productivity had been thwarted by conditions of particularly intense malaria transmission. This could be argued for the sub-Himalayan Terai hill tracts of the United Provinces, and in the northern 'dry zone' of Sri Lanka. However, even in these regions, settlement failed for reasons of inadequate economic support for workers and immigrants to tide over the period of extreme physical demands entailed in initial land clearing and preparation. In the Terai, 'swampy' conditions required extensive and costly drainage operations before soil conditions could permit successful harvests. Sinton himself understood this larger economic context to settlement failures, having officially investigated and documented such questions in his 1931 study of malaria in Spain.[23] As for northern Sri Lanka, the region historically had once supported a thriving Indic civilization;[24] but sufficient investment required to return the land to prosperous cultivation had not been forthcoming under colonial rule.

Such areas moreover represented only a very small portion of the malarious regions of the subcontinent.[25] Where land was being lost it was generally due to water-logging, often related to neglect of surface drainage in relation to canal and transportation development, and here debilitating malaria was a secondary effect to human impoverishment. In this case effective remedial action was not anti-larval measures but improved drainage or flood control. Indeed, it was well known that canal irrigation, though it often increased malaria transmission levels, generally brought greater prosperity and food production, and declining mortality levels in turn. The argument, in other words, that malaria *per se* was the cause of agricultural impoverishment generally across India was a very hard sell. It clearly required a monumental promotional campaign. Sinton's 194-page literature review, 'What Malaria Costs India,' can be seen in this light,[26] the monograph transparently offered as a resource for 'those workers who have to represent to the financial authorities the necessity, the urgency and the economic importance of anti-malaria measures.'[27]

To be fair, a role for underlying 'economic stress' in malaria's toll was not excluded from the Sinton monograph. Christophers and Bentley's work on the 'Human Factor' in malaria was briefly cited. Economic hardship had a 'marked influence,' Sinton acknowledged, not only on the prevalence of malaria, but also on 'the case mortality among those afflicted.'[28] Yet the monograph's overriding emphasis lay elsewhere. Bengal would be cited as illustrating the 'effects of malaria in *causing* a decline of agricultural prosperity,' an inversion of the relationship documented painstakingly by Bentley over the preceding several decades.[29] In the monograph's final pages all reference to the role of underlying economic factors was omitted, Sinton concluding in rhetorical style to rival the so-called Rockefeller creed that malaria was 'probably the greatest obstacle' to India's development, 'engendering poverty, diminishing the quantity and the quality of the food supply, lowering the physical and intellectual standard of the nation, and hampering increased prosperity and economic progress in every way.'[30]

What explains the Sinton monograph's stunning turnaround in disease theory from that expressed in the *Indian Medical Gazette* 13 years earlier?[31] Answers involve considerable conjecture, but among them, some are inevitably political. For the colonial government, faced with a growing nationalist movement in the early decades of the twentieth century, the thesis of malaria as a major cause of poverty – a postulate referred to in modern historiography as 'malaria as a block to development' (MBD)[32] – offered a near-irresistible alternative explanation (as opposed to colonial misrule) for continuing endemic poverty in British India.[33] For members of the Indian Medical Service facing drastic research and program funding cutbacks post-Inchcape, the temptation to 'sell' the public health costs of malaria transmission in unidirectional economic terms no doubt was equally compelling.[34] But fiscal retrenchment also brought with it another dynamic, setting the stage for beginning reliance on external sources of funding for new 'interventionist' public health programs, including that of malaria transmission control. And as elsewhere in Western imperial domains, the Rockefeller Foundation with its germ-eradication pedagogical framework was there to oblige.

## Rockefeller in India

To what extent did Rockefeller Foundation engagement in India contribute to the reversal in disease paradigms evident by the mid-1920s? Certainly, a narrowed view of the detrimental impact of malaria on colonial economies was already prominent among many malaria workers and sanitarians in India in the lead-up to the 1909 Simla malaria conference. But the abrupt epistemic turnaround in disease causation doctrine in the mid-1920s corresponds temporally with the Foundation's growing presence and influence in the country. By the later 1910s, the Rockefeller Foundation's International Health Board (IHB)[35] had already established a South Asian presence, with prominent anti-hookworm schemes in the tea plantations of Ceylon (Sri Lanka) and southern India.[36] The timing, moreover, of the MBD-esque resolutions at the 1925 Conference of Medical Research Workers coincides with formal initiatives by Indian Medical Service officials to elicit Rockefeller Foundation funding for disease control programs. A funding request by the Director of the newly opened Calcutta School of Tropical Medicine, for example, had already been submitted in 1922 – and turned down – by the IHB, as were several other high-level requests.[37] Thus it was clear that Rockefeller Foundation funding would be forthcoming only for projects closely aligned with Foundation principles and largely under its direction.

Those principles were clear from IHB-funded anti-hookworm work in the 1910s on the Darjeeling and Madras tea plantations, projects that were primarily educational in purpose, geared to demonstrate the economic value of parasite eradication. There had been little IHB funding, by contrast, channelled to existing medical research facilities in India. Research was considered unnecessary apparently, for the answers were already at hand. In the case of ankylostomiasis (hookworm), simple field surveys clearly demonstrated widespread fecal presence of hookworm eggs. The Foundation's central goal instead was the training of a cadre of public health specialists dedicated to eradicating specific microbes and 'creat[ing] demand for protection against disease.'[38]

Despite initial proposal rejections, prospects for Rockefeller funding in India in the early 1920s must still have seemed promising, with the Foundation's public health philanthropy rapidly expanding on other continents. Its global institution-building had begun in 1915 with the Peking Union Medical College, and other projects had rapidly followed, with schools of hygiene and public health in London and Prague in 1921, Warsaw in 1923; Budapest, Zagreb, and Toronto in 1925; Rome, 1930; and Tokyo in 1933. It was the school in London, however, that was of particular importance for the Foundation's pedagogical aspirations by virtue of the British empire's global reach – envisaged by Wycliffe Rose, Director of the International Health Board, to be 'a great dynamo that would vitalise and inspire public health work, not only in the country, but throughout the world.' The $2 million facility would incorporate the existing London School of Tropical Medicine but refashion it to fully embrace 'hygiene' both in name and programmatic commitment.[39] Approval of the London School of Hygiene and Tropical Medicine proposal by the British Cabinet had prompted accolades in the British medical press, the *Lancet* describing the decision as 'a tremendous compliment to our Empire,'

> convey[ing] . . . definite recognition by the United States that the constructive side of British Imperialism can be used to the advantage of the whole world . . . to serve the common needs of the medical services of the Foreign Office, the colonies, the India Office, the combatant forces, and the Ministry of Health, and also those of students, duly accredited from the medical centres of the world.[40]

The effusive 1923 *Lancet* editorial was followed, in stark contrast, by a scathing *British Medical Journal* critique of public health and research cutbacks in India that decried the country's 'rather evil reputation as a reservoir for great epidemic diseases such as cholera and plague,'[41] a rebuke that undoubtedly reverberated throughout the IMS. Several months later, a lead editorial in the *Indian Medical Gazette* compiled a list of Rockefeller Foundation funding elsewhere in the colonial world, including a $10.5 million grant directed to the Peking Union Medical College. These were 'figures,' the editor commented, 'which make the mouth water and show the possibilities for medical education in India.'[42] The prospect of Rockefeller funds filling some of the Inchcape gap in medical funding in India thus had emerged enticingly on the horizon. By December of 1924, the All India Conference of Medical Research Workers had passed a resolution urging the Government of India to issue an invitation to the Rockefeller Foundation to make a survey of medical education and research in India: an initiative that would be embraced by the IHB as a prelude to Rockefeller funding of a new separate training institution, what would become the All-India Institute of Hygiene and Public Health (AIIHPH) in Calcutta.[43] Accounts of the

Foundation's global activities continued to appear regularly in the pages of the *Indian Medical Gazette* through the 1920s, along with enthusiastic updates of the Gorgas campaign in Panama which had led to completion of the canal in 1914.

It seems likely, then, that the groundswell of interest in Rockefeller Foundation funding was, in part, what Forster was reacting against in his Punjab public health reports of 1921 and 1925. In the bleak climate of Inchcape retrenchment, many in the beleaguered Indian medical research community would have been ripe for almost any argument offering prospects of funding, and willing to voice support for the MBD premise, and its broader sweep of disease theory.[44] At the very least, the climate of expectant philanthropy made it that much more difficult for those IMS researchers, hopeful of Rockefeller institutional beneficence, to question the reductive paradigm.

Nonetheless, provincial public health officers during these years still continued to report prices, harvest conditions, and wages in the preamble to their annual reports. In Punjab, Gill repeatedly stressed the distinction between immediate triggers of epidemic malaria mortality and their underlying economic causes. 'Famine,' he wrote in his 1928 *Genesis of Epidemics*, 'is a *predisposing* cause. Excess monsoon rainfall is the *precipitating* cause of regional [malaria] epidemics.'[45] Christophers, too, in this period of epistemological contestation would come to express his own unease with what he saw as an increasingly divisive reliance on external medical expertise. In the concluding remarks of his 1924 critique of funding cutbacks, he urged the maintaining of an indigenous medical research establishment, arguing '[i]t is no question of applying such knowledge only as we now have, nor of purchasing the necessary knowledge from Europe. Europe cannot help, for her problems are different and she knows nothing of India's requirements.'[46] Characteristically oblique in wording, it seems quite possible the new London School of Hygiene and Tropical Medicine was being alluded to within his appellation of 'Europe.'[47]

## Hookworm eradication questioned

The reservations expressly publicly by Forster and Christophers over outside 'expertise' were all the more apt in light of the actual practical results of the International Health Board's work in India at this point. The Board's consultants had had in fact very limited success in galvanizing an hygienic 'revolution' against hookworm in South Asia in the 1920s. There were few examples of project replication of its flagship campaign, even on the tea estates where infection levels were highest and 'pay-back,' in theory, most likely. Instead, many projects lay unreplicated or abandoned.[48] With IHB failure to interest plantation and provincial government authorities in preventive campaigns of latrine construction, India had become instead, some argue, primarily a site for Rockefeller experimental testing of anti-hookworm drugs on 'controlled communities' of human populations (jail populations and tea estate labour lines).[49] By 1927, a 'million' treatments had been given, with carbon tetrachloride considered the least toxic of the chemicals employed.[50] The choice of hookworm as a public health campaign, as in the earlier Rockefeller campaign in the southern U.S., had been based from the beginning not upon its priority as a cause of ill-health, but rather for its instrumental value as a demonstration of rapid interventions and presumed mass instructional impact. As a means of getting 'knowledge into the minds of the people,' J.D. Rockefeller Sr had exhorted early on, '[h]ookworm seemed the best way.'[51] 'Hookworm was a means to an end,' Farley has observed, 'a way to educate the public, physicians, and politicians in public health with the hope that professionally-run public health services would develop.'[52]

Then, in 1928, the results were released of a major epidemiological study into hookworm infection in the country undertaken by the Calcutta School of Tropical Medicine, findings that raised fundamental questions with respect to the central premise underlying the anti-hookworm campaign. Summarizing the study's conclusions, the *Indian Medical Gazette* noted that 'although throughout India hookworm infestation is excessively common, yet heavy infections are rare, and hookworm disease – as apart from infestation – is uncommon.' The study also showed that 'treatment only temporarily reduced the worm load in the body,' re-infection occurring rapidly in the absence of regular use of footwear. Moreover, 'a dry season of from 6 to 8 months ha[d] practically the same effect as mass treatment would have on the population.' 'We have been accustomed for many years to think of hookworm infection as being one of the chief scourges of India,' Asa Chandler, author of the report observed. 'Actually, it is apparently a relatively unimportant cause of disease in this country – except in certain specified areas.' Those areas were primarily the industrial plantations – the tea estates of the Duars and Assam. Elsewhere, 'hookworm disease is practically non-existent in most places,' he concluded, adding that '[o]f course, the vitality and degree of resistance of the patient are important factors in determining whether light infections may give rise to anaemia.'[53] The study questioned in turn policies promoting enclosed latrines, noting their rapid befoulment in the absence of ready water supply. It urged greater hygienic benefit from the rural practice of open areas 'exposed to direct sunlight' and traditional conservancy practices in Bengal employing raised bamboo canes.[54]

Such basic questions had long been evident to many. Rama Rao, a prominent physician in Madras city and member of the provincial legislature, had raised similar concerns seven years earlier,[55] frustrated by the drain of resources and effort directed to an infection of limited significance relative to tuberculosis, and the need instead for access to clean water and anti-malarials. The Chandler findings, in other words, amounted to a clear rebuke of the central Rockefeller paradigm: the assertion that infection *per se* necessarily was the problem.

## Rural malaria vector-control trials

There was another deeply ironic dimension to the IHB anti-hookworm campaign. Of any infection, it was malaria that the Rockefeller Foundation considered the greatest global health burden, not hookworm. Early on it had judged malaria to be 'probably the number one obstacle to the welfare and economic efficiency of the human race.'[56] Yet malaria received negligible attention through the first two decades of Rockefeller involvement in South Asia. Funding requests from the Malaria Survey of India, for example, had consistently been rejected.[57] Not until the mid-1930s did malaria become a focus for the IHB, renamed in 1927 as the International Health Division (IHD), and here funding was directed solely to experimental methods of vector control, with anti-malarial drug research eschewed.[58] In November 1934, Paul Russell, then on Rockefeller assignment in the Philippines, was deputed by the IHD to work with the King Institute of Preventive Medicine in Madras to assess rural malaria prevalence and initiate demonstration control trials.[59]

Preliminary surveys soon led Russell to acknowledge that little scope existed for rural malaria transmission control through existing anti-larval methods, a conclusion not unfamiliar to Indian malaria workers. 'Certainly larval control by oil, Paris green, or drainage is out of the question in most of rural India,' he observed. 'Deaths can be lessened and the duration of malarial attacks shortened by better distribution of drugs. But at present only amelioration and not prophylaxis seems economically possible.'[60] Russell refrained, however, from acknowledging the earlier three decades of studies which formed the basis for such conclusions. With respect to Bengal he concluded '[i]t is likely there will be no real prevention of malaria in Bengal until it is possible to institute a vast scheme of *bonification* which will include regulation of surface waters and improved agriculture,' again leaving Bentley's published studies uncited. As for Punjab malaria, he offered no comment at all, for lack of 'time and space.'[61]

Russell went on to investigate the problems of 'untidy irrigation' in relation to the Mettur-Cauvery irrigation project, a canal system opened in 1933 in the Tanjore district of Madras province. Excessive water usage appeared to be the primary source of heightened malaria transmission, and here he urged greater attention to the anti-malariogenic principles drawn up years before for the irrigation department but left largely ignored.[62] His critique was scathing, highlighting the enormous revenue sums garnered annually by the irrigation administration, and pointing out that 'not a single anna (penny)' from the enormous irrigation revenues had 'ever been used for malaria research.'[63] He went on to devise methods of intermittent irrigation of paddy fields, a technique which appeared to offer 'the only cheap method of [malaria transmission] control.' When it became clear that local authorities were reluctant to promote such methods, however,[64] he turned to a more geographically limited anti-larval project in Pattukottai Town and the neighbouring village of Ennore. Here, too, he met with local resistance for reasons of cost, and in 1939 the IHD transferred its malaria headquarters and laboratory from the King Institute in Madras city to the Pasteur Institute of southern India at Coonoor in Mysore State. There, Russell began investigating hyperendemic malaria in the neighbouring hills of the western Ghats, a region seen to offer increasing potential for plantation development. The choice of these later project sites, however, meant returning to essentially an enclave framework, activities feasible financially only in a limited rural industrial setting.[65]

In his final years of work in India Russell pursued economic arguments for control of rural malaria transmission, initiating in 1939–1940 a 'malario-economic' survey to assess the cost of malarial infection to rural communities. Undertaken in three villages in Pattukkottai taluk neighbouring the recently opened Mettur-Cauvery canal, the study sought to measure the costs of malarial fever in terms of medical care and lost wages. In a community where annual income averaged Rs 36–13–0, the cost of 'fever' illness was estimated to be between Rs 2–2–0 to Rs 3–14–0 per capita annually. The cost of '[s]pray killing' (pyrethrum), by comparison, was estimated at one-half to one rupee per capita annually. More thorough anti-mosquito measures – cleaning and oiling ditches, irrigation channels, and standing water collections – were estimated to cost 'over two rupees' per annum. He concluded that 'these villages could spend at least Re.1–0–0 per capita per year for malaria control and if the control measures succeeded, they would be financially better off.' Ultimately, however, he acknowledged that the prospects of raising such funds by direct taxation were 'practically *nil*,' calling instead for government funding of such work through revenues from irrigation tax revenues.[66]

Published in 1942, Russell's malario-economic study is important as one of the first attempts in South Asia to estimate the economic costs to a rural population of a major endemic disease. But its importance lies also as an illustration of the analytic limitations flowing from a narrow microbiologic focus to such calculations. Left unexplored were alternative approaches to addressing the economic costs of seasonal malaria debility. Assured access to quinine treatment could have substantially reduced the extent of lost wages in addition to saving lives, and at a much smaller cost. Indeed, it could be argued the study demonstrated instead the key importance of reliable and affordable quinine access. Moreover, as a study ostensibly concerned with agricultural development, one might also have expected at least passing attention to the comparative costs of malaria transmission control in relation to other factors holding back agricultural productivity, constraints such as lack of affordable credit and security of tenure. For in addition to illness costs of malarial infection, the study also found that interest payments on debt, land rent, and taxes averaged Rs 8–1–0 per capita annually, or between 15 and 30 per cent of total household income.[67] With the study constructed narrowly as a problem of plasmodia, other sources of 'wages lost' were invisible, including recurring seasonal un- and under-employment, and thus also other causes of, and solutions to, agricultural underdevelopment. Finally, as a public health study, it is puzzling that no discussion was directed to the mortality data collected over the course of the study. In two of the three malarious study villages, infant mortality and crude death rates were considerably lower than in the two non-malarial study villages in a neighbouring deltaic taluk. These data however failed to warrant comment.

This critique of the 'malario-economic' study's conclusions is not to ignore the human costs of endemic malaria infection, nor to dismiss the potential value of enviro-entomological techniques of transmission control. Rather, it highlights the limitations of health analysis framed narrowly with a singular focus on infection *transmission*, and at that, on a single infection. But it highlights, as well, the highly tenuous character of the MBD argument that would be advanced several years later in post-WW2 deliberations on the economic benefits of malaria eradication – a thesis argued in no small part, it appears, on the basis of Russell's 1942 study, as we will consider in chapter six. The Pattukkottai study, in this sense, encapsulates many of the concerns of public health officials such as Forster over the limitations of the narrow sanitationist model that increasingly dominated deliberations within the Indian Medical Service.

## The germ-transmission paradigm ascendant

In a recent overview of the activities of the International Health Division in India, Kavadi concludes that the tutelary 'model' of hygiene promoted by Rockefeller Foundation activities had 'only a marginal impact' on colonial government policy and program.[68] This was the case, he suggests, even in regard to the All-India Institute of Hygiene and Public Health (AIIHPH).[69] More problematic, arguably, was the Foundation's approach to public health 'modelling.' Amrith notes the proliferation of demonstration projects that only rarely expanded beyond the 'pilot' stage – a practice, he observes, of 'making "policy" out of myriad isolated "pilot projects" and "demonstrations", a model which the WHO [later] took to India, and elsewhere in Southeast Asia, as a first step in reorienting the discourse and practice of public health.'[70] Kavadi notes that of the seven demonstration units initiated under the IHD, only one was even moderately successful.[71] To at least some within the existing public health administration, the pursuit of disease control programs through 'education,' in isolation from basic curative health services and broader subsistence security, was transparently unrealistic.[72]

Indeed, failure was privately acknowledged within the Rockefeller Foundation itself. In internal reports to the New York office, IHD consultants referred to work in India as 'a big disappointment. . . . [T]here is not a single good example of [disease] control work to be demonstrated,' one official concluded.[73] Responsibility for the failures was directed unsurprisingly not to the Foundation itself, but laid at the feet of the Government of India, and to disinterest and incompetence among provincial public health officials. It is a view that has tended to colour modern historiographic analysis as well, with colonial government recalcitrance ('unwilling[ness] to learn') interpreted in terms of official 'defeatism' or purely cynical 'profit motivated' jettisoning of health responsibility.[74]

Undoubtedly, there were elements of both. But there was a great deal more lying behind medical and governmental unresponsiveness to the IHB/IHD model projects. In the case of the hookworm campaign, as we have seen, there were good reasons for scepticism. As for malaria, reluctance on the part of the Government of India with respect to IHD programs is hardly comprehensible without taking into account the larger context of pre-1920 British Indian experience and research into malaria mortality. That body of epidemiological research on Punjab and Bengal malaria provided deep insights into practical remedial measures and, crucially, where priorities should lie. This earlier experience would be largely ignored however in the activities of the IHD consultants. As to 'native apathy,' the record of local rural response to malaria control initiatives was also clear: where programs addressed economic conditions such as surface water drainage operations and land reclamation, they generally were embraced with alacrity by rural cultivators in Punjab. Assumptions of 'native apathy,' in other words, merit considerably closer scrutiny as well.

One area of IHD achievement widely cited in post-Independence public health literature lay in the 1946 *Report of the Health Survey and Development Committee* (popularly referred to as the Bhore Committee Report), a document that, as we have seen in chapter three, laid the groundwork for post-Independence rural health care organization.[75] A leading figure behind the Bhore report was John Black Grant, a Rockefeller consultant deputed to take over the directorship of the troubled AIIHPH in 1939 following his nearly two decades of work at the Peking Union Medical College in China. Arguably, however, the need for basic rural health infrastructure was already self-evident to the post-colonial government. Moreover, in prioritizing primary health care (*viz.* basic curative care along with preventive), the Bhore report was itself quite unrepresentative of most previous Rockefeller policy. At the same time, in the absence of strong advocacy for fundamental agricultural reforms, the report largely steered shy of concrete economic recommendations that could begin to address the deep poverty underlying much ill-health, or for that matter the political conditions necessary to ensure accountability of the rural health services recommended.[76]

## Epistemic success

One is tempted, from this history, to dismiss the Rockefeller Foundation's impact in South Asia as largely inconsequential, not least because what it offered institutionally in terms of paramedical training was to a certain extent already in place through smallpox vaccinators and 'field' Sanitary Inspectors. Nevertheless, its pedagogic influence was real. In the immediate term, it helped nourish within sectors of the Indian Medical Service a technological view of health both in medical thought and broader public programs. In Madras province IHB officials as early as 1925 were reminding government officials that their 'province was the main source of [hookworm] infection spreading to foreign lands . . . [and] that they had an international obligation to control it.'[77] At the central government level, Rockefeller influence was evident in a Government of India directive to provincial public health departments for anti-hookworm educational and treatment programs, with special medical officers appointed to supervise mass carbon tetrachloride 'preventive' treatment camps.[78] Despite questions of treatment risk, and far greater priorities, Punjab officials obliged, though it was manifestly evident to many in the field that, without latrines, there was little prospect of preventing re-infection.[79]

With respect to malaria, one can wonder how the credibility of the 'malaria-blocks-development' thesis was sustained through this period. That it was, however, is evident in the pages of the 1945 Bengal Famine Commission Report. At a time when famine had just claimed 2 million lives – the largest proportion of deaths triggered by malaria primed by starvation – the Famine Commission pointed to Russell's 1941 *Indian Medical Gazette* analysis of the obstacle to malaria prevention in India as primarily 'a social as much as a technical problem.'[80] Yet the 'social' dimensions detailed in the Russell article pertained not to economics and hunger, but rather to the 'absence of a sufficient weight of public opinion' in favour of vector control, a situation where '[t]he average individual in India . . . has not the remotest feeling of social responsibility for the control of the disease.' Characterizing malaria as an 'insidious enemy, producing . . . lethargy and destroying initiative and ambition,' the 1945 Famine Commissioners' report urged a 'most vigorous attack on both urban and rural malaria . . . after the war,' concluding that '[m]alaria control . . . is essential to the satisfactory development of the country's agricultural resources.'[81] In other words, the Rockefeller Foundation's influence on perception of the malaria problem in India appears to have been substantial at the highest levels of the colonial administration.

Certainly Russell's technical skills in malaria *transmission* control were innovative, his anti-larval field work painstaking, and his recommendations on 'untidy' irrigation welcome, if directed to entomological concerns rather than economic. Yet in all his South Asian writing, save his initial 1936 overview, socio-economic dimensions of the malaria problem in India were scrupulously set aside – a bias manifest, as we have seen, in his 1941 assertion that 'well fed soldiers in perfect physical condition go down with malaria as rapidly and as seriously, with as high a death rate as average villagers.'[82] Five years later these same words would re-appear in a prominent malaria text, *Practical Malariology*, with Russell as primary author.[83]

In the medical climate of 1946, Paul Russell's dismissal of the role of hunger in South Asia's malaria burden went seemingly without remark within the malaria research community. This, though it contradicted the entire body of research on malaria linking much of the malaria lethality in the subcontinent to human destitution, epidemiological experience which in the early post-WW1 days had led the League of Nations' Malaria Commission (LNMC) to the shores of the Indian subcontinent. Here we return briefly to that parallel perspective on India's 'malaria problem' as documented by the League's Malaria Commission less than two decades earlier.

### The League of Nations Malaria Commission circumvented

As seen in chapter one, an alternate view of the malaria problem, one contrary to the MBD paradigm, was clearly evident internationally in the early work of the League of Nations Malaria Commission in the 1920s. The Commission's frank articulation of broader determinants underlying the malaria problem in Europe, however, had only fanned disagreement amongst Western malaria workers, discord that the Commission had been established, in part, to moderate. Packard describes the divide thus: one group, 'influenced by American and British scientists,'

> view[ed] malaria narrowly as a problem of vector control. The other group, following the lead of Celli in Italy (and influenced by Virchow's social medicine in Germany), [saw] malaria as a problem of social uplift and thus intimately tied to social and economic conditions like rural housing, nutrition, and agricultural production.[84]

Frustrations would erupt publicly in 1930, in Malcolm Watson's response to an address by S.P James to the Royal Society of Medicine a year earlier. A prominent member of the League's Malaria Commission, James had suggested in his talk that malaria, like tuberculosis, was largely a disease of poverty. Where 'the level of wages is low, work is scarce,' measures directed to socio-economic improvement offered the primary route to control, he had argued.

> The sources of malaria are not eradicated by these [bonification] schemes, but as the people live in better houses, have more and better food and are within easy reach of medical aid, they are not

infected so frequently, and the disease, when it occurs, is quickly and effectively treated and overcome. Thus severe and fatal cases become rare and, after a time, the disease ceases to be of great importance as a cause of sickness and death.[85]

Watson, who had worked to reduce malaria transmission on the Malaysian rubber plantations through drainage and jungle clearing, countered that the designation of malaria as a 'social disease' was a defeatist stance, 'in effect, 'amount[ing] to waiting until people acquire an active immunity to malaria, . . . [which is] not likely to arise for thousands of years.' 'Was it right,' he asked, revisiting the acrimonious Mian Mir debate two decades earlier, 'that, on such flimsy evidence one of the most illuminating and revolutionary discoveries in medicine should have been condemned and thrown on the scrap-heap as useless to humanity?'[86]

For Watson, acknowledgement of economic dimensions to the malaria problem appeared to threaten progress on vector control efforts. But the 'social disease' designation likely was also read as a slight on the technical skills themselves, a professional affront. If so, Watson was hardly alone. Earlier in 1929 an even more heated refutation of the Malaria Commission's 'social' perspective on the world malaria problem had come from septuagenarian Ronald Ross, in a letter to the editor of the *Journal of Tropical Medicine and Hygiene*.

An absurd notion has been ventilated in the lay press to the effect that the way to prevent malaria fever is to feed the natives more copiously. We should all like to see them better fed, but doubt much whether they will acquire malaria any less in consequence than before. . . . The present propaganda . . . [can] be seen to be sufficiently ridiculous when we remember that the Europeans and soldiers in the tropics acquire much malaria in spite of being very well fed as a rule. One wonders how such notions obtain any entry into the British Press at all. The cost of a 'free breakfast table' for all the natives in any colony would probably exceed the cost of any anti-mosquito campaign a hundred times.[87]

By the late 1920s, in other words, the two streams of malaria workers were at loggerheads, and as in India two decades earlier, disagreement was now also spilling over into the public domain.[88] Once again, the analytic fault line lay in the definition of the malaria 'problem' – infection (transmission) versus 'pernicious' malaria morbidity – a line that generally distinguished those workers with years of experience in colonial service who were responsible for malaria policy in large administrative areas 'for the long haul' and required a broad epidemiological approach, and those who held roles as short-term technical advisors on specifically limited assignments.[89]

Inevitably perhaps, the Malaria Commission reports would be criticized by vector control researchers as biased against anti-mosquito programs.[90] The charge, however, was open to question. In the case of the 1930 report on malaria in India, for example, the Malaria Commission had unequivocally recommended anti-larval programs in areas where considered technically and financially feasible: in urban areas and industrial sites. Indeed, its one area of pointed criticism of malaria control efforts in India had been directed to insufficient funding for larval-control programs in the major urban centres of the country, citing the failure of the anti-*An. stephensi* campaign in municipal Bombay.[91] Vector control clearly was not being ignored, but nor were observations on the significance of economic conditions.

Working in an institutional setting where diplomatic consensus was imperative, however, meant that members of the Malaria Commission were reluctant to allow economic conclusions, deemed by critics as 'political,' to jeopardize the ongoing functioning of the League of Nations Health Organisation (LNHO), and above all its largest single source of funding, the Rockefeller Foundation.[92] Subsequent reference to economic dimensions of the malaria burden would be expressed in ever more nuanced ways, now within the more abstract rubric of 'social medicine.'[93] At the same time, those very voices increasingly were being replaced by younger cohorts from newly established institutions of hygiene and tropical medicine but often without extended rural epidemiological experience. Work within the Malaria Commission itself through the 1930s was directed largely to the not unimportant field of anti-malarial drug research. Moreover, by the later 1930s, the Italian approach of 'bonaficazione,' Litsios suggests, came to be ' "classified" as fascist and, thus an inappropriate model,'[94] a taint which overlooked the fact that the dramatic decline in malaria death rates in much of the country associated with quinine distribution and economic reclamation work under Celli had predated Mussolini's statist drainage of the Pontine marshes south of Rome.[95] Meanwhile, the umbrella Health Organisation of the League of Nations had turned its attention through the Depression years to questions of dietary quality, as we have seen, and away from issues of quantitative hunger. By 1949 the first comprehensive malaria textbook, *Malariology*, edited by M.F. Boyd, contained only two passing references to the existence of the League of Nations Malaria Commission. In neither case were its study tour reports mentioned, nor any aspect of their content.[96] Among the compendium's 1,500 pages, only a single contributor sought to bring the historical experience of 'fulminant' malaria into analytic view, in a chapter contributed by Christophers himself.[97]

Curiously, the work of the League of Nations Malaria Commission has continued to receive little historiographic attention, despite the professional prominence and extensive field experience of many of its study tours' participants.[98] The Malaria Commission is remembered instead largely in terms of the professional divisions between malaria workers on different sides of the Atlantic, rather than the epidemiological content of its study tour observations from which those differing opinions arose. Moreover, its assessment of malaria work in India remains virtually invisible historiographically, a reflection perhaps of how little attention in general has yet been directed to the South Asian colonial malaria literature[99] – and to malaria mortality history more generally.[100]

As for the malaria-blocks-development thesis itself, it would rise again phoenix-like from the ashes of WW2 destruction and into the halls of the emergent World Health Organization, now freed of the 'social medicine' constraints of an abandoned League of Nations Health Organisation. Ironically enough, in this resurgence, Russell's brief malaria work in India in the later 1930s would come to play a pre-eminent role, despite the limited track record of Rockefeller malaria control work in India. More ironically still, it would be Russell himself who carried, for reasons of timing and war-time geopolitical circumstance, the mantle of South Asian malaria experience, now MBD-transformed, into the WHO's Expert Committee on Malaria, an account of which is traced in the chapter that follows.

## Notes

1 A. Balfour, and H.H. Scott, *Health Problems of the Empire: Past, Present and Future* (New York: Henry Holt, 1924), 195, 232.
2 *Annual Report of the Public Health Commissioner with the Government of India*, 1924, 99, 102.
3 I. Galdston, 'Humanism and Public Health,' *Bulletin of the History of Medicine*, 8, Jan. 1940, 1032–1039; E. Ackerknecht, 'Hygiene in France, 1815–1848,' *Bulletin of the History of Medicine*, 22, 1948, 117–155.
4 Anon. ['from a special correspondent'], 'The Need for a Public Health Policy for India,' *Indian Medical Gazette*, Oct. 1927, 575–582, at 575 [hereafter, *IMG*].
5 The disability-adjusted life year is a measure of overall disease burden, an estimate of years lost due to ill-health, disability, or early death. See, e.g., the 1993 World Development Report; World Bank, *Investing in Health* (New York: Oxford University Press, 1993) for application of DALY methodology. For critique of underlying assumptions of the measure, see, e.g., M. Rao, *Disinvesting in Health: The World Bank's Prescriptions for Health* (Delhi: Sage, 1999).
6 Anon., 'The Need for a Public Health Policy,' 575.
7 Editorial, 'The Economic Factor in Tropical Disease,' *IMG*, 57, Sept. 1922, 341–343. See above, ch. 1, at note 17.
8 Anon. 'The Need for a Public Health Policy.'
9 W. King, 'Sanitation in Politics,' *Science Progress [in the Twentieth Century]*, 18 (1923/24), 113–125, at 123–124.
10 S. Zurbrigg, *Epidemic Malaria and Hunger in Colonial Punjab* (London and New Delhi: Routledge, 2019), ch. 8.
11 R. Ross, *The Prevention of Malaria*, 2nd ed. (London: John Murray, 1911).
12 The doctrine, according to later Rockefeller Foundation president Raymond Fosdick, was articulated by Frederick Gates, principal administrative aide to the Foundation; R. Fosdick, *History of the Rockefeller Foundation* (New York: Harper Bros., 1952), 23.

13 Regarding the exceptional entomologic conditions giving rise to holoendemic malarial transmission in areas of sub-Saharan Africa, see J.L.A. Webb, *Humanity's Burden: A Global History of Malaria* (New York: Cambridge University Press, 2009), 27–41.

14 R. Senior White, 'Studies in malaria as it affects Indian railways,' Indian Research Fund Association, Technical Paper, No. 258 (Calcutta: GOI, Central Publication Branch, 1928).

15 S.R. Christophers, and C.A. Bentley, *Malaria in the Duars. Being the Second Report to the Advisory Committee Appointed by the Government of India to Conduct an Enquiry Regarding Blackwater and Other Fevers Prevalent in the Duars* (Simla: Government Monotype Press, 1909), 12. The measure of 'prosperity' intended here of course was one belonging to a pre-modern era where the definitional bar was set low: conditions where birth rates exceeded death rates. It did not mean there was no mortality attributable directly to malaria.

16 W.H.S. Jones, *Malaria: A Neglected Factor in the History of Greece and Rome* (London: Macmillan, 1907). Baron and Hamlin highlight overt racial dimensions to Western analysis of the 'great malaria problem'; C. Baron, and C. Hamlin, 'Malaria and the Decline of Ancient Greece: Revisiting the Jones Hypothesis in an Era of Interdisciplinarity,' *Minerva*, 52, 2015, 327–358, at 331.

17 See ch. 1, note 17.

18 Great Britain, *Report of the Royal Commission on Agriculture in India* (London: HMSO, 1928), 481–482; Appendix III, 155[hereafter *RCAI*].

19 *RCAI*, 492–493.

20 J.A. Sinton, 'What Malaria Costs India, Nationally, Socially and Economically,' *Records of the Malaria Survey of India*, 5, 3, Sept. 1935, 223–264 [hereafter, *RMSI*]; Sinton, *RMSI*, 5, 4, Dec. 1935, 413–489; Sinton, *RMSI*, 6, 1, Mar. 1936, 92–169.

21 Sinton, 'What Malaria Costs India,' *RMSI*, Sept. 1935, 225.

22 Sinton, 'What Malaria Costs India,' *RMSI*, Dec. 1935, 424.

23 J.A. Sinton, League of Nations. Health Organisation, 1932. Document No. CH./Mal.202; reprinted in 'Rice Cultivation in Spain, with Special Reference to the Conditions in the Delta of the River Ebro,' *RMSI*, 3, 3, June 1933, 495–506. Sinton's 194-page 'What Malaria Costs India' monograph includes three pages on anti-malarial 'bonification' work; *RMSI*, Mar. 1936, 131–133.

24 'Malaria is very intense in the Terai, which is the belt of low, swampy, forest ground at the foot of the Himalaya mountains . . . [with] silted-up beds and debouchures of rivers . . . land in which watercourses have been obstructed'; Sir Joseph Fayrer, *On the Climate and Fevers of India* (London: J&A Churchill, 1882), 23, 41; T.W. Tyssul Jones, 'Malaria and the Ancient Cities of Ceylon,' *Indian Journal of Malariology*, 5, 1, Mar. 1951, 125–134.

25 In 1961, Indian officials enthusiastically pointed to an additional 130,562 acres brought under agricultural production in Punjab following initiation of the DDT malaria eradication program, an area of 14 miles square representing 0.2 per cent of the plains of pre-Partition Punjab; *Malaria Eradication in India* (New Delhi: Indian Central Health Education Bureau, GOI Press, 1961), 15, as cited in A.L.S. Staples, *The Birth of Development: How the World Bank, Food and Agriculture Organization, and World Health Organization Changed the World, 1945–1965* (Kent, OH: Kent State University Press, 2006), 172.

26 Soper employed a similar strategy, R. Packard and P. Gadelha suggest, by representing the arrival of *An. gambiae* in Brazil as a threat to all of the Americas, a claim subsequently disputed by leading Brazilian entomologist Dr. Leonidas Deane; 'A Land Filled with Mosquitoes: Fred L. Soper, the Rockefeller

Foundation, and the *Anopheles gambiae* Invasion of Brazil,' *Parassitologia*, 36, 1–2, 1994, 197–213.

27  Sinton, 'What Malaria Costs India,' *RMSI*, Sept. 1935, 224.

28  Ibid., 252–255.

29  J.A. Sinton, 'What malaria costs India,' *RMSI*, Dec. 1935, 457, 459–460 [emphasis added]. Curiously, Sinton cites his Spain study only once, in relation to problems of quinine cost but not to his key insights into migrant labour conditions and need for economic support for workers during extension of cultivation; 'Rice Cultivation in Spain,' 142.

30  J.A. Sinton, 'What Malaria Costs India,' *RMSI*, 6, 1, Mar. 1936, 91–169, at 159.

31  Editorial, 'The Economic Factor in Tropical Disease.' A 1924 *IMG* editorial hints at the shift in process. Listing malaria as the leading 'scourge of India,' it concluded that '[t]hough it is true that poverty begets disease, and that disease again begets further poverty, yet the general economic condition of the masses in India is to-day distinctly in advance of what it was fifteen years ago'; 'On the Seven Scourges of India,' *IMG*, July 1924, 351–355.

32  P.J. Brown, 'Malaria, Miseria, and Underpopulation in Sardinia: The "Malaria Blocks Development" Cultural Model,' *Medical Anthropology*, 17, 3, May 1997, 239–254.

33  King's 1924 treatise on malaria as key obstacle to India's economic development was phrased explicitly in terms of the 'drain upon India'; 'Sanitation in Politics.' His critique offered the British Raj a more convenient explanation of the 'drain' on India's economy, a 'natural' one of vectors and ecology, rather than the fiscal drain of revenues [tribute] back to London stressed in earlier anti-imperial tracts such as Dadabhai Naoroji's *Poverty and Un-British Rule in India* (London: Swan Sonnenschein & Co, 1901); Romesh Chunder Dutt, *The Economic History of India under Early British Rule* (London: Kegan Paul & Co., 1906).

34  David Rieff describes a similar dynamic in modern-day humanitarianism: 'the contest for limited resources and contracts feeds the imperative to "trumpet" . . . worst-case scenarios . . . for acquiring a substantial "market share" of each humanitarian crisis'; *A Bed for the Night: Humanitarianism in Crisis* (New York: Simon & Schuster, 2003), 228.

35  Rockefeller Foundation international public health work was undertaken by the International Health Commission (1913–1916), renamed the International Health Board (IHB) in 1916 and the International Health Division (IHD) in 1927.

36  S.N. Kavadi, *The Rockefeller Foundation and Public Health in Colonial India, 1916–1945, A Narrative History* (Pune and Mumbai: Foundation for Research in Community Health, 1999).

37  Kavadi's detailed account of the Rockefeller Foundation's involvement in British India notes IHB rejection of an official Bengal funding request for anti-malarial activities by the Central Cooperative Anti-Malarial Society of Calcutta. In 1926, Christophers's request for assistance in locating malaria personnel to join the Central Research Institute for malaria work in India was also rejected; Kavadi, *Rockefeller Foundation and Public Health*, 76–78. See also J. Farley, *To Cast Out Disease: A History of the International Health Division of the Rockefeller Foundation, 1913–1951*, (New York: Oxford University Press, 2004).

38  Kavadi, *Rockefeller Foundation and Public Health*, 16, 18–50, 53.

39  D. Fisher, 'Rockefeller Philanthropy and the British Empire: The Creation of the London School of Hygiene and Tropical Medicine,' *History of Education*, 7, 2, 1978, 129–143, at 129, 130, 136, 142, 143. By 1937, the LSHTM was providing teaching or research facilities for 422 students from 27 countries. In this way,

Fisher observes, 'the Foundation helped preserve both life and capital in Britain and her Empire and laid the ground for the increasing investment of American capital in the underdeveloped world'; ibid., 129, 142–143.

40 Editorial, 'An Imperial School of Hygiene,' *The Lancet*, Mar. 4, 1922, 441. The appointment of Andrew Balfour as the new school's first director was a perfect match: malaria, he pronounced in 1924 was 'sapping life and energy' from colonial populations; Balfour, *Health Problems of the Empire*, 232. His admiration for the Foundation's anti-hookworm campaigns was unabashed:

> Even when it began to dawn upon the medical world that hookworm disease was a foe to be fought upon a large scale, the various British Governments did next to nothing, and it was left to the Americans to conceive the idea of a world campaign against the insidious enemy, and, furnished with the sinews of war by John Rockefeller, to embark upon one of the most remarkable enterprises recorded in the history of hygiene; ibid., 195.

The text was written, Harrison suggests, 'largely to convince British and colonial administrations of the economic utility of medical intervention'; M. Harrison, *Public Health in British India: Anglo-Indian Preventive Medicine 1859–1914* (Cambridge: Cambridge University Press, 1994), 3.

41 Editorial, 'Public Health and Medical Research in India,' *British Medical Journal*, Apr. 14, 1923, 640.

42 'We need not humble ourselves and go hat in hand as beggars, all that is needed is to invite the Foundation to send a commission to enquire into the needs of India. . . . the conditions attached to the gifts are such that countries like England have not hesitated to take full advantage of the benefactions of the Foundation'; Editorial, *IMG*, Apr. 1924, 195–196.

43 Kavadi, *Rockefeller Foundation and Public Health*, 94.

44 See note 32, above.

45 C.A. Gill, *The Genesis of Epidemics and the Natural History of Disease* (London: Bailliere & Co, 1928), 93 [emphasis in original].

46 S.R. Christophers, 'What Disease Costs India' – Being the presidential address at the Medical Research Section of the Fifth Indian Science Congress, *IMG*, Apr. 1924, 196–201, at 200.

47 Ramasubban highlights the impact of the post-WW1 fiscal predicament in shifting medical research back to tropical medicine institutes in Britain, a legacy which continues with the 'tendency . . . to rely on foreign and international agencies'; R. Ramasubban, *Public Health and Medical Research in India: Their Origins under the Impact of British Colonial Policy* (Stockholm: SIDA, 1982), 42–43.

48 Kavadi, *Rockefeller Foundation and Public Health*, 32; S. Hewa, 'The Hookworm Epidemic on the Plantations in Colonial Sri Lanka,' *Medical History*, 38, 1994, 73–90, at 84–87.

49 Kavadi observes 'a carbon tetrachloride-chenopodium mixture was known to be efficient but it was not known to be safe'; *Rockefeller Foundation and Public Health*, 47, 136; S.N. Kavadi, ' "Wolves Come to Take Care of the Lamb": The Rockefeller Foundation Hookworm Campaign in the Madras Presidency, 1920–29,' in E. Rodríguez-Ocaña, ed., *The Politics of the Healthy Life: An International Perspective* (Sheffield: European Association for the History of Medicine and Health, 2002), 89–111.

50 Kavadi, *Rockefeller Foundation and Public Health*, 50.

51 V. Heiser, in *A Doctor's Odyssey: Adventures in Forty-five Countries* (London: Jonathan Cape, 1937), as quoted in Kavadi, *Rockefeller Foundation and Public Health*, 16.

52 Farley, *To Cast Out Disease*, 27.

53 Editorial, 'Hookworm in India,' *IMG*, May 1928, 261–265, at 261–262; Asa Chandler, 'The Prevalence and Epidemiology of Hookworm and Other Helminth Infection in India, *Indian Journal of Medical Research*, 15, Pt. XII, 1928, 695–743.

54 Editorial, 'Hookworm in India,' 264–265.

55 Kavadi, *Rockefeller Foundation and Public Health*, 40. For parallel critique of the Rockefeller Foundation hookworm and malaria campaigns in Latin America, see Marcos Cueto, 'The Cycles of Eradication: The Rockefeller Foundation and Latin American Public Health, 1918–1940,' in Paul Weindling, *International Health Organisations and Movements, 1918–1939* (Cambridge: Cambridge University Press, 1995), 222–243, at 228; M. Cueto, *Cold War, Deadly Fevers: Malaria Eradication in Mexico, 1955–1975* (Baltimore: Johns Hopkins University Press, 2007); M. Cueto, and S. Palmer, *Medicine and Public Health in Latin America: A History* (New York: Cambridge University Press, 2015). A larger goal, Rockefeller officials acknowledged, was convincing the public 'that the government has a real interest in [their] welfare, health and happiness. Tuberculosis control, on the other hand, was routinely rejected because "it takes too many years to show results"'; A.-E. Birn, and A. Solórzano, 'The Hook of Hookworm: Public Health and Politics of Eradication in Mexico,' in A. Cunningham, and B. Andrews, eds., *Western Medicine as Contested Knowledge* (Manchester: Manchester University Press, 1997), 147–171, at 163.

56 *Annual Report, 1915* (New York: Rockefeller Foundation, 1915), 12; cited by S. Franco-Agudelo, 'The Rockefeller Foundation's Antimalarial Program in Latin America: Donating or Dominating?,' *International Journal of Health Services*, 13, 1, 1983, 51–67, at 54. S.P. James, too, would ponder the irony of Rockefeller Foundation anti-malarial projects in 39 areas of eastern and southern Europe 'when so much has been left undone in the tropics'; in Presidential Address, 'Advances in Knowledge of Malaria Since the War,' *Transactions of the Royal Society of Tropical Medicine and Hygiene*, 31, 3, Nov. 1937, 263–280, at 274.

57 See note 37.

58 Malaria pharmacotherapeutic research within the LNMC also was ignored by the Rockefeller Foundation; James, 'Advances in Knowledge of Malaria,' 274.

59 Kavadi, *Rockefeller Foundation and Public Health*, 78; Kavadi, 'Wolves Come to Take Care,' 104.

60 P.F. Russell, 'Malaria in India: Impressions from a Tour,' *American Journal of Tropical Medicine*, 16, 6, 1936, 653–664, at 663. Twelve years earlier Balfour had also acknowledged the costliness of anti-mosquito measures that in many areas did 'not justify the expense,' recognizing that such measures were feasible only in enclave settings; *Health Problems of the Empire*, 237, 249. See also Kavadi, *Rockefeller Foundation and Public Health*, 81. In 1942 Russell would qualify his 'pessimism' based on later work with pyrethrum . . . at per capita costs around $0.08 per year; P. Russell, F.W. Knipe, and T.R. Rao, 'Epidemiology of Malaria with Special Reference to South India,' *IMG*, 77, 1942, 477–479.

61 Russell, 'Impressions from a Tour,' 661.

62 Proceedings of the Water-logging Board, Punjab, Dec. 6, 1930, 'Principles to be observed in the preparation of canal projects and in their execution,' *RMSI*, 3, 2, Dec. 1932, 269–270; P.F. Russell, 'Malaria due to defective and untidy irrigation,' *Journal of the Malaria Institute of India*, 1, 4, 1938, 339–349; W.C. Sweet, 'Irrigation and malaria,' *Procs. Nat. Inst. Sci. Ind.*, 4, 1938, 185–189.

63 Russell, 'Malaria due to Defective and Untidy Irrigation,' 342.
64 It would later be acknowledged that the technique 'may interfere with the growth of rice crops and the question is one which requires further investigation'; *Famine Inquiry Commission (1945) Report on Bengal*, Pt. II (New Delhi: GOI, 1945), ch. 6, 'Malaria and Agriculture,' 170–175, at 173.
65 Russell, 'Impressions from a Tour,' 662.
66 P.F. Russell, and M.K. Menon, 'A Malario-economic Survey in Rural South India,' *IMG*, 77, Mar. 1942, 167–180, at 179.
67 Causes of unemployment in 1946–1947 for West Bengal agricultural labourers were estimated at 3.1 per cent for sickness, 8.2 per cent for 'want of work' and 9.1 per cent for 'miscellaneous'; 1951 *Census of India*, VI West Bengal, Pt. I-A, 98. At the same time, the Russell study was silent on the possibility that access to irrigation substantially reduced seasonal hunger and may well have outweighed the wages lost due to more frequent malaria infection. Unconsidered as well was the likelihood of labour inefficiencies entailed with wage levels often below subsistence levels, or that debt-servicing costs are likely to have been highly skewed against the poorest households.
68 Kavadi, *Rockefeller Foundation and Public Health*, 92.
69 Ibid., 94, 109. Unlike in China where the limited presence of Western medical institutions allowed a free hand to the Foundation in establishing Peking Union Medical College, in India negotiations would drag on for years over how such public health training would be integrated into existing medical training facilities and who would be in control. Proposed initially in 1923 by the All-India Conference of Medical Research Workers, and recommended in 1927 by the IHD as a teaching and research institute, the institute was inaugurated only in December 1932. Thereafter relations were fraught with administrative dissatisfaction on both sides. On intra-professional tensions between European and Indian membership on the AIIHPH Governing Body, see D. Arnold, 'Colonial Medicine in Transition: Medical Research in India, 1910–47,' *South Asia Research*, 14, 1, 1994, 10–35, at 27–28.
70 S. Amrith, *Decolonizing International Health: India and Southeast Asia, 1930–65* (Basingstoke: Palgrave Macmillan, 2006), 104.
71 Kavadi, *Rockefeller Foundation and Public Health*, vi, 94, 109.
72 In the case of mosquito control programs, Amrith notes gently satirical reaction to such projects in Phanishvarnath Renu's 1954 novel, *Maila Anchal. The Soiled Border* (Delhi: Chanakya Publ., 1991); *Decolonizing International Health*, 122.
73 Kavadi, *Rockefeller Foundation and Public Health*, 92, citing R.B. Watson of the Rockefeller Foundation in his 1946 India tour. See also V.R. Muraleedharan, and D. Veeraraghavan, 'Anti-malaria Policy in the Madras Presidency: An Overview of the Early Decades of the Twentieth Century,' *Medical History*, 36, 1992, 290–305.
74 Kavadi, *Rockefeller Foundation and Public Health*, 92, 137.
75 GOI, *Report of the Health Survey and Development Committee* (New Delhi: GOI Press, 1946), vols. 1 & 2.
76 See also ch. 3 at note 15 for the influence of the Rockefeller-funded AIIHPH on 'nutritional' thought. Perhaps the most valuable IHD work in India was in nurse training, a health field of otherwise markedly low status, although here too public health nursing appears to have been directed primarily to disease-transmission interventions and maternal (behavioural) education.
77 Kendrick to Sawyer, October 28, 1925, cited in Kavadi, *Rockefeller Foundation and Public Health*, 49–50.
78 Kavadi, *Rockefeller Foundation and Public Health*, 50. In 1929, 489 Punjab villages were treated with carbon tetrachloride; *PPHA 1929*, 2; *PPHA 1934*,

19. This, though Forster had testified one year earlier that the 'hookworm is not a disease of any consequence in Punjab' (*RCAI*, vol. 8, 524), a conclusion supported by the Chandler study that had found a 'fairly high incidence (60 to 70%) of very light infections . . . along the eastern and northern borders of the Punjab . . . but infections severe enough to be of pathogenic significance are practically unknown'; Chandler, 'The prevalence and epidemiology of hookworm,' 717.

79 Kavadi, *Rockefeller Foundation and Public Health*, 44.

80 P.F. Russell, 'Some Social Obstacles to Malaria Control,' *IMG*, Nov. 1941, 681–690.

81 GOI, *Famine Inquiry Commission (1945) Report on Bengal* (New Delhi: GOI, 1945), Pt. II. 'Death and Disease in the Bengal Famine,' ch. VI 'Malaria and Agriculture,' 170–175, at 171.

82 P.F. Russell, 'Some Aspects of Malaria in India,' Jul. 5, 1941, as cited in Farley, *To Cast Out Disease*, 123.

83 P.F. Russell, L.S. West, and R.D. Manwell, *Practical Malariology* (Philadelphia: W.B. Saunders, 1946), 541.

84 R. Packard, and P.J. Brown, 'Rethinking Health, Development, and Malaria: Historicizing a Cultural Model in International Health,' *Medical Anthropology*, 17, 1997, 181–194, at 184. Patrick Zylberman similarly describes the 'widening gulf' that had emerged between what he has termed 'American malariology' and the 'social malariology of a European ilk'; 'A Transatlantic Dispute: The Etiology of Malaria and Redesign of the Mediterranean Landscape,' in S.G., Solomon, L. Murard, and P. Zylberman, eds., *Shifting Boundaries of Public Health: Europe in the Twentieth Century* (Rochester: University of Rochester Press), 2008, 269. According to Lewis Hackett's notes to the Rockefeller Foundation, the 33 attendants at a June 1928 'special meeting of critics and advocates' of the second Malaria Commission report quickly fell into two groups: 'mitigators' and 'eradicators'; as cited in H. Evans, 'European Malaria Policy in the 1920s and 1930s: The Epidemiology of Minutiae,' *ISIS*, 80, 1989, 40–59, at 51. Hackett similarly described the gulf as between 'the Anglo-Saxons' and the 'Europeans'; 'Address by Dr. Lewis W. Hackett,' *Proceedings of the Fourth International Congress on Tropical Medicine and Malaria* (Washington, D.C., May 10–18, 1948), 10–15.

85 S.P. James, 'The Disappearance of Malaria from England,' *Proceedings of the Royal Society of Medicine*, 23, 1929–30, 71–87, at 84–85.

86 M. Watson, 'The Lesson of Mian Mir,' *Journal of Tropical Medicine and Hygiene*, Jul. 1, 1931, 183–89 at 189. On the Mian Mir 'debate' and its significance for colonial malaria policy, see Zurbrigg, *Epidemic Malaria and Hunger*, 12–13, 210–212; W.F. Bynum, 'An Experiment that Failed: Malaria Control at Mian Mir,' *Parassitologia*, 36, 1994, 107–120.

87 R. Ross, 'Malaria and Feeding,' *Journal of Tropical Medicine and Hygiene*, May 1, 1929, 132.

88 Zurbrigg, *Epidemic Malaria and Hunger*, 242–245.

89 Litsios describes Fred L. Soper, a quintessential Rockefeller vector 'eradicationist,' as one who 'prided himself on having made the word eradicate "respectable once more" . . . . His world was a world of action . . . there was little room in that world for "esoteric" issues such as the relationship between malaria control and agriculture. He believed in getting a specific job done with the conviction that job would contribute to the wider good, however "good" was defined'; *The Tomorrow of Malaria* (Wellington, NZ: Pacific Press, 1996), 78. Worboys also notes in early twentieth-century Britain the 'relative decline in the influence of epidemiology signalling declining interest in social factors, as disease was

constituted in relations between bacteria and individual bodies'; M. Worboys, *Spreading Germs: Disease Theories and Medical Practice in Britain, 1865–1900* (Cambridge: Cambridge University Press, 2000), 285.

90 P.F. Russell, *Man's Mastery of Malaria* (London: Oxford University Press, 1955), 202, 204–205. In his generally appreciative summary of the work of the LNMC, L. Bruce-Chwatt also interpreted its reports as 'prejudice[d] . . . show[ing] a regrettable neglect of anti-anopheline methods of control'; 'History of Malaria from Prehistory to Eradication,' in W.H. Wernsdorfer, and I.A. McGregor, eds., *Malaria: Principles and Practice of Malariology* (Edinburgh: Churchill Livingstone, 1988), vol. 1, 1–60, at 41.

91 LNMC, *Report of the Malaria Commission on its Study Tour of India* (Geneva: League of Nations, 1930), 74 [hereafter, LNMC, India report].

92 For details on Rockefeller Foundation funding of the LNHO, see M.D. Dubin, 'The League of Nations Health Organisation,' in Weindling, *International Health Organisations*, 56–80, at 72. Already in the case of the 1927 U.S. study tour, where deep differences in perspective existed between the socio-economic and vector control interpretation of malaria decline in the country, a compromise of sorts had resulted in no official report being issued; James, 'Advances in Knowledge of malaria since the War,' 266. Yet even within the Rockefeller Foundation itself there were individual consultants who by the late 1920s had come to address a broader economic understanding of the malaria burden. I.J. Kligler's study of malaria in Palestine, for example, pointed clearly to the primacy of economic conditions in malarial epidemiology. 'Malaria may be classified among the social diseases of a country,' he concluded, 'most prevalent and of greater severity in countries of low social and economic status'; *The Epidemiology and Control of Malaria in Palestine* (Chicago: University of Chicago Press, 1928), 12.

93 W. Schüffner, 'Notes on the Indian Tour of the Malaria Commission of the League of Nations,' *RMSI*, 11, 3, Sept. 1931, 337–347, at 339. Yet the central importance of economic and agrarian conditions in relation to the malaria health burden would continue to be documented; J.A. Sinton, 'Rice cultivation in Spain.' For an overview of 'social medicine' thought of this period, and its subsequent sidelining in the early years of the WHO, see J. Farley, *Brock Chisholm, the World Health Organization, and the Cold War* (Vancouver: University of British Columbia Press, 2008), 111–118.

94 Litsios, 'Malaria Control, the Cold War,' 267.

95 Malaria deaths declined from an estimated 16,000 per year in 1900 to 2,045 in 1914; F. Snowden, *The Conquest of Malaria: Italy, 1900–1962* (New Haven: Yale University Press, 2006), 89, 120. Malaria mortality appears to have declined from the later nineteenth century, along with general death rates. Nájera shows funding for 'land reclamations' to have begun as early as 1901 and that for mass quinine distribution in 1904; ' "Malaria Control" Achievements, Problems and Strategies,' *Parassitologia*, 43, 2001, 1–89, at 12; A. Celli, 'The restriction of malaria in Italy,' in *Transactions of the Fifteenth International Congress on Hygiene and Demography, Washington, September 23–28, 1912* (Washington, D.C., 1913), 516–531, at 529–530.

96 M.F. Boyd, ed., *Malariology: A Comprehensive Survey of All Aspects of This Group of Diseases from a Global Standpoint* (Philadelphia: W.B. Saunders, 1949), 22, 698, 1470. In his 1955 text, Russell devotes 10 pages to the LNMC's anti-larval work, expresses regret over the Commission's emphasis on 'epidemiology and drugs,' and in a single-sentence reference to the India study tour report points to inadequate urban anti-mosquito measures; *Man's Mastery of Malaria*, 198–208.

97 S.R. Christophers, 'Endemic and Epidemic Prevalence,' in M.F. Boyd, ed., *Malariology* (Philadelphia: W.B. Saunders, 1949), ch. 27, 698–721.

98 Siddiqui notes the India study tour report but mirrors Russell's 1955 assessment of the LNMC; *World Health and World Politics*, 128. Litsios provides perhaps the most specific account of the LNMC policy dispute; *The Tomorrow of Malaria*, 56–69. Curiously, in a later overview of pre-eradication era malaria control work, the LNMC is omitted; S. Litsios, 'Malaria Control and the Future of International Public Health,' in E. Casman, and H. Dowlatabadi, eds., *The Contextual Determinants of Malaria* (Washington, D.C.: Resources for the Future, 2002).

99 Among the few references to the India study tour report, William Bynum notes its 'striking' conclusions regarding the 'economic and social dimensions' to the malaria problem in both Bengal and Punjab; 'Malaria in inter-war British India,' *Parassitologia*, 42, Jun. 2000, 25–31, at 29–30. Gordon Harrison refers to the European and U.S. study tours of the LNMC but not that to India, interpreting LNMC reluctance to embrace the anti-mosquito approach as 'defeatist,' 'pessimis[tic],' and 'close-minded,' and overlooking the Italian success in 'removing the terror' of malarial infection; *Mosquitoes, Malaria, and Man: A History of the Hostilities since 1880* (London: John Murray, 1978), 185.

100 An important exception appears in the work of José A. Nájera, where the decline in the 'pernicious' form of malaria well in advance of the DDT era is discussed for a number of regions in Europe; J.A. Nájera, *Malaria Control: Achievements, Problems and Strategies* (Geneva: World Health Organization, 1999), 10–31. See also, Farley, *To Cast Out Disease*, 114–118.

# 6

# MALARIA AND THE W.H.O.

## The 'Human Factor' set aside

The seminal role played by malaria activities in shaping the nascent World Health Organization following the Second World War has been highlighted in recent historiography of the agency. This important work has explored the backgrounds of key medical figures selected in early 1947 as initial members of an Expert Committee on Malaria (ECM), as well as the larger geopolitical context and interests underlying the choice of malaria as an initial focus for the emergent organization.[1] Several key questions within this work however remain largely unexplored: how decisions regarding expert input came about in the formative deliberations taking place in late 1946; the empirical evidence underlying inclusion of global malaria transmission control within the initial mandate of the new organization; and above all for the purposes of this study, what pre-existing epidemiological understanding of malaria was set aside in the process. How was it that the wealth of earlier insights arrived at by the League of Nations Malaria Commission into the socio-economic determinants of malaria's global 'burden' – a good portion derived from South Asian epidemiological experience[2] – came to be circumvented in the two-year interval leading up to the convening of the first World Health Assembly in June 1948? This chapter considers the events of this formative period of the World Health Organization that, beginning in late 1946, constitute the final stage of the abandonment of the 'Human Factor' in twentieth-century Western malaria thought.

## Beginnings: UNRRA and the Interim Commission

In the wake of the dissolution of the Geneva-based League of Nations and its Health Organisation over the course of WW2, public health advisors from 18 member countries of the fledgling United Nations Economic and Social Council (ECOSOC) met in Paris in March 1946 to establish a successor global health organization.[3] A provisional body, the Interim Commission (IC), was constituted in July of that year,[4] tasked with setting out a structure and preliminary program of work for the new agency while awaiting final ratification by member countries and formal inauguration as the World Health Organization in 1948. One of the first tasks of the Interim Commission was the establishment of an Epidemiology and Quarantine Committee, mandated to assume the international epidemic surveillance work which the United Nations Relief and Rehabilitation Administration (UNRRA) had taken over from the League of Nations Health Organisation (LNHO) in 1944 at the invitation of the U.S. government.[5] This was quickly followed by deliberation on the global health issues to be taken up by the organization on a priority basis.

Among the several issues selected by the Interim Commission was a DDT-based anti-malaria program.[6] Widespread media reporting of war-time successes in typhus control employing the new 'miracle' insecticide (dichloro-diphenyl-trichloro-ethane) had already fanned professional aspirations for global extension of malaria control. DDT had become 'one of the heroes of the war, heralded and praised in as many as twenty-one thousand newspaper articles by the end of the war . . . reportedly saving some five million lives by 1950.'[7] By early 1947, preliminary success with DDT-based malaria control in U.S.- and UNRRA-funded demonstration projects in Venezuela, Italy, and Greece had won over many Interim Commission delegates to the possibility of eradicating the disease globally. Adding to the euphoria was a general sense of optimism engendered by the new medical technology developed during and leading up to the war: among the 'magic bullet' discoveries were synthetic anti-malarial medicines, antibiotics such as penicillin, and in 1943 the anti-tuberculosis antibiotic, streptomycin.

But acceptance of malaria control as an urgent priority for WHO derived also, it is argued in this chapter, from a carefully constructed strategy on the part of the handful of malaria workers already engaged in the above anti-malarial projects. The initial proposal for an Expert Committee on Malaria was submitted at the second meeting of the Interim Commission on November 6, 1946 by Arnoldo Gabaldón, director of the DDT-based malaria program initiated under U.S. direction in Venezuela. From the earliest days Gabaldón had aspired to the goal of malaria eradication for his country. But he also recognized that effective control required eradication well beyond its borders, a realization that likely underlay his enthusiasm for a global program.[8]

More crucial, still, in the Interim Commission's acceptance of the malaria control mandate was the role of UNRRA as initial funding source for the provisional WHO. The agency had been proposed in June 1943 by U.S. President Roosevelt, anxious to pre-empt a replay of the mass starvation, epidemics, and revolution that had followed in the wake of WW1.[9] Established as a temporary body in late 1943 by the 44 non-occupied Allied Nations, UNRRA provided $3.8 billion in food and medical supplies to liberated populations in the final days of WW2 and immediate post-war period to help alleviate widespread hunger and typhus, venereal disease, and tuberculosis epidemics among the war-torn regions of Europe and China.[10] Its activities were funded by member countries at the rate of 1 per cent of GDP. However, given the size of the U.S. war economy and the catastrophic economic destruction in the war theatres of Europe, the agency's activities were highly dependent on U.S. contributions, funding that was itself conditional on year-to-year Congressional approval. UNRRA staffing was headed by the New York State Governor, Herbert H. Lehman, as Director General, while the key post of Director of the Health Division was held by Wilbur A. Sawyer, former Director of the International Health Division of the Rockefeller Foundation. Under Sawyer, health funding was directed to short-term relief, sufficient to avert 'disease and unrest,'[11] rather than to longer-term economic reconstruction.[12]

With the establishment of the Interim Commission in June 1946, the UNRRA administration announced its intention to wind down its activities and to transfer all the agency's remaining funds to the new emerging UN institutions.[13] The decision presented the Interim Commission with the urgent obligation of assuming, in addition to UNRRA's epidemiological surveillance functions, its ongoing medical operations. Despite objections from some IC delegates that 'only the epidemiological work of UNRRA should be assumed by the Commission,' UNRRA officials made the transfer of its funds conditional on maintaining all of the agency's existing health activities 'without interruption.'[14]

During the final years of the war, experimental DDT malaria control activities had been conducted in military theatres in southern Italy and the Pacific, undertaken by the Allied military command.[15] At the close of the war, UNRRA, under Sawyer, immediately extended DDT-based malaria control programs to civil war–torn Greece,[16] and to Sardinia in April 1946.[17] Thus, included in the UNRRA mandate handed to the fledgling Interim Commission in mid-1946, alongside tuberculosis and venereal disease control activities were civilian DDT spray programs in several countries.

Up to this point, malaria does not appear to have figured prominently in initial Interim Commission discussions on global epidemic conditions. Nor was malaria included among the diseases listed by the Interim Commission in early November 1946 as requiring 'expert missions to countries with special needs.'[18] Indeed, at a subsequent IC meeting on November 13, the Norwegian delegate queried spending so much of the Commission's very limited resources on one disease, and the French and British delegates questioned the urgency, and the idea itself, of eradicating malaria in the world.[19] But with much of Europe and the Soviet Union preoccupied with relief and reconstruction, U.S. influence in the shaping of the new UN institutions in these early post-WW2 days prevailed.[20] U.S. delegate to the IC, A. Doull, also a former senior UNRRA official, strongly urged formation of a special expert malaria committee, to be financed through UNRRA funds, while Sawyer opined that 'the malaria programme [in Greece and Italy] had been extremely popular and that eventually complete control might be possible.'[21]

In the event, in addition to assuming ongoing responsibility for the existing DDT-based malaria control programs, other conditions came attached to the offer of a portion of the UNRRA funds being directed to the Interim Commission. Activities 'would be limited to countries already receiving UNRRA assistance,'[22] with additional but very limited funding going to finance small groups of 'consultative' experts as envisaged in Gabaldón's 'nuclear' malaria committee. Sawyer also stipulated that '[n]either UNRRA nor the Interim Commission should be responsible for financing the importation or purchase of supplies.'[23] Thus, all supplies required for malaria activities undertaken by WHO would require external funding through bilateral arrangements, ultimately occurring primarily through U.S. government agencies.[24] A minimalist size and framework to the Expert Committee on Malaria was ensured by the total level of funding, $1.5 million, offered for continuation of all UNRRA health activities, a sum representing barely 10 per cent of the annual UNRRA health program expenditures for 1946. Of this, less than one-tenth was allocated to malaria 'consultations and assistance.'[25] The bulk of residual UNRRA funds was channelled instead to the newly created United Nations International Children's Emergency Fund (UNICEF).[26]

With the WHO charter still awaiting U.S. ratification, there appeared to be little choice but to accept the UNRRA terms if the Interim Commission was to continue to function. On November 6, 1946, Gabaldón presented a formal proposal for the establishment of an expert committee on malaria, to 'speed up the diffusion of new methods of control' for a disease that 'remained a scourge.'[27] Although few details on the post-war priority of malaria were included in the Gabaldón proposal,[28] the Committee on Epidemiology and Quarantine one week later 'agreed unanimously that the problem of malaria was sufficiently urgent and important to warrant immediate action' and the decision was taken to 'appoint a Sub-committee of five experts to study and advise on the important problem . . . and submit a report.' On December 31, 1946, UNRRA officials formally handed over responsibility for its 'field health activities,' and assigned US$1.5 million to the Interim Commission.[29]

The 'nuclear' committee on malaria[30] so formed in the early days of 1947 would soon be named the Expert Committee on Malaria (ECM), and would formally meet for the first time in April 1947. But well before its first official meeting, the future WHO had already been placed on an institutional course that would lead nine years later to the global Malaria Eradication Program (MEP). In the process, the precedent of purely 'technical assistance' and a narrowly constituted expert advisory framework for the new organization had also been established.

## The Expert Committee on Malaria

Scant details appear in the official records of the Interim Commission regarding the selection process of initial members of the Expert Committee on Malaria. Even less clear is the basis upon which Emilio Pampana himself came to be elected as convenor and secretary of the Expert Committee on Malaria. Described as 'an exceptional administrator,' Pampana had served as a staff member of the Health Organisation of the League of Nations, and more recently as Health Bureau Director of the U.S. League of Red Cross Societies. His epidemiological malaria experience however appears to have been primarily industrial-enclave in nature, as medical officer to a Colombian mining population in the mid-1920s.[31] Nonetheless in the early weeks of 1947, with his strong 'pro-DDT sentiments' and 'staunch' support of eradication plans,[32] Pampana was appointed to the permanent WHO. IC Secretariat as secretary to what would soon formally become the Expert Committee on Malaria, his first task that of 'suggest[ing] names for a pre-paratory [malaria] group.'[33]

The five members of the ECM appointed included Paul Russell of the Rockefeller Foundation, Arnoldo Gabaldón, N. Hamilton Fairley (UK), a senior military officer during the war in charge of testing new synthetic anti-malarial drugs among Allied troops, and Mihai Ciuca, a Romanian malaria researcher and former Secretary to the League of Nations Malaria Commission. A fifth seat was reserved for a USSR representative who had 'not yet been appointed.' Officially, Expert Committee members were cho-sen by the Executive Director of the Interim Commission, Brock Chisholm. As a psychiatrist, however, Chisholm was hardly in a position to question the candidacy of prominent figures such as Russell and Gabaldón who were among the few malaria workers with substantial DDT experience. Before transferring funds to the Interim Commission, UNRRA officials had stip-ulated that ECM members be chosen 'for their technical proficiency and experience.'[34] On leave from the Rockefeller Foundation during the final years of WW2, Russell as Chief Malaria Officer for the Allied Forces had coordinated the initial DDT-based malaria and typhus control programs in southern Italy and the Pacific, experience that made him a leading candi-date for appointment to the new committee. In recommending candidates for ECM membership, Pampana consulted with Dr Melville Mackenzie of the U.K. Ministry of Health, and with Dr Thomas Parran, U.S. Surgeon-General and former General of the U.S. Army, the latter also likely to strongly support candidates committed to global DDT-based eradication plans.[35]

Organizationally, the structure and functioning of the ECM – its small size and requirement that members be 'free to attend' twice yearly meetings[36] – also favoured independently funded figures such as Russell. Funded by the International Health Division of the Rockefeller Foundation, Russell was not bound by demanding national official responsibilities – arguably a situ-ation inherently favouring candidates working in corporate philanthropic agencies. J. Jackson offers detailed insights into the backgrounds and per-sonalities of each of the members of the Expert Committee on Malaria (the 'epistemic community'), as well as the limits imposed from the beginning on

ECM deliberations. He describes a 'forsaking [of] research,' a 'ridiculing' of alternative (earlier) approaches to malaria control, and notes how 'the epistemic community used their individual prestige to insert the DDT gospel into the technical forums of the WHO.'[37]

At its first formal meeting in April 1947, four of the five members of the new committee were in attendance, the absence of a USSR representative possibly one of the early casualties of the rapidly emerging Cold War: one month earlier, President Truman had announced the U.S. doctrine of Communist 'containment.'[38] Gabaldón was elected as Chairman, with Pampana as Secretary to the committee. Listed as 'also present' at the April 1947 ECM sessions were J.M. Vine, UNRRA medical director in Greece and author of a report on the recent DDT anti-malaria operations there,[39] and N.M. Goodman, former UNRRA Director of the European Health Division, and now Director of Field Services, WHO.

The official report of the first meeting of the Expert Committee on Malaria, held April 22–25, 1947, set out a spare description of the future functions and organization of the Committee. Prefaced with a description of malaria as 'one of the world's greatest afflictions,'[40] malaria was presented as an urgent priority, threatening 'doubtless . . . severe epidemics,' and 'the greatest obstacle in the way of the objective of the World Health Organization.' But with the new insecticides and anti-malarials, the report stressed, 'malaria epidemics can be stopped effectively and quickly when a suitable organization and the supplies are available': the advent of 'new era' technologies meant that 'malariology has come of age.'[41] Few data however accompanied the report's assessment of malaria as 'the world's greatest affliction,' an omission only marginally made up a year later in a 'Note by the [IC] Secretariat.' The latter cited, unreferenced, a global figure of 3 million malaria deaths a year and an estimated 1 per cent case mortality rate for malaria,[42] alongside a 1936 statement by J.A. Sinton, former Director of the Malaria survey of India, that malaria cost India 'unbelievable millions of pounds Sterling each year.'[43]

Missing also from the ECM proceedings was a definition of what 'malaria control' constituted: whether it meant reduction or global elimination of malaria transmission (infection), or illness (morbidity), or malaria mortality.[44] Though a question central to the work of the League of Nations Malaria Commission only 15 years earlier, and to malaria policy in India before that, by mid-1948 such distinctions appeared to many as no longer relevant: the dramatic power of DDT to interrupt malaria transmission was already evident in Greece and Italy, as well as U.S.-funded programs in Venezuela. Thus in skirting discussion of the meaning of malaria 'control' in these formative years, deliberations foreclosed the possibility of epidemiological experience informing post-war malaria policy.[45]

## First meeting of the ECM, April 1947

A sense of how basic decisions were made within the Expert Committee on Malaria can be gleaned from 'summary minutes' of the first meeting, the only ECM session for which minutes of the proceedings appear to be available.[46] A dominant theme to the proceedings quickly emerged. Earlier approaches to malaria control were now outdated. 'In the past,' Fairley noted, 'it was customary for malariologists to be satisfied with a state of premunity in malarious countries; their aim was to prevent the devastating mortality of epidemics. Now it is different.'[47] Previous policy of the League of Nations Malaria Commission (LNMC) that had focused on preventing severe illness and mortality from malaria was explicitly set aside. Limiting goals to mortality prevention was now imbued with a tone of professional negligence. The new tools had opened up possibilities for 'malaria control and even of practical eradication . . . unthinkable in pre-war days.'[48] A subsequent 'Note by the [IC] Secretariat,' perhaps penned by Pampana, suggested that the 'new synthetic drugs and insecticides have . . . revolutionized malaria control . . . [and] raised hopes of the complete eradication of the disease – even of anopheles – from entire countries.'[49]

Moreover, with Gabaldón's November 1946 proposal 'taken as a basis for the discussion,'[50] the agenda for the first meeting of the Expert Committee on Malaria had evidently been set in advance. From the outset, demonstration and dissemination of DDT-based control methods was assumed to be the centrepiece of WHO malaria activities. Through the course of the three days of meetings, Ciuca would attempt to incorporate perspectives from earlier LNMC research activities in areas such as chemotherapeutics and local entomological studies of insecticide efficacy. But in each case his suggestions were dismissed or left unanswered in the recorded minutes, Russell at one point opining that 'the present Malaria Committee should not necessarily take over the functions of the old League of Nations Malaria Commission but should determine its own policy in relation to present conditions.'[51] Dr N. Goodman, former UNRRA official and an observer to the meeting, urged attention instead be directed to the 'really urgent work . . . such as getting out publications and reports in relation to DDT for the benefit of those countries which had been out of touch with the latest developments.'[52]

Ciuca also advocated for a larger membership for the Expert Committee, arguing that 'the various problems [associated with malaria] are so different that it was necessary to choose the members according to their competence in the matters discussed,' reminding his colleagues that the LNMC had been made up of 'some 50 members.' Here too, however, Russell prevailed, recommending a six-member committee for the first two years, with subsequent expansion to nine members.[53]

Most perplexing perhaps for Ciuca, given earlier emphasis on the risk of post-war malaria epidemics, was the response of the committee to his resolution requesting supplies of anti-malarial medication for an epidemic in the

Tulcea district of Romania, the single example of post-war epidemic conditions cited by committee members in earlier discussion of malaria urgency.[54] His request, relegated to the final ('Miscellaneous') agenda item, elicited tepid interest. When the Committee secretary suggested Ciuca present more details at the subsequent meeting of the Interim Commission set for the following September, Chisholm as IC Executive Secretary and an observer to the April 1947 ECM meeting, interceded. '[I]t was not necessary to wait,' he suggested, and offered the services of his office to vouch for an application to the League of Red Cross Societies for anti-malarial drugs.[55] But by this point any confidence Ciuca might still have had in the Expert Committee's interest in malaria control beyond DDT is likely to have been shattered. A narrow DDT framework to the remainder of the deliberations was ensured by the Committee 'proceeding point by point' through Gabaldón's DDT-framed proposal.[56]

In the event, the second meeting of the Expert Committee on Malaria convened only in April 1948. Again, the USSR chair was vacant, but this time so also was that of the Romanian delegate, Ciuca.[57] Without specific expertise in DDT there now seemed perhaps little purpose to participation.[58] Even in relation to basic chemotherapeutics, ECM policy was constrained. Ciuca would go on to conduct clinical trials of chloroquine and paludrine in the epidemic area of his country with the drugs supplied by the Red Cross. But despite the inclusion in the first ECM report of a thorough overview by Fairley of the efficacy of recent synthetic anti-malarial drugs and a detailed outline of further drug trials required, no action on drug testing was taken by the ECM, '[o]wing to the absence of funds for the purpose.'[59] By the following year's meeting, Fairley had resigned from the Expert Committee, and priority had unequivocally been accorded anti-mosquito work over therapeutics: 'the primary consideration in the communal control of malaria,' the Committee asserted, 'is interruption of transmission *at the mosquito level*.'[60] At its third meeting, in 1949, the ECM formally advised leaving anti-malarial drug research to 'existing institutions,' an area of malaria research consistently eschewed also by the Rockefeller Foundation in its inter-war malaria work in India.[61] In the meantime, a new Expert Committee on Insecticides had been formed in response to the emerging problem of vector resistance, a potential problem flagged as early as January 1948 in Greece with observed DDT-resistance among houseflies.[62]

Thus in the earliest days of the formative WHO, the Expert Committee on Malaria assumed an organizational and programmatic structure that lent little space to broader views and approaches to the malaria problem.[63] Earlier epidemiological perspectives on underlying determinants of the malaria burden explored earlier by the LNMC were expressly set aside, and along with them, the colonial South Asian literature as well.[64] Several Interim Commission delegates had attempted earlier on 'to ensure representations of various schools of thought and experience' in the formation of expert committees, but this recommendation subsequently was deleted at the suggestion of the

Indian and Mexican delegates.[65] Here, added irony attaches to the fact that Ciuca, as Secretary to the former LNMC, had participated in the Commission's study tour of India less than two decades earlier and had co-authored its ensuing report.

Even with respect to DDT, the purpose of the program drawn up by the ECM in these early years was intended solely as demonstration. Funding was limited to expert consultancy costs. Like the Rockefeller Foundation before it, the goal was one of paradigm building, not service or supplies provision. The role of the WHO and its Expert Committee on Malaria was one of disseminating technical advice, with most funding coming through bilateral agreements. Such funds, coming almost entirely from the U.S. at this point, were directed largely to regions of the world aligned with its strategic interests.[66] 'In postwar history,' James Gillespie observes, 'UNRRA has been relegated to a footnote, written off as a temporary experiment in international enthusiasm, of interest mainly as the site of some of the opening manoeuvres of the cold war.' To the contrary, he suggests,

> UNRRA's Health Division was the theatre for a complex battle over the future direction of international health work. . . . UNRRA's field operations, especially in health, drew on models developed by the Rockefeller Foundation's International Health Division during the interwar years, and became the progenitor of fieldwork in the UN system. . . . International health became one arm of the struggle by the United States and its allies to build stable, politically sympathetic regimes on the periphery.[67]

It was a legacy destined to continue.

## The 1948 U.S. proposal

At the second meeting of the Expert Committee on Malaria in May 1948, membership had expanded to include D.K. Viswanathan, then intensely involved in DDT-spray operations in Kanara district, India, and M.A. Vaucel, of France; with Gordon Covell, a former director of the Malaria Survey of India, now a U.K. delegate, taking the place of N.H. Fairley. At this meeting, too, the agenda had largely been set in advance. Four months earlier, a 'US Proposal' had been presented to the Interim Commission by U.S. delegate H. Van Zile Hyde that added a new dimension to the argument for urgent malaria control, one that framed the WHO malaria task in much more explicit terms of malaria as a block to economic development.[68] Aside from being the 'the prime world health problem' in itself, the proposal asserted that

> the direct suffering caused by malaria is multiplied by the hunger and malnutrition resulting from lowered food production in

malarious areas. Malaria is a direct and important contributing cause of the current world food shortage. . . . This situation is *being allowed to continue* in the face of new discoveries of major importance in the field of malaria control.[69]

The Van Zile Hyde submission concluded that 'the WHO should direct a major share of its energy and resources during its first years to the application of [malaria control] measures to . . . the major food-producing areas afflicted by malaria.'[70]

Dated January 23, 1948, the U.S. proposal contained other advisements. The Interim Commission, it suggested, 'should seek the opinion' of the Food and Agriculture Organization (FAO) in selecting agricultural regions for demonstrating the impact on agricultural productivity of a 'mass attack' on malaria, and went on to recommend a collaborative joint FAO-WHO Working Party on Food Production and Malaria Control.[71] Three days later, the IC Secretariat embraced the proposal's arguments, submitting a draft resolution in near identical language for consideration by the World Health Assembly at its inaugural meeting the following June. Concurring that malaria 'impoverishes the world,' the Secretariat urged that '[a]t a time when the world is poor, it seems that control of malaria should be the first aim to achieve in order to increase agricultural output, . . . [and] entrusts to its Expert Committee the study of a general plan for world malaria control.' It further recommended that 'a major share in the WHO's energy and resources during its first years be directed [to malaria],'[72] and endorsed the U.S. proposal for ECM collaboration with the FAO. Included was a detailed budget for joint ECM-FAO 'malario-economic surveys' in selected areas to document the health and economic benefits of malaria control.[73] 'Everybody knows,' the draft resolution suggested, ramping up the professional onus, 'what has been achieved in selected areas of such countries, once malaria has been controlled.'[74] Thus well before the second meeting of the ECM, the U.S. proposal had pre-emptively framed malaria as a major contributing cause of world hunger and 'block' to global development.

As the single malaria worker on the Secretariat of the Interim Commission, it seems likely Pampana played a major role in shaping the Interim Commission's response to the U.S. January proposal – though it is unclear where the procedural precedents lay for this direct submission of a proposal to the Interim Commission by a single member government rather than through the Expert Committee on Malaria. Nonetheless, the ECM at its second official session in May 1948 'heartily endorse[d]' the view that malaria 'directly contributes to the world shortage of food.' To the U.S. proposal's argument for urgent anti-malarial action, the expert committee added 'wide-spread . . . mental and physical deterioration . . . [and] serious loss of working efficiency.' One week earlier, in his address to the Fourth International Congresses on Tropical Medicine and Malaria held in Washington,

D.C., U.S. Secretary of State George Marshall had added a further argument for urgent action on malaria control: the 'profound' impact of the disease in undermining of 'any hopes of social stability.'[75]

The relationship between the May 1948 Malaria Congress in Washington and the ECM is an interesting one. At the first ECM meeting one year before, Russell had piloted a resolution ensuring an invitation for ECM members to attend the 1948 Congress, with the Committee's second malaria meet scheduled to follow one week later.[76] Indeed, the U.S. 'proposal' in January 1948 specifically called on the ECM to seek advice 'in consultation' with the International Congress on Malaria, part of the larger conference where Marshall, soon to unroll what would come to be known as the Marshall Plan, gave the opening address,[77] and where DDT-based malaria control practitioners, including Indian delegate D.K. Viswanathan, reported their initial results.[78] With Sawyer as Executive Secretary of the Malaria Congress and still actively directing the anopheles eradication campaign in Sardinia, the portion of the Congress agenda devoted to malaria not surprisingly was heavily weighted toward recent experience with DDT.[79]

But the January 1948 U.S. proposal contained yet a further directive. It requested a clear 'statement of commitment' from the ECM 'in regard to such an attack [on malaria].'[80] It is difficult to read the request as stemming from doubts on the part of the U.S. IC delegates about the technical merits of the DDT 'demonstration' projects proposal. More likely, broader 'commitment' to an insecticide-based global malaria control program was being sought by U.S. members in the face of lingering doubts amongst other national delegations about the priority and feasibility of such a plan. At the sixth meeting of the Fifth Session of the Interim Commission, on January 27, 1948, the Soviet representative, for example, had called for 'speedy case-finding' and treatment of malaria cases alongside spray programs and 'hydraulic sanitation.' British and French delegates had in turn warned of the 'danger . . . of giving the impression that the Organization was attempting world control of malaria. That was quite impossible.'[81] With the WHO constitution still awaiting U.S. ratification, endorsement by the U.S., along with its funding contribution, appears to have hinged upon unequivocal commitment by Interim Commission member states to the vector eradication approach to malaria control in advance of the first official meeting of the World Health Assembly set for the following June.[82]

Included also within the U.S. proposal, moreover, was a request for endorsement of collaboration with the Food and Agriculture Organization. By this point the FAO, inaugurated in 1945, was already involved in a major global campaign to increase food production. As Litsios highlights, it was 'politically expedient' on the part of the ECM to garner support from the increasingly UN-prominent FAO, collaboration that would enhance both the scientific credibility of the MBD thesis underlying the WHO's call for urgent malaria control, and the humanitarian profile of the WHO. Short on analytic or methodological detail, the only empirical evidence the U.S. proposal cited for its argument that malaria was a barrier to global food production and development was Russell's 1942 South Indian malario-economic study.[83] Evidence to the contrary was ignored. In the case of Punjab, for example, the malaria transmission associated with canal irrigation across the colonial period had not 'blocked' cultivation expansion where basic care was taken to avoid waterlogging.

The FAO delegate on the joint FAO-WHO Working Party on Food Production and Malaria Control would be W.R. Aykroyd, recently appointed to head the FAO's nutrition division. Familiar with at least some of the larger dimensions of the hunger problem in India through his earlier work in India at the Coonoor nutrition laboratory, Aykroyd expressed some doubts about malaria eradication as a major route to increased food production, suggesting 'other hindrances to efficient production' such as 'lack of capital or credit . . . [and] systems of land tenure and taxation.'[84] Nevertheless, the joint WHO-FAO study proposal was adopted on February 5, 1948, by the Interim Commission at its Fifth Session.[85] Some governments no doubt were swayed by Marshall's promise of 'social stability' through removal of the malarial 'brake' on food production. Others, it appears, were reluctant to jeopardize U.S. engagement in the new WHO. U.S. cooperation in purely technological programs at least, would foster, it was hoped, the 'habit' of participation in the wider UN process and advance prospects for world peace.[86] Thus in June 1948 at the first World Health Assembly of the newly ratified WHO, a global 'demonstration' program of malaria control based on residual insecticide spraying was formally endorsed.[87]

In the event, little visibility would accrue to the project's subsequent failure to document any substantive evidence regarding the impact of malaria control on agriculture.[88] The FAO quietly withdrew from the joint study in 1953 and the project withered away – though not before the MBD thesis arguably had helped derail the pre-WHO momentum within the new UN institutions for addressing deeper structural causes of poverty, global hunger, and food insecurity.[89]

## Post-war hunger politics

That an urgent international food crisis existed in the final years of WW2 and immediate post-war days is beyond dispute. But it was not one induced by malaria. Depression unemployment had already brought hunger concerns to the fore in the committee halls of the League of Nations Health Organisation and the ILO through the 1930s, as we have seen.[90] With the outbreak of war at the end of the decade, war-induced hyperinflation dramatically compounded difficulties in food access globally, triggered by military foodgrain demand throughout the European and colonial theatres of war, as witnessed so catastrophically in India in 1942 and 1943. Even before the 1943–1944 Bengal famine, Roosevelt was acutely attuned to a possible repeat of the starvation, epidemics, and revolution triggered in the aftermath of WW1, as seen with the establishment of UNRRA. In a further effort to pre-empt similar events, Roosevelt had invited Allied governments in 1943 to a conference at Hot Springs, Virginia, to deliberate on coordinated efforts, beyond emergency relief measures, to '[p]revent . . . speculative and violent fluctuations in the prices of food . . . [and] conditions of scarcity that appear certain to prevail after the war.' In addition to formation of UNRRA, the Hot Springs initiative laid the groundwork for establishment of the FAO in 1945.[91]

Earlier LNHO concern over global conditions of agriculture and hunger with the Depression already had been directed primarily to issues of supply (foodgrain availability) and micronutrient quality of foodstuffs rather than to structural determinants of low productivity, or inadequate and insecure *access* to available staple foods. Crisis conditions during the war, however, had forced far more explicit acknowledgement of the consequences of unregulated foodgrain markets in terms of price volatility and epidemic mortality.[92] Resolutions coming out of the Hot Springs conference in 1943 stressed 'the dominant role played by *adequate* food in the reduction of sickness and death rates,' in turn warning that 'the most fundamental necessity . . . required to promote freedom from disease . . . [was] adequate food.' Proposed solutions lay overwhelmingly in the sphere of increased purchasing power, it was argued. This was to be achieved through expansion of 'the whole world economy.'[93]

> It is useless to produce more food unless men and nations provide the markets to absorb it. There must be an expansion of the whole world economy to provide the purchasing power sufficient to maintain an adequate diet for all. With full employment in all countries, enlarged industrial production, the absence of exploitation, an increasing flow of trade within and between countries, an orderly management of domestic and international investment and currencies, and sustained internal and international economic equilibrium, the food which is produced can be made available to all people.[94]

Issues of 'social security' also were raised at the Hot Springs meet, as were underlying structural issues such as control of global foodgrain speculation, the need for buffer grain stocks, agricultural credit, and land reform. Clearly, the Hot Springs deliberations were an ideological battle ground. Ultimately, however, the measures adopted were set largely in neo-liberal terms of free trade, 'enlarged industrial production,' and scientific advances in agriculture and promotion of 'protective foods,' a technological framework that would largely come to shape the subsequent work of the FAO.

In its final recommendations the 1943 conference acknowledged that '[a]gricultural productivity and efficiency and the well-being of the tiller of the soil depend largely upon the system of land tenure and conditions of farm labour'; but these were qualified as voluntary or short-term measures, the report advising 'each nation . . . [to] make a careful survey of existing systems of land tenure . . . to ascertain whether changes in these systems and conditions are necessary or desirable.'[95] Nevertheless, the Hot Springs conference marked a moment of exceptional political (and professional) transparency, one where the curtain was pulled back on the primacy of hunger in determining epidemic mortality[96] – akin in one sense to the publication of *Malaria in the Punjab* three decades earlier in British India.

Recognition of the importance of public policy on foodgrain regulation was of course a matter of acknowledging facts on the ground. Over the course of the war the dire food crisis had forced governments to take unprecedented measures to control foodgrain prices and ensure access by public rationing. Food distribution policies had been embraced in Britain and in many other countries at war, if tragically belatedly in India. Such wartime conditions had also prompted calls for permanent measures to insulate populations from the vagaries of international grain markets through a world system of buffer foodgrain stocks. On October 16, 1945, 42 countries met in Quebec City to create the Food and Agriculture Organization on the basis of the resolutions from the Hot Springs conference. John Boyd Orr, a leading U.K. nutritionist responsible for Britain's school-milk program, was appointed founding director-general, Western delegates perhaps assuming him to be a 'moderate' head for the agency. The dire late- and post-war food situation[97] however had turned Orr's attention sharply from dietary qualitative issues to the glaring question of staple food sufficiency (acute hunger). Riding a tide of deep public anxiety, Orr recommended a policy of global foodgrain reserves as a central goal for the FAO, one that would give the emerging 'united nations' system the capacity to actively buffer international foodgrain price fluctuations and then-rampant commodity speculation. The call for an international buffer foodgrain system (World Food Bank) however would soon be overridden by U.S. and U.K. delegates who together succeeded in limiting Orr's tenure to a two-year term as FAO director-general.[98]

It was in this mid-1940s period of extraordinary international engagement in, and contestation over, questions of global food security that the WHO (IC) was also taking shape. With the backdrop of unparalleled political and economic failings – the 'unprecedented carnage'[99] of two European imperial wars, a world-wide economic depression, and decolonization and revolution ushering in sweeping shifts in global political relationships – it was thus also a point where, for Western governments, ideological hegemony and boundaries had appeared seriously vulnerable: a period of political contestation within countries as much as between them.[100] The wars and the

Great Depression had left North Atlantic societies ripe for alternate symbols of accomplishment and sources of belief.

But the same wars had also thrown up dramatically powerful new technologies. 'Good news' in the ashes of 1945 lay in the optimistic promise of science. With DDT, here was a demonstration of science and technology used for social good, to advance civilization, decrease suffering and deaths, and to relieve the tedium and exhaustion of laborious work. Thus by enjoining the FAO to collaborate with the WHO in documenting the economic benefits of DDT-based malaria control, the U.S. joint-study proposal in January 1948 in effect was attempting to harness the tide of Western scientific humanism to the malaria eradicationist cause via MBD.[101]

Paul Russell may not have been closely conversant necessarily with the fierce contest between Orr and the U.S.-British delegates within the FAO. But positioned at the centre of the new UN institutional processes, it is unlikely he could have been unaware. By engaging the FAO with the DDT campaign, the Expert Committee on Malaria was able to finesse the global food crisis issue at the close of the war. Appropriating the prevailing sense of crisis to the cause of DDT-malaria control, it strategically harnessed the FAO's new profile of competency to buttress the malaria eradicationist argument as an alternate route to food production security,[102] thereby redirecting attention away from the underlying structural determinants of hunger and related ill-health.

## Global eradication questioned: the Kampala Conference, 1950

A food security rationale to the Expert Committee on Malaria's global eradication project arguably was necessary for other reasons as well. For as momentum for malaria control drew to its 'logical' conclusion[103] of ultimate global eradication, the ECM faced an even more awkward question. Such a vision inevitably hung on eradication also in the exceptionally intense (holoendemic) malaria transmission areas of west and central sub-Saharan Africa. In this region, the prime mosquito vector, *Anopheles gambiae*, feeds almost exclusively on humans rather than animals, resulting in almost daily infective bites in many areas. Such extreme inoculation rates induce high levels of protective *acquired* immunity among the adult population, but intense infection rates in the as yet non-immune infants and young children, amongst whom the malaria mortality impact is considerable. Attempts at control of malaria transmission in this context thus raised serious questions: among them, the possible consequences of undermining high levels of acquired immunity in regions where permanent eradication could not be guaranteed for reasons of prohibitive long-term costs and likely re-introduction of infection from surrounding rural tracts.[104]

In November 1950, members of the Expert Committee on Malaria, now nine in number, joined colonial malaria workers with extended African malaria experience to debate in Kampala, Uganda, the wisdom and feasibility of extending the WHO malaria control program to include holoendemic Africa. Deliberations between the two groups, not surprisingly, were marked by intense disagreement. As something of a compromise, an experimental malaria transmission control project was agreed upon for the Pare-Taveta region of Tanzania and bordering Kenya: the goal to assess the impact on mortality levels of transmission control, and of subsequent malaria 'rebound' with discontinuation of spray operations in a population where acquired immunity levels likely had declined.[105] Yet without waiting for the results of the trial, the ECM continued to argue for a 'global' eradication program,[106] and its proposal would subsequently be endorsed at the Eighth World Health Assembly in 1955.[107]

The many complex ethical and technical questions raised by the early trials of residual insecticide spray operations at Pare-Taveta and other hyper- and holoendemic regions of Africa, at the time unresolved, involve a subject well beyond the scope of this study. They have recently, however, begun to be revisited in historiographic analysis.[108] Here, one can simply note the considerable irony at play in Russell's strong advocacy at Kampala, alongside Macdonald's, for residual-insecticide malaria eradication efforts in Africa – policy that could be predicted to reduce protective levels of acquired immunity – while in contemporaneous academic writing both workers continued to interpret the 'notorious' malaria epidemics in India to be a function of declining acquired immunity.[109]

## The 'Human Factor' set aside

The reductive triumph of the Expert Committee on Malaria within the nascent World Health Organization between 1946 and 1948 lay in two spheres. First, international malaria policy formation was divested of any lingering association with the 'social medicine' leanings of the former League of Nations Health Organisation, the latter based on understanding of the role of hunger as a major determinant of malaria's lethality burden. The global Malaria Eradication Program thus came at the expense of any serious consideration of alternate, or additional, approaches to malaria 'control' such as ensuring access to effective anti-malarial medication and addressing subsistence and livelihood precarity.[110]

Second, through the joint FAO-WHO project that framed malaria as a block to agricultural development, the Expert Committee on Malaria had succeeded in wresting institutional attention to hunger away from its structural determinants and the para-United Nations agencies attempting to address issues of livelihood.[111] It would thus leave health advocacy solidly in the technological and behavioural domains rather than in the economic arena of working conditions, resource disparities, and international grain markets, issues the ILO and a minority of FAO members were attempting to address. The joining of WHO-FAO in a malaria-agriculture alliance in the earliest days of the IC-WHO effectively sealed the technological framework to post-war international cooperation in the field of health, and a U.S. prominence within it.

Like the Rockefeller Foundation before it, the ECM agenda involved paradigm building, not service or supply provision. The opportunity to forge a practical and encompassing approach to malaria globally thus would be deferred a half-century. Also deferred was the possibility of turning human subsistence, and the foodgrains upon which it depended, from a tool of geopolitical influence[112] and coercion to an expression of common humanity and tool of peace.[113] Staples observes that with regard to removing global foodgrain supply from economic power politics, 'this road was not taken. . . . Instead, the countries of the world slid into the Cold War, and food remained just another trade commodity, just another weapon in the superpowers' arsenal.'[114] By 1949, she notes, the issue of land tenure was sidelined from the FAO's agenda, as also rural agricultural credit for small farmers, and supplanted by largely voluntary and often equally abstract 'community development.'[115] Amrith describes parallel efforts of the U.S. to remove health as an enforceable 'right' within the UN's Commission on Human Rights, leaving 'technical assistance . . . as a *substitute* for rights,'[116] and the definition of human health in the covenants of the WHO shorn of socio-economic context.

The reductive triumph in understanding of human health that took place within the formative World Health Organization was not wholly attributable to the Expert Committee on Malaria. Nor was Russell alone in viewing malaria, and health more generally, as simply a technological problem. A parallel shift was taking place in many academic realms, as seen in the emergence of nutritional science. Yet in his long-term influence on the Expert Committee, Russell nonetheless played a distinctive role in shaping its policies and exerted a dominant influence in the sidelining of a broader perspective on the malaria burden and approaches to malaria 'control.'[117] Though membership was notionally on a rotating basis, Russell would sit on the committee throughout the 1947–1956 period until commitment to a program of global malaria eradication was assured, the only member to do so; Gabaldón was a delegate to four of the six meetings.

Moreover, with respect to the central question of this study, Russell also played a pivotal role in the obscuring of the rich epidemiological literature from colonial South Asia on determinants of malaria lethality.[118] In his 1946 text, *Practical Malariology*, Christophers's study of the 1908 Punjab epidemic was accorded a cameo appearance, but without reference to preceding harvest failure and 'scarcity.' Russell recounted Christophers's observations on the characteristic 'sudden onset' of the epidemic in Amritsar city, but interpreted its lethality in terms of the epidemic 'upset[ting] . . . the entire routine of the city. . . . Food was difficult to obtain and prices became prohibitive,' thus inferring scarcity prices were a consequence of malaria transmission rather than of preceding harvest failure.[119] While secondary debility no doubt was a later aspect to the 1908 Punjab epidemic, such a reading leaves out the key dimension Christophers identified as underlying malaria fulminancy in the province: epidemic (semi-)starvation.[120] Elsewhere in his 1946 text Russell claimed that the commonplace association of epidemic malaria with famine could be explained by ecological conditions triggering enhanced transmission, repeating his earlier assertion that '[a]rmies of well-fed, robust individuals go down with malaria to all appearances just as rapidly and as seriously as any other group.'[121] Nine years later, Russell would publish his influential *Man's Mastery of Malaria*, a history of malaria research and control efforts. Indian malaria research would figure prominently in the accompanying 24-page bibliography. Yet among the more than 500 references listed, both *Malaria in the Punjab* and *Malaria in the Duars* were missing, as also Bentley's studies on malaria and agriculture in Bengal – though the collection did include two 1866 *Indian Medical Gazette* articles on the use of cobwebs to treat malaria fever.[122]

It stretches credulity that Russell had not come across the earlier work of Bentley, or was not aware of the economic content of *Malaria in the Punjab*, findings cited in much of the Indian malaria literature through to the late 1930s. One can only speculate about the reasons that impelled him to omit Christophers's economic conclusions, and in the case of Bentley his entire body of epidemiological analysis of malaria and agriculture in Bengal.[123] Russell may have genuinely believed that the omissions were justified in the belief that 'social' science was not true science – though here one might have expected that cobweb treatment of malaria might have merited similar omission. Whatever the reasoning for Russell personally, within the span of a single generation of malaria workers, recognition of an historical role for hunger in shaping the mortality burden of malaria had essentially vanished from the post-WW2 medical literature.[124]

## 'Not a policy to be recommended'

Even in the earliest days of DDT-euphoria in the new World Health Organization, there were many who were uneasy with a purely microbiological understanding of the malaria problem and who warned against reliance on the singular approach to malaria 'control' emerging within the WHO. One of the more prominent sceptics in India was V. Venkat Rao, a leading malaria researcher whose own career was devoted to devising local, often naturalist, measures of transmission control. In December 1949, Venkat Rao published 'a critical review' of chemical-spray control measures employed to date in the subcontinent, a paper that identified 'a large number of problems' with DDT requiring 'further study,' among them the question of DDT-resistance.[125] Warning against sole reliance on DDT, he argued that 'though eminently suitable for emergencies and during periods in which permanent or biological measures are under way, [DDT] cannot constitute by itself an economic long-term policy of malaria control, even if meanwhile the vector insects do not develop chemico-resistance against its action.'[126] It was a view that presciently predicted present-day Indian policy where chemical spraying increasingly is reserved for serious outbreaks and specific areas of hyperendemic transmission.[127]

But it is in his attention to agricultural conditions that Venkat Rao's broadest insights lay, noting that entomological conditions favourable to malaria transmission were generally associated also with agricultural decline. Here he pointed to the moribund rivers tracts of lower Bengal, and to the waterlogged soils of the Terai, reminding readers that malaria was mainly a disease of poor and economically backward countries: 'a disease of waste land, waste water and waste men.' 'Bonification measures,' he stressed, 'are the best and most effective in the long run as they do not involve the use of chemical larvicides but, on the other hand, include works which gradually raise the economic level of the people and increase their resistance to disease.'[128] Such works were costly, he acknowledged, yet their potential longer-term impact relative to initial costs clearly warranted careful consideration.

In the final paragraphs of his overview, Venkat Rao went further, questioning Russell's dismissal of the importance of 'nutrition' as a factor in the epidemiology of malaria. 'A study of most epidemics,' he pointed out, 'indicates the presence of this economic factor.'

> The great epidemic of 1917 in the U.S.S.R. followed widespread famine caused by a total breakdown of agriculture after the revolution. In Ceylon, failure of the south-west monsoon, which must affect the delicately balanced economy of the people, was the prime factor of the 1934 epidemic. The famines of Bengal and the North Madras Coast in 1942–43 were quickly followed by large-scale epidemics in the affected areas. The chronic low economic conditions of the inhabitants of most hyperendemic areas is too well known to require emphasis. One cannot, therefore, entirely agree with Russell *et al.*, (*loc. cit.*) that susceptibility to infection is not dependent on the state of nutrition.[129]

He concluded by urging 'a fresh approach to the problem of malaria control,' adding '[i]f this paper dispels even to some extent, the popular notion that, after the advent of D.D.T., malaria research has become a luxury and all that needs to be done is only periodical spraying of D.D.T. on the walls, its purpose is served and . . . the author is amply rewarded.'[130]

In his concern over the rush to chemical-based malaria eradication Venkat Rao was not alone. Several delegates at the Interim Commission deliberations, as we have seen, had also questioned, for perhaps varying reasons, the urgent priority directed to eradication of malaria transmission. Six years later, in August 1955, at the height of eradication enthusiasm, an 82-year-old Christophers submitted a characteristically thoughtful article to the *Indian Medical Gazette* highlighting a number of insights gained from malaria control work in the Indian subcontinent. Beginning with a brief section on 'Economic Status' aspects, the paper quietly hinted at key questions missing from the global malaria eradication program about to be embraced formally by the World Health Assembly the following month, and warned against 'smash and grab' approaches to malaria control.[131]

> It is not usually that a country is uniformly malarious, or even that there are not extensive areas where malaria is not a serious problem. . . . On these accounts the urgency or even the desirability of taking action under such conditions has been considered by some authorities to be doubtful. . . . Without some system of ascertaining what areas and communities are in need of action to be taken, wide-scale institution of some particular method of control is not a policy to be recommended.[132]

Christophers had retired from the Indian Medical Service 24 years earlier, and as professor of 'Malaria Studies' at the London School of Hygiene and Tropical Medicine he had gone on to pursue research on malaria chemotherapeutics, quinine, and the new synthetic anti-malarials, an area of malaria research consistently eschewed by the Rockefeller Foundation. Reluctant as ever to directly contradict his medical colleagues, his 1955 paper nonetheless conveyed a deep concern with malaria policy direction.

Here we return, then, to consider at broader levels why the thesis of malaria as a 'block to development' remained so compelling, even in colonial South Asia with its well-documented history of malaria in relation to destitution.

## Notes

1 S. Amrith. *Decolonizing International Health: India and Southeast Asia, 1930–65* (Basingstoke: Palgrave Macmillan, 2006); J. Siddiqui, *World Health and World Politics: The World Health Organization and the UN System* (London: Hurst, 1995); J. Farley, *Brock Chisholm, the World Health Organization, and the Cold War* (Vancouver: University of British Columbia Press, 2008); J. Jackson, 'Cognition and the Global Malaria Eradication Programme,' *Parassitologia*, 40, 1998, 193–216; S. Litsios, 'Malaria Control, the Cold War, and the Postwar Reorganization of International Assistance,' *Medical Anthropology*, 17, 1997, 255–278; R.M. Packard, 'Malaria Dreams: Postwar Visions of Health and

Development in the Third World,' *Medical Anthropology,* 17, 1997, 279–296; R.M. Packard, ' "No Other Logical Choice": Global Malaria Eradication and the Politics of International Health in the Post-War Era,' *Parassitologia,* 40, 1998, 217–229; J.A. Gillespie, 'Social Medicine, Social Security and International Health, 1940–60,' in E. Rodríguez-Ocaña, ed., *The Politics of the Healthy Life: An International Perspective* (Sheffield: European Association for the History of Medicine and Health, 2002), 219–239; A.-E. Birn, 'Backstage: The Relationship between the Rockefeller Foundation and the World Health Organization, Part I: 1940s–1960s,' *Public Health,* 128, 2014, 129–140. For an historical overview of the establishment of the Rockefeller Foundation and early decades of its international health activities and influence, see A.-E. Birn, 'Philanthrocapitalism, Past and Present: The Rockefeller Foundation, the Gates Foundation, and the Setting(s) of the International/Global Health Agenda,' *Hypothesis,* 1, 12, 2014, 1–27, at 1–8.

2  In 1938, for example, the League's Malaria Commission re-published, in full, the Punjab Public Health Department's 1937 policy report on epidemic forecasting, as well as an accompanying memorandum on 'naturalist' anti-malaria measures employed in Punjab. In the province's forecast calculation based on 'quantum of infection' and 'immunity in the population,' the latter was based on child spleen rate and 'state of nutrition as calculated from availability of staple articles of diet in any year'; LNMC, 'Report on The Method of Forecasting the Probably Incidence of Malaria in the Punjab,' Geneva, 28 May 1938, C.H./Malaria/258.

3  The term 'United Nations' was first used in the 'Declaration by United Nations of 1 January 1942' when representatives of 26 nations pledged their governments to continue fighting together against the Axis Powers.

4  World Health Organization, *Official Records of the World Health Organization,* No. 2, 110–12 [hereafter *WHO OR*]. For a concise history of the institutional origins of the Interim Commission and WHO in relation to preceding organizations of the League of Nations Health Organisation and UNRRA, see 'Historical Introduction,' *WHO OR,* No. 9, 20–27. See also Farley, *Brock Chisholm,* 7–26, 48–57.

5  Amrith, *Decolonizing International Health,* 64; N. Howard-Jones, *International Public Health between the Two World Wars – The Organizational Problems* (Geneva: World Health Organization, 1978), 75–79.

6  For discussion of other infective diseases addressed initially, see Farley, *Brock Chisholm,* chs. 8–11.

7  K.S. Davis, 'Deadly Dust: The Unhappy History of DDT,' *American Heritage,* 22, Feb. 1971, 44–47; A.L.S. Staples, *The Birth of Development: How the World Bank, Food and Agriculture Organization, and World Health Organization Changed the World, 1945–1965* (Kent, OH: Kent State University Press, 2006), 162.

8  *WHO OR,* No. 5, 52; P.F. Russell, *Man's Mastery of Malaria* (London: Oxford University Press, 1955), 161; *WHO OR,* No. 8, 9. See also J.A. Nájera, 'Epidemiology in Strategies for Malaria Control,' *Parassitologia,* 42, 2000, 9–24, at 15.

9  'Historical Introduction,' *WHO OR,* No. 9, 23. China under the Kuomintang government was the largest beneficiary, Amrith observes, of UNRRA medical supplies ($117 million); *Decolonizing International Health,* 56. Weindling details parallel interest in 'prevent[ing] socialist uprisings' underlying the American Relief Administration's food aid to central Europe immediately post-WW1; 'The Role of International Organizations in Setting Nutritional Standards in the 1920s and 1930s,' in H. Kamminga, and A. Cunningham, eds., *Science and Culture of Nutrition* (Atlanta, GA: Rodopi, 1995), 319–32 at 320.

10  For the official history of UNRRA, see G. Woodbridge, *UNRRA: The History of the United Nations Relief and Rehabilitation Administration* (New York: Columbia University Press, 1950), 3 vols.

11  UNRRA Papers, British Library of Political and Economic Science (LSE), Committee for Coordination in Far East (44), 11, Sept. 28, 1944, 'Relief Requirements for Certain Areas in the Far East,' quoting a report by the British War Cabinet's Official Committee on Supply Questions in Liberated and Conquered Areas SLAO/ER (44) 16; cited in Amrith, *Decolonizing International Health*, 55–56.

12  J. Gillespie notes that '[a]t the first UNRRA Council, at Atlantic City in 1944, ILO observers, supported by the British delegation, urged that social security organizations, which have survived remarkably intact in all occupied territories except Poland, would be the most efficient method of distributing medical supplies and services. All references to this proposal were dropped however in the final report "in deference to the views of the State Department members of the United States delegation"'; 'Social Medicine, Social Security and International Health, 1940–60,' in E. Rodríguez-Ocaña, ed., *The Politics of the Healthy Life*, 221–222. See also, J. Gillespie, 'International Organisations and the Problem of Child Health, 1945–1960,' *Dynamis: Acta Hispanica Ad Medicinae Scientiarumque Historiam Illustrandam*, 23, 2003, 115–142, at 130. Also, Amrith, *Decolonizing International Health*, 84.

13  T. Patterson, *On Every Front: The Making and Unmaking of the Cold War* (New York: W.W. Norton, 1992), 85, as cited in Litsios in 'Malaria Control and the Cold War,' 269. Farley traces the geopolitical manoeuverings underlying this decision; *Brock Chisholm*, 67–68.

14  *WHO OR*, No. 4, 104–109, 154.

15  Snowden describes '[m]assive welfare spending' of a billion dollars by the Allies and UNRRA in Italy between 1943 and 1947, 'hoping to prevent epidemics, restore the shattered Italian economy, and forestall an outburst of revolutionary activity'; F. Snowden, *The Conquest of Malaria: Italy, 1900–1962* (New Haven: Yale University Press, 2006), 204.

16  M.J. Vine, 'The Malarial Campaign in Greece,' *Bulletin of the WHO*, 1, 1947, 197–204.

17  J. Farley, 'Mosquitoes or Malaria? Rockefeller Campaigns in the American South and Sardinia,' *Parassitologia*, 36, 1994, 165–173. Snowden relates that proceeds from the sale of UNRRA goods provided free to the post-war Italian government were used to fund the DDT spray program (ERLAAS) in Sardinia; F.M. Snowden, and R. Bucala, eds., *The Global Challenge of Malaria: Past Lessons and Future Prospects* (Hackensack, NJ: World Scientific Publishing, 2014), 80.

18  *WHO OR*, No. 4, Minutes of the Second Session of the IC, 4–13 Nov. 1946, 112. The three-volume official history of UNRRA makes only brief reference to DDT use for malaria control in southern Italy and post-war Greece, although extensively used for typhus control; Woodbridge, *UNRRA: The History*, vol. 2, 134–135, 281.

19  IC, Fifth Session, *WHO OR*, no. 7, 23–25. See also Farley, *Brock Chisholm*, 229.

20  Farley, *Brock Chisholm*, 23, 63.

21  *WHO OR*, No. 4, 65, 107.

22  *WHO OR*, No. 4, 108. In June 1946, UNRRA-directed health programs were heavily weighted in a handful of countries: of 353 Class 1 professional health personnel in the field, 54 were in Italy, 114 in Greece, and 174 in China; Woodbridge, *UNRRA, the History*, 22–23.

23  *WHO OR*, No. 4, 108.

24 'Congress,' Gillespie observes, 'remained reluctant to meet its budgetary commitments to WHO and other multilateral agencies, while providing generous funds to aid programmes that were more closely controlled by the United States. A senior U.S. Public Health Service member of the American delegation to WHO complained bitterly that: "It is difficult for many people to understand the attitude of a Government which, having worked for the establishment of international machinery to deal with these problems . . . nevertheless restricts use of this machinery to minimum activities while at the same time setting up its own or different international machinery, to which it contributes liberally to carry out activities which an international organization like the WHO was created to perform"'; 'Social Medicine, Social Security,' 233–234.

25 *WHO OR*, No. 4, 111, 157–158.

26 Farley, *Brock Chisholm*, 68.

27 *WHO OR*, No. 4, 60, 21, 164–166.

28 Ibid., 168; *WHO OR*, No. 5, 52. In referring to UNRRA's work in controlling epidemics 'aggravated by the war,' malaria is not specified, although elsewhere the DDT campaigns in Greece and Italy are mentioned; ibid., 109, 112.

29 *WHO OR*, No. 4, 27, 108, 115, 168.

30 Nuclear Committee on Malaria, First Session: Geneva, April 21–24, 1947, Draft Agenda; *WHO OR*, No. 4, 160.

31 Jackson, 'Cognition,' 206, 208.

32 Jackson, 'Cognition,' 206. Pampana's support for eradication goals continued, despite being already aware of the possible emergence of insect resistance to DDT in 1947 from his tour of spray operations in Greece and Italy; 'Jackson, 'Cognition,' 206, as detailed in his ECM report, *Report on Dr Pampana's Mission to Greece and Italy*, WHO.IC/Mal/8.

33 Jackson, 'Cognition,' 209.

34 *WHO OR*, No. 4, 160. 'A technical committee must be made up of a small number of real experts,' their competency based upon 'knowledge of the health techniques concerned'; Note by the Secretariat, 'Appointment of Expert Members of Technical Committees,' Oct. 21, 1946, in *WHO OR*, No. 4, 158. An UNRRA memorandum to the IC advised that '[m]any experienced members of the staff of the UNRRA Health Division will soon be released, and among them there should be a considerable number who would be useful in the programme of the Interim Commission. Every assistance will be given . . . in helping the officers of the Commission to make contacts with such personnel and to learn of their qualifications'; *WHO OR*, no. 4, 112. Birn describes UNRRA as 'a pipeline for WHO's first generation of personnel'; 'Backstage,' 131.

35 Jackson, 'Cognition,' 209.

36 ECM, Summary Minutes of the First Session, April 22–25, 1947, WHO.IC/Mal./6, 21, 27; Jackson, 'Cognition,' 209.

37 Jackson, 'Cognition,' 193.

38 Farley, *Brock Chisholm*, 60–63. The Soviet delegate to the Epidemiology and Quarantine Committee, Dr Fedor Krotkov, repeatedly expressed 'apprehension . . . about the creation of too many committees' and urged more attention to responding to specific post-war relief needs 'as judged by individual governments'; *WHO OR*, No. 4, 18, 20.

39 Vine, 'The malarial campaign in Greece.' The DDT program in Greece was directed by Colonel D.R. Wright, a Rockefeller consultant engineer, 'lent' to the IC, who had begun his career with Gorgas in Panama; G. Harrison. *Mosquitoes, Malaria and Man: A History of the Hostilities Since 1880* (New York: E.P. Dutton, 1978), 230–231; *WHO OR*, No. 9, 31.

40 ECM, Report on the First Session, Geneva, April 22–25, 1947, WHO.IC/Mal./4, 3.

41 Ibid., 5.

42 *WHO OR*, No. 7, Minutes and Documents of the Fifth Session of the IC, 22 Jan – 7 Feb. 1948, Annex 44, 223.

43 Ibid., 223; J.A. Sinton, *Health Bulletin*, No. 26 (Simla: GOI, Malaria Bureau, 1939), 13; J.A. Sinton, 'What Malaria Costs India,' *Records of the Malaria Survey of India*, Dec. 1935, 418.

44 The third ECM Session in 1949 suggested 'the ultimate aim of WHO should be to eliminate this disease as a public-health problem from the world,' though this too skirted the definitional question of 'problem'; WHO *Technical Report Series*, No. 8, ECM, Report on the Third Session, Aug. 10–17, 1949, 7.

45 'Malariologists in the United States,' however, Nájera observes, 'continued to equate malaria control with anopheline control'; J.A. Nájera, 'Malaria Control: Achievements, Problems and Strategies,' *Parassitologia*, 43, 2001, 1–89, at 21.

46 ECM, 'Summary Minutes,' 22–25 April 1947. As of August 1947, it was noted at the fifth meeting of the IC, 'documents of Technical Committees are not printed in the *Official Records*'; WHO OR, No. 5, 128.

47 ECM, 'Summary Minutes,' 14–15. 'Premunity' refers to a sufficient level of naturally acquired immunity where clinical symptoms from continuing re-infection are limited or nil.

48 *WHO OR*, No. 8, 9.

49 *WHO OR*, No. 7, 224; ECM, 'Extract from the Report on the First Session, Note by the Secretariat,' *Bulletin of the WHO*, 1, 1, 1948, 21–28, at 23.

50 ECM, 'Summary Minutes,' 13.

51 Ibid., 6, 16, 24. On U.S.-UK 'hostility' to the LNHO, see Gillespie, 'Social Medicine, Social Security,' 222. Nájera describes the functioning of the subsequent WHO Malaria Eradication Program in similar terms, as involving 'the establishment of a central power, which recruited and trained its own peripheral cadres . . . [and] took over and displaced previous antimalarial services, and the early dissociation of operational planning from research, including epidemiological and field research'; in 'Malaria Control: Achievements, Problems,' 5.

52 ECM, 'Summary Minutes,' 11.

53 Ibid., 17, 19, 32.

54 *WHO OR*, No. 8, 9.

55 ECM, 'Summary Minutes,' 39–41. Ciuca's request for a three-week fellowship for two Romanian entomologists to acquire field experience with DDT residual spraying to assist in malaria control in the country also was turned down for lack of funds; *WHO OR*, no. 7, 84–85.

56 ECM, 'Summary Minutes,' 14.

57 In an April 27, 1948, memorandum submitted in advance of the second ECM meet that he would not attend, Ciuca urged 'WHO's aid' in covering costs of 'anti-malarial products (medicaments and insecticides)' for non-producing countries through the UN and co-ordination of their distribution through the Economic and Social Council (ECOSOC); WHO.IC/Mal.24. Siddiqui notes concerns by Eastern European member states that distribution of WHO funding did not 'correspond to actual needs,' and the larger 'political' manoeuvering around such issues as Chinese membership; *World Health and World Politics: The World Health Organization and the UN System* (London: Hurst, 1995), 104–116.

58 With the 20 states of Latin America now under a Soper-headed Pan American Health Organization (PAHO) and voting as a bloc, Soviet views routinely were outvoted. Farley details Soviet objections to the direction in which the Executive

Board was taking WHO, prompting its withdrawal from the organization in February 1949, returning only in 1956; Farley, *Brock Chisholm*, 80–93. For a detailed account of U.S. influence in opposing integration of the Pan American Sanitary Bureau and the WHO, see, ibid., 97–110.

59 *WHO OR*, No. 8, ECM, *Report on the First Session*, 8–16, at 11.

60 WHO OR, No. 11, 59 [emphasis added].

61 *WHO OR*, No. 8. ECM, Report on the Third Session, 39–40; S.P. James, 'Advances in Knowledge of Malaria Since the War,' *Transactions of the Royal Society of Tropical Medicine and Hygiene*, 31, 3, Nov. 1937, 263–280, at 266.

62 *WHO OR*, No. 7, 224.

63 For general discussion of the restrictive character and functioning of UN agency expert committees, see K.J. Carpenter, *Protein and Energy: A Study of Changing Ideas in Nutrition* (Cambridge: Cambridge University Press, 1994), 227–228. Reliance on the authority of the expert committee was exemplified at the Jan. 27, 1948 (5th) session of the IC with the Brazilian member and vice-president suggesting with reference to the joint WHO-FAO study proposal 'that the [Interim] Commission was not the appropriate body to enter into technical discussions about the recommendations submitted by experts'; *WHO OR*, No. 7, 24.

64 A photo of the 34 delegates to the 1928 LNMC conference offers an interesting contrast to the size of the ECM; *International Public Health between the Two World Wars*, 63.

65 *WHO OR*, No. 4, 22. Amrith points out how India 'played a central role in shaping consensus around "modern" technological methods of disease control,' presenting a willing and 'ideal ground for "pilots projects" [and] demonstration areas,' an outlook which 'after 1945 accorded closely with the assumptions of India's new technocratic elite'; *Decolonizing International Health*, 12–13. Administratively, Bombay was considered to provide a model of malaria control organization as the work of Viswanathan was expanded to cover the whole state; *WHO OR*, No. 11, 45. Lee notes that it was only in the early 1970s with China's entry into the World Health Organization that complete reliance on the Western medical model and on technical aid was challenged with a 'call to a new politicization, based not on global transfers of wealth but on the reordering of domestic political priorities'; Sung Lee, 'WHO and the Developing World: The Contest for Ideology,' in B. Andrews, and A. Cunningham, eds., *Western Medicine as Contested Knowledge* (Manchester: Manchester University Press, 1997), 24–45, at 36.

66 Litsios observes, 'The Cold War' [political contest] . . . led to a distortion of the priorities of global programs being carried out under the various UN agencies. Preference was given to countries where the threat of communism was judged to be greatest. Preference was also given to more quickly achieved results that placed anti-communist governments in a "good light" '; 'Malaria Control and the Cold War,' 271.

67 J. Gillespie, 'Europe, America, and the Space of International Health,' in *Shifting Boundaries Boundaries in Public Health: Europe in the Twentieth Century* (Rochester: University of Rochester Press, 2008), 117–119. Gillespie suggests a larger U.S. concern with disease control lay with enhancement of trade. 'According to the new approach to international public health associated with the American architects of WHO, the first tactic against disease was eradication at its source. International quarantine, with its restrictions on movements of people and commerce, must finally be supplanted by programs that drew on UNRRA's experience – namely, vertically driven disease-eradication programs'; 'Social Medicine, Social Security,' 127. Indeed, from its first meeting onward, the

ECM agenda included anopheline quarantine measures for air traffic 'to prevent the inadvertent transportation of malaria vectors across national boundaries'; *WHO OR*, No. 8, ECM, *Report on the First Session*, 10. See also E. Pampana, 'Malaria as a Problem for the World Health Organization,' in U.S. Department of State, *Proceedings of the Fourth International Congress on Tropical Medicine and Malaria*, Washington, D.C., May 10–18, 1948, vol. 2, 940–946, at 644.

68 For discussion of the wider application of the thesis, see P.J. Brown, 'Malaria, Miseria, and Underpopulation in Sardinia: The "Malaria Blocks Development" Cultural Model,' *Medical Anthropology*, 17, 3, May 1997, 239–254.

69 'Malaria Programme: Proposal from the Representative from the United States of America,' Jan. 23, 1948, in *WHO OR*, No. 7, 222–223 [emphasis added].

70 Ibid.

71 Ibid.

72 'Note by the Secretariat' *WHO OR*, No. 7, 223–225.

73 Ibid., 224–226; subsequently adopted by the IC on Feb. 3, 1948; ibid., 254.

74 Ibid., 223.

75 Report on the Second [ECM] Session, May 19–25, 1948, *WHO OR*, No. 11, 44, 48.

76 'Summary Minutes,' 26.

77 United States. Department of State. 'Address of welcome by the honorable George Marshall, Secretary of State,' *Proceedings of the Fourth International Congresses on Tropical Medicine and Malaria*, Washington, D.C., May 10–18, 1948, vol. 2, 1–4 [hereafter, *Proc. 4th Int. Cong. Mal.*].

78 Viswanathan would report the rapid decline in malaria incidence that followed 1946 initiation of the Kanara district DDT spray trial; D.K. Viswanathan, 'Activities of the Bombay Province Malaria Organization, 1942–27,' *Proc. 4th Int. Cong. Mal.*, 873–880. But discussion of the study's finding of limited mortality impact awaited a final report published in 1949; D.K. Viswanathan, 'A Study of the Effects of Malaria Control Measures on Population and Vital Statistics in Kanara and Dharwar Districts as Compared with the Rest of the Province of Bombay,' *Indian Journal of Malariology*, 3, 1, Mar. 1949, 69–99 [hereafter, *IJM*].

79 Of the 37 malaria papers presented, 17 were authored by U.S. malaria workers, 3 by U.K. delegates, and a further 7 by delegates of other countries already actively engaged in DDT-based campaigns.

80 *WHO OR*, No. 7, 222.

81 Ibid., 23–24. Amrith recounts the serious questions raised by the Liberian delegate to the 1955 World Health Assembly, Dr Togba, regarding feasibility of eradication in Africa; *Decolonizing International Health*, 118–119. Nájera suggests serious misgivings were 'voiced in private talks' by many World Health Assembly delegates, despite a large majority vote in favour'; 'Malaria Control: Achievements, Problems and Strategies,' *Parassitologia*, 43, 2001, 1–89, at 35.

82 Gillespie, 'Social Medicine, Social Security,' 225. Litsios reports that 'Soper claimed that it was the lack of this money that gave him time, as the Director of the Pan American Sanitary Bureau, to mobilize such an important regional program, as to preclude the PASB [Pan American Sanitary Bureau] being absorbed by WHO'; 'Malaria Control, the Cold War,' 273.

83 *WHO OR*, No. 7, 223; P.F. Russell, and M.K. Menon, 'A Malario-economic Survey in Rural South India,' *Indian Medical Gazette*, 77, Mar. 1942, 167–180. For details, see ch. 5 above. A comprehensive 1978 bibliography of economic aspects of malaria includes few documented examples of rural economic

benefits; J. Sotiroff-Junker, *A Bibliography on the Behavioural, Social and Economic Aspects of Malaria and its Control* (Geneva: World Health Organization, 1978). A Rockefeller-assisted 1951 study in Mysore State estimated an 'annual per-family lost earnings attributed to malaria' of Rs 656 was reduced to Rs 68 'post-DDT'; S.R. Bhombore, C. Brooke Worth, and K.S. Nanjundiah, 'A Survey of the Economic Status of Villagers in a Malarious Irrigated Tract in Mysore State, India, before and after D.D.T. Residual Insecticidal Spraying,' *IJM*, 6, 4, Dec. 1952, 355–366; C.S. Narahari Rao, and S.R. Bhombore, 'A Survey of the Economic Status of Villages in a Malarious Tract in Mysore State (India) after residual insecticide spraying,' *Bull. Nat. Soc. Ind. Mal. Mosq. Dis.*, 4, 1956, 71–77. These figures are puzzling, however, given that annual income for 60 per cent of surveyed households was less than Rs 500.

84 'Memorandum prepared by FAO at the request of the Expert Committee on Malaria,' *WHO OR*, No. 11, 60.

85 Report of the Fifth Session of the IC, 5 February 1948, *WHO OR*, No. 7, 254.

86 Amrith notes that the British government viewed U.S.-UNRRA engagement as key to ensuring American participation in a future international health organization, co-operation that officials believed otherwise 'might be very difficult to obtain' after the war; *Decolonizing International Health*, 68. Siddiqui also suggests a functionalist purpose in the preamble to the WHO's constitution that begins, 'the health of all peoples is fundamental to the attainment of peace and security and is dependent upon the fullest cooperation of individuals and states'; *World Health and World Politics*, 45, 51, 42. See also Staples, *The Birth of Development*, 169.

87 *WHO OR*, No. 13, 300, 306; *WHO OR*, No. 10.

88 Litsios, 'Malaria and the Cold War,' 259–260. Packard recounts Russell's subsequent whitewashing of the absence of data on economic benefits of malaria eradication in a 1959 presentation to the WHO Director-General; R.M. Packard, 'Malaria Dreams: Postwar Visions of Health and Development in the Third World,' *Medical Anthropology*, 17, 1997, 279–296, at 285. For a more recent critique, see R. Packard, '"Roll Back Malaria, Role in Development"? Reassessing the Economic Burden of Malaria,' *Population and Development Review*, 35, 1, 2009, 53–85. Amrith observes that '[w]hen it could not be shown that malaria control was transforming agricultural productivity, particularly as the Indian economy moved towards agrarian crisis in the 1960s, or when other inventions – viz., population control – seemed more "cost-effective", support for malaria control ebbed'; 'Political Culture of Health in India: A Historical Perspective,' *Economic and Political Weekly*, Jan. 13, 2007, 114–21 at 118.

89 Litsios, citing E. Goldman, *The Crucial Decade and After: America, 1945–60* (New York: Alfred A. Knopf, 1960), details the profound impact that political ('anti-communist') concerns within the ' "troubled American mind" ' had in shaping malaria and broader health policies of the WHO and FAO through this formative period; 'Malaria and the Cold War,' 267–271.

90 LN, *Final Report of the Mixed Committee of the League of Nations on the Relation of Nutrition to Health, Agriculture and Economic Policy* (Geneva: LNHO, 1937); ILO, 'Workers' Nutrition and Social Policy,' Studies and Reports (Social and Economic Conditions), No. 23 (Geneva: ILO Office, 1936); E. Burnet, and W.R. Aykroyd, 'Nutrition and Public Health,' LN, *Quarterly Bulletin of the Health Organisation*, 4, 2, June 1935, 323–474.

91 'United Nations Conference on Food and Agriculture: Text of the Final Act,' *American Journal of International Law*, 37, 4, Supplement: Official Documents, Oct. 1943, 159–192, Resolution XIII, 172–173. The FAO was the single UN organization the USSR did not join, though Soviet delegates attended the 1943 Hot Springs conference. In 1946 an unofficial American Famine Mission under T.W. Schultz visited India to assess foodgrain supply adequacy; Indian Famine Emergency Committee, *India's Hunger: Report of the American Famine Mission to India* (New York, 1946), as cited in H. Knight, *Food Administration in India 1939–47* (Stanford: Stanford University Press, 1954), 253.

92 Zurbrigg, *Epidemic Malaria and Hunger*, ch. 12.

93 'Conference on Food and Agriculture,' 163, 166, 171, 173.

94 Ibid., 163.

95 Ibid., 163, 175, 177, 183, 184–185.

96 In January 1946 'Montgomery reported to the cabinet that the existing ration in Germany was only 1500 kilocalories per person per day, which was a bare minimum to prevent starvation and disease. . . . The army was making arrangements for handling an epidemic; Montgomery believed that if it occurred it would probably spread to Britain'; J. Perkins, *Geopolitics and the Green Revolution: Wheat, Genes, and the Cold War* (New York: Oxford University Press, 1997), 128.

97 Zurbrigg, *Epidemic Malaria and Hunger*, 390.

98 On Jan. 24, 1947, the final report of the FAO's preparatory committee 'recommended creation of the World Food Council and emphasized industrial development, full employment, and self-help,' signaling defeat of the World Food Bank proposals; Staples, *Birth of Development*, 78–81, 94.

99 S.G. Solomon, L. Murard, and P. Zylberman, *Shifting Boundaries of Public Health: Europe in the Twentieth Century* (Rochester: University of Rochester Press, 2008), 1.

100 See also, Packard ' "No Other Logical Choice",' 227. As the Eighth World Health Assembly delegates gathered in Mexico City in 1955, they realized, Packard observes, 'that they had only two choices, they could jump on the eradication train or get out of the way. Eradication was rapidly being adopted by national malaria programs whether or not WHO adopted it'; ibid., 228.

101 D. Porter, 'Social Medicine and the New Society: Medicine and Scientific Humanism in mid-Twentieth Century Britain,' *Journal of Historical Sociology*, 9, 2, June 1996, 168–187.

102 Present as 'Counsellor' at the Second ECM session on 'Agriculture and Malaria' was Frank McDougall, co-architect of the 1930s 'marriage of health and agriculture' efforts within the LNHO's 'Mixed' Nutrition Committee that interpreted global hunger as principally a problem of inadequate extension of modern agro-technology. See above, ch. 3, at note 67.

103 Packard, ' "No Other Logical Choice".'

104 The extreme efficiency of the main vectors (*An. gambiae*) in many regions of central and west Africa (several hundred infective bites per person per year) led to acquired immunity levels so high as to leave most of the population clinically asymptomatic, a state referred to as 'premunition,' except among young children.

105 For detailed accounts of the Kampala conference and larger issues raised, see M.J. Dobson, M. Malowany, and R.W. Snow, 'Malaria Control in East Africa: The Kampala Conference and the Pare-Taveta Scheme: A Meeting of Common and High Ground,' *Parassitologia*, 42, 2000, 149–166; Farley, *Brock Chisholm*, 159–169. The study would proceed through the years

1954–1966, ultimately with inconclusive results regarding mortality impact of initial transmission control and subsequent rebound, in part due to confounding effects of drug treatment; Dobson, et al., 'Malaria Control in East Africa,' 160–164.

106 Ibid., 150.

107 WHO, 'Minutes of Discussion of Committee on Programme and Budget, Eighth World Assembly, 105, as cited in Packard, ' "No Other Logical Choice",' 228. 'As a group,' Packard observes, World Health Assembly 'members were not in a position to seriously question the proposal's scientific merit. They could and did raise questions concerning the feasibility of the proposal in terms mostly of finances and the underdeveloped state of much of the world within which malaria was a problem. But that was all. Few had first hand experience combating malaria. Those who did, as noted above, were among the most vocal critics of the proposal'; ibid., 224.

108 J.L.A. Webb, 'The First Large-Scale Use of Synthetic Insecticide for Malaria Control in Tropical Africa: Lessons from Liberia, 1945–1962,' *Journal of the History of Medicine and Allied Sciences*, 66, 3, July 2011, 347–376; J.L.A. Webb, *The Long Struggle Against Malaria in Tropical Africa* (New York: Cambridge University Press, 2014), 88–95; M. Graboyes, *The Experiment Must Continue: Medical Research and Ethics in East Africa, 1940–2014* (Athens, OH: Ohio University Press, 2015), 155–186.

109 Webb suggests that the severe 1958 malaria epidemic in the Ethiopian highlands, among a famished population with limited acquired immunity levels, dampened advocacy for malaria eradication in tropical Africa; J.L.A. Webb, *Humanity's Burden*, 166; R.E. Fontaine, A.E. Najjar, and J.S. Prince, 'The 1958 Malaria Epidemic in Ethiopia,' *The American Journal of Tropical Medicine and Hygiene*, 10, 795–803.

110 The influence of the malaria eradication program on the early WHO is reflected in the fact that 'five of the six WHO regional directors were ex-malariologists, alongside the Director-General Candau himself'; M.A. Farid, 'The Malaria Programme – from Euphoria to Anarchy,' *World Health Forum*, 1, 1–2, 1980, 8–33, 12.

111 For discussion of inter-agency competition through this period, see also, Gillespie, 'Social Medicine, Social Security.' Gillespie notes that the International Labour Office (ILO) was 'the only significant survivor from the wreckage of the LN to become the main international force in social and health policy. . . . With a strong prewar record of support for reform of labor conditions in dependent territories the ILO argued that the new standards of "social security" developed for postwar Europe and America must apply equally in their colonial possessions'; 'Europe, America,' 127–129. See also P. Weindling, 'Social Medicine at the League of Nations Health Organisation and the International Labour Office compared,' in P. Weindling, ed. *International Health Organisations and Movements, 1918–1939* (New York: Cambridge University Press, 1995), 134–153, at 138–141; P. Weindling, ed., *The Social History of Occupational Health* (London: Croom Helm, 1985).

112 For discussion of the impact of surplus food 'dumping' on rural African agriculture and livelihood, see e.g., E. Boserup, 'The Primary Sector in African Development,' in M. Lundahl, ed., *The Primary Sector in African Development* (London: Croom Helm, 1985), 43–55; E. Holt-Giménez, and R. Patel, *Food Rebellions: Crisis and the Hunger for Justice* (Cape Town: Pambazuka Press, 2009), 37–49; M. Ishii-Eiteman, 'Perspectives on the IAASTD Report,' *Development*, 5, 14, 2008, 570–573.

113 Susan George recounts how in 1965–1966 when India was in the throes of the Bihar famine U.S. Food for Peace shipments 'were suddenly placed on a month-to-month basis and threatened with curtailment . . . India had no choice but to accept America's terms for resuming the Food for Peace programme. These conditions consisted largely of greater freedom for US private investment . . . and for the American management of India's fertilizer industry'; *How the Other Half Dies* (Harmondsworth, England: Penguin Books, 1977), 118; D. Morgan, *Merchants of Grain* (New York: Viking Press, 1979), chs. 10–12.

114 Staples, *Birth of Development*, 96; Litsios, *Malaria Control, Cold War*, 269. On the eve of yet another 'great' war, Nagendranath Gangulee in 1939 decried the use of hunger as among the most coercive weapons of war, describing post-WW1 policies of 'embargoes, war debts, [and] financial restrictions' by the victorious Powers as 'victory with vengeance' and rued 'the supreme illusion of the post-war world . . . that armed conflict alone is war'; *Health and Nutrition in India* (London: Faber and Faber, 1939), 20.

115 Staples observes that 'the preamble to the [FAO] constitution was not as forth-right as the Hot Springs declarations had been. Instead of calling for freedom from hunger, it merely called on all signatories to better standards of living and nutrition'; *Birth of Development*, 78.

116 Amrith, *Decolonizing International Health*, 88–89 [emphasis in original].

117 Jackson highlights Russell's particular role in controlling the ECM agenda; 'Cognition,' 207.

118 In a 1980 WHO article, for e.g., the subject of epidemic forecasting dealt exclusively with entomological variables, with no reference to the human host; E. Onori, and B. Grab, 'Indicators for the Forecasting of Malaria Epidemics,' *Bulletin of the WHO*, 58, 1, 1980, 91–98.

119 P. Russell, L.S. West, and R.D. Manwell, *Practical Malariology* (Philadelphia: W.B. Saunders, 1946), 375. This reading by Russell may well be the source for recent accounts of the 1908 epidemic where high prices are interpreted as secondary to malarial debility; I.A. McGregor, 'Malaria and Nutrition,' in W.H. Wernsdorfer, and I.A. McGregor, eds., *Malaria: Principles and Practice of Malariology* (London: Churchill Livingstone, 1988), 754–777, at 754. See Introduction, at note 9.

120 Russell, et al., *Practical Malariology*, 374–375.

121 Ibid., 541. See above, ch. 2 at note 116. Russell conceded that famine possibly influences relapse rate of malaria infection, yet qualified even this admission with a behaviouralist hue: famine victims 'attempt[ing]to work before they are fit'; ibid. Missing was any reference to the massive malaria mortality in famine-stricken 1943–1944 Bengal in the absence of any change in entomological conditions; Zurbrigg, *Epidemic Malaria and Hunger in Colonial Punjab*, ch. 12.

122 *Man's Mastery of Malaria*. Only one of Christophers's 215 published articles and reports is included in Russell's 1955 bibliography: a paper co-authored with J.A. Sinton; 'The Correct Name of the Malignant Tertian Malaria Parasite,' *British Medical Journal*, 3, Dec. 2, 1938, 1130. Three decades earlier, Andrew Balfour's single reference to Christophers's malaria research would appear in a passing general phrase as 'pioneer work on mosquitoes'; A. Balfour, and H.H. Scott, *Health Problems of the Empire: Past, Present and Future* (New York: Henry Holt, 1924), 78.

123 Nor, in Pampana's 1933 overview of LNMC epidemiological research, is mention made of the 1930 India Study Tour report, though earlier European 'tours of investigation' reports are discussed: E.J. Pampana, 'Malaria Research and the Malaria Commission of the League of Nations,' *Annals of Tropical Medicine and Parasitology*, 28, 1, 1934, 63–65.

124 '[U]nder the all powerful gaze of the western eradicator,' Packard observes, 'local knowledge of malariologists built up over decades of experience became irrelevant'; 'Malaria dreams,' 290. For on-going influence of the Rockefeller Foundation and World Bank in shaping of the WHO, see T. Brown, M. Cueto, and E. Fee, 'The WHO and the Transition from International to Global Public Health,' *American Journal of Public Health*, 96, 1, Jan. 2006, 62–72. Interestingly, in the 1963 second edition of Russell's *Practical Malariology*, the section on 'regional epidemics' is rewritten, much of the content replicating an article previously published by G. Macdonald, now a fourth co-author to Russell's collaborative text. Here, brief reference to *Malaria in the Punjab* did include acknowledgement of pre-existing economic hardship in relation to fulminant epidemic malaria conditions; P. Russell, L.S. West, R.D. Manwell, and G. Macdonald, *Practical Malariology* (London: Oxford University Press, 1963), 473.

125 Already, he pointed out, there were reports of vector resistance 'from Italy and other countries including India,' and that mud surfaces of village houses absorbed 70 to 90 per cent of the DDT applied; also the problem of exophily: the mosquito habit of resting outdoors after a human blood meal rather than inside, in the case of some important vector species; V. Venkat Rao, 'A Critical Review of Malaria Control Measures in India,' *IJM*, 3, 4, Dec. 1949, 313–326, at 317–318. Venkat Rao was not among the 15 Indian delegates to attend the May 1948 Malaria Congress in Washington.

126 Venkat Rao, 'A Critical Review of Malaria Control,' 319 [emphasis added].

127 In 1999, V.P. Sharma reported that DDT coverage in India in 1996 extended to a population of 56 million, with another 7 to 10 million protected with synthetic pyrethroids, the aim 'to substantially reduce morbidity and mortality and control malaria without contaminating the environment, and therefore wherever feasible insecticides are being phased out'; 'Current Scenario of Malaria in India,' *Parassitologia*, 41, 1999, 349–353. For an overview of recent malaria control policy based on early diagnosis, prompt treatment, and alternate vector control methods including larvivorous fish, wherever feasible, see L.M. Barat, 'Four Malaria Success Stories: How Malaria Burden was Successfully Reduced in Brazil, Eritrea, India, and Vietnam,' *American Journal of Tropical Medicine and Hygiene*, 74, 1, 2006, 12–16, at 13.

128 Venkat Rao, 'A Critical Review of Malaria Control,' 314, 322–323.

129 Ibid., 324.

130 Ibid.

131 S.R. Christophers, 'Policy in Relation to Malaria Control,' *IJM*, 9, 4, Dec. 1955, 297–303, at 299.

132 Ibid., 300. In 1969, several U.S. malaria workers would rue 'the diminishing number of "malariologists" and proliferation of "eradicationists"'; R. Scholtens, R. Kaiser, and A. Langmuir, 'An Epidemiological Examination of the Strategy of Malaria Eradication,' *International Journal of Epidemiology*, 1, 1, 1972, 15–24, at 23.

# 7

# ALLURE AND LEGACIES OF THE GERM PARADIGM

Tropical Hygiene . . . [can] give us a complete knowledge of the dynamics of infections of all types and thus enormously concentrate our powers of prevention . . . [a] strategy of disease prevention which would give us complete power over virtually all communicable diseases.

> —— G. Macdonald, 'On the Scientific Basis of Tropical Hygiene,' Presidential address, *Transactions of the Royal Society of Tropical Medicine and Hygiene* (1965), 59, 618–619

We do a disservice to the weight of evidence, past and present, on social inequalities in health if we suggest that what chiefly hampers efforts to promote social equity in health is a lack of knowledge.

> —— N. Kreiger, 'Historical Roots of Social Epidemiology,' *International Journal of Epidemiology*, 30, 4, Aug. 2001, 899–900.

## The allure of eradication

For medical scientists and practitioners in the post-1897 era, attraction to a narrowed biomedical model of malaria – and the promise of the parasite's eradication – lay in myriad realms. Most basic was the common-sense maxim that prevention is better than cure. Eradication's appeal in turn lay also in its inherent democratic aura. Interrupting malaria transmission meant eradication for everyone, including for the poor who suffered most. Conversely, to question the eradication approach could open oneself to the professional opprobrium of depriving those same poor of such benefits: 'unwarrantably attacking proven prophylactic measures,' Ronald Ross would urge in 1909, constituted 'a very grave scientific crime.'[1]

Through the 1920s the eradicationist promise was fuelled by triumphalist accounts of malaria control in the Panama Canal zone. No other sanitary campaign exemplified the heroic motif so powerfully, the challenge defined overtly as a 'battle' against nature, an enthusiasm that would culminate with U.S. Surgeon General William Gorgas's knighthood in Britain. This, despite evident questions about the broader applicability of the Panama example in relation to cost and the confounding contributions to malaria mortality decline in the canal zone of unlimited quinine and 'a well-fed labour force' – despite, in other words, its enclave and imperially funded character.[2] The Panama campaign, nevertheless, would continue to serve as reference point for vector eradication advocacy, no more so than within the Rockefeller Foundation's International Health Board as it turned away from hookworm and embraced malaria in the 1920s as the new microbiological enemy of global development.[3]

Across this same period, momentum for a war on malaria was building also at the institutional level as tropical medicine schools proliferated. '[I]n the scramble for imperial power and wealth,' Bynum observes, 'schools of tropical medicine . . . represented tangible monuments to the power of medicine and medical research,'[4] a common central plank within the intra-Western imperial contest. 'Before the outbreak of World War I,' he notes, 'there were schools of tropical medicine in Germany, France, Belgium, the Netherlands, and the United States, in addition to research stations in India, Indochina (now Viet Nam), the Sudan, and Malaysia.' Increasing cohorts of graduates through the 1920s and 1930s were trained in ever more sophisticated entomological and anti-larval techniques, imbued with the challenge of the Gorgas example and Ross's exhortation that 'malaria has done more than anything else to prevent the settlement and civilization of the vast tropical areas which would otherwise be most suitable for the human race.'[5] In time, medical historians contributed to nourishing the heady heroic appeal, with dramatic accounts of the discovery of new vectors and extirpation campaigns incidentally offering a 'darn good story.'[6]

The allure of malaria eradication was fuelled at a quite different level, by the complexity of the microbe's transmission cycle as a vector-borne disease. Recognition of the fragility of that cycle, and of the numerous points at which it potentially could be broken, endowed each new entomological discovery with the promise of a technological breakthrough around the corner. The tropical (colonial) world with its 'wealth . . . of pathogenic organisms,' in Manson's terms,[7] offered unlimited research possibilities, Worboys notes, for 'stak[ing] out new professional territory.'[8] One of the more promising entomological developments in the 1920s was identification of the different feeding habits of *Anopheles* vectors: the observation that some anopheline species such as *An. culicifacies* fed mainly on animals (zoophilic) rather than humans. This helped to explain the perplexing phenomenon of 'anophelism without malaria,' but also suggested that interruption of transmission might be more feasible in regions where the main vector was zoophilic. This entomological advance ultimately failed to bring about the hoped-for breakthrough in vector control in most endemic regions, but it did rekindle and reinvigorate confidence in an entomological solution.[9]

Arguably, however, it was the rise of private 'public health' philanthropy that ultimately gave financial legs to the reductive trajectory in the case of malaria work, greatly expanding enthusiasm for the idea of vector-control and development of related technical skills. Corporate funding, most prominent in relation to the Rockefeller Foundation, made possible the convenient format of the short-term expert consultant, allowing heroic aspirations to flourish. Very quickly the new medical subdiscipline of 'malariology' was being shaped by professionals whose expertise lay primarily in laboratory training or circumscribed anti-larval field trials, technical experts who had little in-depth epidemiological experience of malaria in human populations, or indeed none at all.[10] More and more, Packard observes, the 'problem of malaria' was coming to be defined in terms of the tools the professional 'malariologist' had for dealing with the disease, 'as a case with a positive blood smear, of plasmodia seen on a microscope slide . . . an infection by a microorganism transmitted by anopheline mosquitoes.'[11]

For many of the new malaria professionals, agricultural development ('bonification') was a less attractive malaria control strategy than sharply defined, if painstaking, anti-larval campaigns. The former was not their mandate, an arena where there was little interest or comfort, and even less skill. To younger cohorts, the experience in Italy under Celli – where land reclamation had left vectors and infection levels still abundant – appeared to leave malaria workers without a role, except for perhaps the seemingly undignified task of confirming that malaria transmission levels were unchanged, though the 'terror' of that transmission had largely vanished.[12] Such a job description hardly conjured up the heroic victories epitomized by the Panama Canal campaign: a role antithetical to the 'action man.' Nor, Amrith notes, did 'the patient, unglamorous task of building up local health services.'[13] For some like Lewis Hackett, a prominent Rockefeller consultant pursuing anti-larval trials in Italy through the 1920s, the Malaria Commission's gravitation to a 'social disease' definition of malaria was viewed as a professional threat, 'doom[ing] . . . the medical field malariologist . . . to extinction in Europe.'[14] Hackett for his part would acknowledge a role for poverty in malaria's toll, conceding at one point that '[i]gnorance, poverty, and disease constitute the vicious triangle of human social inadequacy. An attack on any one of them helps to dissipate the other two.' Yet ultimately, he urged, the most practical point of intervention in that vicious cycle was an attack on the infective agent, arguing that

> the causes of malaria, at least, are in the main independent of the ignorance and poverty of its victims and can be separately handled. It is easier to believe that release from the burden of malaria will

help to bring prosperity and knowledge than that a higher standard of living and education must precede the eradication of malaria.[15]

There is a disarming candour to Hackett's expression of belief. Still, it begged the question: 'easier' for whom? As public health physicians one might expect some acknowledgement – if not satisfaction – from Hackett and Rockefeller colleague, Paul Russell, that by the 1920s the malarial 'terror' of the Pontine marshes had largely been lifted, though transmission of the *Plasmodium* parasite remained. Instead, it was as if the two perspectives, microbial and social, were in competition. And here, for experts such as Hackett and Russell, there was no contest.

But the socio-economic route for malaria control was unattractive for other reasons as well. Addressing economic determinants was frankly impossible within the time-frame imperatives set for overseas consultancy. 'Probably time has been wasted by assumptions that malaria is a sociological rather than sanitary problem,' Russell would argue, adding 'it would probably be *a good deal quicker* and cheaper to induce prosperity through malaria control.'[16] In very concrete ways, in other words, public health approaches to malaria control were being moulded to conform to the time constraints of that new institutional entity, the short-term international expert. In the process, understanding of the malaria problem – indeed its very definition – was being reshaped as well.

## Myriad conveniences

A malaria model shorn of conditions of the human host was convenient at other levels. For local elites, the prospect of malaria eradication offered relief from fear of contamination from the poor, that unlimited reservoir of disease. For the British Raj in the context of 1920s fiscal retrenchment, formal embracing of the doctrine of malaria as a block to development also held out the prospect of Rockefeller funding for programs that could be pointed to as 'doing something,' 'managing a problem or crisis.' Many writers have also highlighted broader corporate interests in the promotion of a unidirectional view of malaria as a principal cause of world poverty.[17] 'The International Health Division,' Farley observes,

> played a crucial role in saving the Rockefeller name from almost universal condemnation. In 1913 the American public associated his name with the very worst features of brutal, unbridled, unprincipled capitalism; today that is no longer the case. . . . Through the Health Division in particular, the Rockefeller Foundation gained a worldwide reputation for medical benevolence and enhanced the reputation of the Rockefeller name.[18]

Indeed, the public relations value of the anti-hookworm campaign was articulated unabashedly in private proceedings in the formative years of the Foundation.[19]

Such broader interests did not exclude genuine belief in the doctrines of germ sanitation, as Ettling has pointed out.[20] Indeed, a good deal of the force of the reductive sanitary model lay in the ardent conviction of its field-level advocates. But that conviction in the case of Rockefeller philanthropy was inseparable from the ideological: a notion of the Western civilizing mission, cultural supremacy expressed quintessentially in 'Western' science, above all medical science.

Moreover, ideological beliefs were inseparable from the geopolitical: expanding markets for goods, ensuring raw materials access and opportunities for investing capital; thus fashioning compliant relations with governments in regions of the world of strategic and corporate interest.[21] Such broader conveniences were openly acknowledged, Randall Packard points out, by prominent U.S. public health figures[22] such as James S. Simmons, Dean of the Harvard School of Public Health who urged in a 1950 address to the conference of Industry and Tropical Health that the 'health and manpower of the free nations of the world are now the most vital resources in our fight against Communism.'[23] In the context of the post-WW2 accelerating Cold War and nationalist movements in many regions of the developing world vowing to ensure food and land for the poor and malaria-afflicted, an urgent need existed on the part of Western powers to be offering alternative 'solutions' to disease and underdevelopment in place of the structural and political reforms sought by revolutionary movements.[24] In this political contest, international health and development agencies became a central *champs de bataille*.[25] Russell himself in 1955 described malaria as 'a factor that, among others, helps to predispose a community to infection with political germs that can delay and destroy freedom.'[26] In the task of winning hearts and minds the promise of an immediate fix was an essential tool.

In the case of DDT, the value of eradication was two-fold: powerfully reinforcing the technological paradigm; but also planting the donor's flag of goodwill and beneficence in regions of particular economic interest or political concern. From its earliest days, WHO funding, as we have seen, was both extremely limited and highly insecure, with most of the actual funding of DDT 'demonstration' programs coming instead through U.S. bilateral aid in the case of southern Europe, Iran, Venezuela, and of course India, regions of strategic U.S. interest.[27] As D.K. Viswanathan described:

> If you take a DDT drum with the stars and stripes on one side and the tricolour on the other side to each of the forty million homes in the country . . . the psychological impact would be so great that public opinion would swing back again in favour of democracy.[28]

Ideological aspirations did not preclude the possibility of local benefits along the way for some among recipient populations. But it did mean that the needs of the poor could never be the central informing purpose of Rockefeller work, nor inform understanding of the broader roots to the disease problem.

The political convenience of malaria eradication could of course apply as well to recipient governments. 'Alongside the redemptive narrative of malaria eradication,' Amrith observes, 'stood a militarised, disciplinary narrative that presented malaria eradication as an assertion of the state's power, its technology and its sovereignty.' In post-Independence India, he observes,

> The [DDT] programme found ritual expression in a way that underscored the state's presence in the lives of its citizens. To commemorate 'World Health Week' in 1955, for example, 'two planes of the India Air Force dropped leaflets' on malaria eradication on Hyderabad and Secunderabad . . . just seven years after Hyderabad was subject to forcible incorporation into independent India by 'police action.'[29]

## The larger sanitationist dilemma

Yet as politically and professionally convenient as the reductive view of malaria as a block to development proved to be, interpreting the exclusion of the 'Human Factor' in malaria analysis in such terms alone is unsatisfying on a further level. The inherent power of the sanitationist paradigm merits analytic consideration on its own terms: the practical dilemma faced by the individual public health worker charged with applying *preventive* germ policies where understanding of disease etiology was narrowed conceptually by the turn of the twentieth century to external, and invisible, pathogens – or vectors. This is demonstrated in the case of South Asian malaria history in the ardent defence, by a local British Indian civil surgeon, A. Hooton, of Ronald Ross's advocacy of vector sanitation at the Bombay Medical Congress in 1909. 'Is there a Civil Surgeon in the country,' he would ask, 'who does not – if only in his own compound – undertake anti-mosquito operations?'[30] Once vector information was available, the onus upon individual sanitary officers was real. In sight of potential breeding sites, individual local officials post-1897 were obliged to act, in situations where it was generally not possible to tell if the 'dangerous' specific vector was present, or could be, with every fresh rainfall – and if so, if any might be infective. In the absence of a broader predispositionist context of malaria lethality, the quandary the new knowledge of malaria presented to those working 'on the ground' was inescapable – unless another voice was also present, reminding of other approaches: ensuring treatment access, and addressing a key lethality risk factor, human destitution. It was precisely this quandary that made the eradicationist argument so appealing: interruption of malaria transmission, once and for all.

Moreover, the dilemma is seen at government levels as well, the narrow germ paradigm posing an equally inescapable, if different, bind. Unable to acknowledge the larger, predisposing determinants of the malaria burden in India, the British Raj soon came to see that it had little choice but to publicly embrace vector extirpation, despite having little intention of, or practical capacity to, follow through as general policy.[31]

## Parallels and legacies

In the demise of the 'Human Factor' in malaria epidemiology, many parallels exist with the 'uncoupling' of disease and destitution one century earlier in industrializing Britain. Where nineteenth-century sanitarians sought to fix public gaze exclusively on environmental (neighbourhood) filth, the gaze one century later was directed to the plasmodium parasite and its anopheline vector. As in the nineteenth century where the sanitary promise was fuelled by the possibility of real benefits, so too a goal of malaria eradication offered the practical possibility of reducing periodic malarial fever and incapacity, at least for some. As in 1840s Britain, advocates of species sanitation a century later would portray malaria control policy in oppositionist terms: optimists 'versus' pessimists – the latter term referring to those who appealed to include socio-economic measures, thereby misguidedly depriving the poor of immediately available technical benefits, 'the Luddhites of public health.'[32] And as a century earlier, rejection of this false dichotomization came from within the medical community and from its most experienced and insightful medical members.

In both eras, too, there were much larger propelling concerns in the background. The 1842 Sanitary Report, Hamlin suggests, was to a major extent a political document. What was originally presented as a managerial strategy for summoning financial commitment to necessary public infrastructure was also a strategy of covering up unpleasant, inconvenient economic realities, 'divert[ing] attention from the charges . . . that the new Poor Law itself bore responsibility for fever. . . . At risk were the survival of the state in the face of revolution, and the grand question of whether the class relations of liberal industrial society could work.' The Sanitary Inquiry, he concludes, not only advanced Chadwick's personal career 'by inventing a field in which he could be the authority,' but also 'helped the hated Poor Law Commission to survive,' an agency which under his stewardship was markedly reducing relief to the destitute.[33]

In this much larger political drama, Chadwick, in his parallel role as Poor Law Commission secretary, was but a single actor. Nonetheless, his contribution included a studied excising of hunger from medical debate, literally removing 'starvation' as a cause of death category from the vital registration system.[34] In doing so, he helped remove not just incriminating statistics, but a concept, and indeed vocabulary, central to the predispositionist argument, making it that much more difficult to engage in broader health debate. As for Ross or Russell, this hardly means the sanitary doctrine, or Chadwick's belief in it, was a fraud.[35] But nor need it deter historians, Hamlin urges, from considering the consequences of its limitations. For in both cases there were costs.

In both eras, the role of carefully selected technical experts made questioning of broader economic roots of the epidemic disease problem difficult, as seen above with the WHO's early Expert Committee on Malaria.[36] As Hamlin observes with respect to the miasma thesis of urban typhus, '[t]he mode of investigation' by Chadwick's selected medical commissioners through summary tours of England's fetid industrial slums 'put a premium on what could be seen or smelled and counted on a *brief stay*. . . . The epidemiologists's searching inquiries or the casual conversations that lead the ethnographer or journalist to sense the tapestry of social relations were impossible.'[37] One century later the phenomenon of the 'international' health consultant would be institutionalized under private corporate philanthropic agencies where short-term assignments similarly lent themselves to narrowly constructed expertise.[38] The resulting constraints led predictably to limited 'demonstration' projects, or to enclave activities, such as the anti-malarial field work of the Ross Institute in India that remained 'chiefly occupied with industrial malaria in tea gardens.'[39] As Gordon Harrison has observed, such a 'crusade for human life, organized selectively, could easily become a defence of the privileged.' He adds that 'it is hard to see how the first [malaria] fighters could otherwise have retained the optimism to act at all and so to keep alive the possibility of extending the fight later on.'[40] Indeed, but this was surely the point. The external expert was inherently caught within a short-term framework where 'success' if it were to happen at all depended on a limited technological approach.

Yet South Asian colonial malaria history suggests – as does the Italian – that a very different framework for action *was* possible, as was a different basis for 'optimism.' The choice was not to extirpate or do nothing. Christophers, Rama Rao, Gangulee, Bentley, and Venkat Rao were all 'acting.' Another choice existed: to assess, articulate, and address determinants of lethality by advocating action on broader levels, alongside factors of transmission where appropriate.

Reliance on external public health philanthropy was problematic not just in terms of content of the programs promoted, however. It was problematic also for the absence of accountability: of the consultant institution, of the models offered, and of the central paradigm itself. Unlike government-based public health services where an obligation for accountability existed at least notionally, the question of whether a philanthropic scheme or pilot project worked or not was hardly an issue. It was enough that the project bore the mantle of modern medical science, though in practice the scientific content applied in the case of much Rockefeller Foundation work in India was often limited simply to confirming the presence of a specific microbe in a population. For the funding agencies themselves, it concretely did not matter if a project was flawed, or failed entirely. In the wake of the failure of its anti-hookworm campaign in Sri Lanka and southern India, the Rockefeller Foundation could quietly move on to another disease, another experimental 'field' study or 'demonstration' project, in another area. And did. In the case of India, the Foundation ultimately turned to malaria in the 1930s. Once malaria eradication was in place within the World Health Organization however, in 1951 it would again move on to seek technological solutions to what Rockefeller directors viewed as the new and more pressing threat to geopolitical stability and global business: population growth and foodgrain production.[41] The Foundation thus stepped away from malaria just when serious research attention was required to face the emerging problems of insecticide, and soon chloroquine, resistance.

In both Chadwick's England and post-1920 British India, endemic undernourishment continued, if in South Asia accompanied by acute hunger in endemic form as well. Increasingly however the new science of dietetics would interpret such hunger in behavioural terms as bad personal dietary habits, or in Britain, 'inefficient mothers,' and sideline underlying causes of deep poverty: insecure, irregular, ill-paid, and exhausting conditions of work and living. In the narrow application of nutritional science, the poor in India would lose any authority to speak of their hunger.[42] Officials sitting on the Royal Commission on Agriculture in India would rail against the vexatious ignorance of the poor who understood little of the new theory of nutrition and insisted on eating too much bulky rice. Lectures and tonics would be offered in the place of structural reforms, and common experience was lost or ignored. With disease and hunger now in the domain of the microbiologic, there was no longer common authority to speak.

But there was another equally problematic 'cost' side to short-term expert consultancy and related unaccountability: a general absence of scientific testing.[43] Moreover, the operative paradigm made it seemingly unnecessary. Where microbes were equated with disease burden, and their absence defined as health and economic productivity, quantitative measurement of the impact of eradication of particular microbes or their vectors on mortality rates could be seen as superfluous. In the case of malaria, the eradication of the protozoa responsible was an incontrovertible good: proof enough. Indeed, the frequent absence of scientific testing with the embrace of modern sanitary science was perhaps the most deeply ironic of all the parallels with the nineteenth-century British experience. In his 1842 Sanitary Report, Chadwick simply assumed, incorrectly, a miasmic explanation of the fever (typhus) epidemics he had been commissioned to investigate.[44] Subsequent decline in typhus outbreaks likewise was assumed attributable, also inaccurately, to sanitation measures (clean streets, eliminating environ- mental human waste, i.e., sewage disposal and water supply).[45] One century later, in the case of South Asia, elimination of vector transmission of malaria has been assumed responsible for post-WW2 decline in mortality from the disease. In this latter case, however, the absence of empirical assessment is even more puzzling because the opportunity for tracking such relationships through vital registration records was that much greater. Yet in the rush to act, elementary scientific practice was set aside.[46] Did it matter, after all, when eradication of the malaria plasmodium was by any standards a cat- egorical good?

Here we turn to this largely neglected question of the mortality impact of malaria transmission control in mid-twentieth-century South Asia, an issue that casts light on both the continuing power of the germ paradigm and the enduring invisibility of hunger in contemporary health history analysis.

## South Asian post-WW2 mortality decline revisited

Within global malaria historiography, assessment of the impact of DDT- based malaria control programs on mortality levels in post-WW2 South Asia has been remarkably limited. Analysis undertaken by Western commenta- tors has often focused on the experience in Sri Lanka, with DDT assumed early on to be responsible for the notable decline in mortality levels in the immediate post-war years. Particularly influential in this literature was the reading offered by Kingsley Davis, a prominent U.S. historical demographer of South Asia. 'The main cause of the spectacular decline of mortality in Ceylon is well known. It was the use of D.D.T.,' he argued in 1956.[47] That death rates for all disease categories over this period had declined as sharply as that for fever was acknowledged by Davis, but was attributed to malar- ia's debilitating effect, 'mak[ing] people susceptible to other diseases.'[48] Very likely the Davis assessment reflected recent remarks from members of the World Health Organization's Expert Committee on Malaria. One year ear- lier, Paul Russell had described the results of the DDT program in Ceylon as 'astonishingly good,' pointing to plummeting malaria prevalence indices and infant mortality rates that by 1951 'had fallen to about half what they were in 1938,' inferring a causal relationship.[49] At a regional World Health Organization conference in Bangkok in 1953, summary proceedings con- tained a similar causal inference.[50]

In the case of India, highly influential commentary on DDT's impact in the country appeared in 1958 within a larger study of India's economic and demographic 'prospects' by U.S. demographer, Ansley Coale, and economist, Edgar M. Hoover.[51] Here, the two authors arrived at an estimate of 2 mil- lion lives saved annually by the National Malaria Eradication Programme

(NMEP) through the 1950s. Their estimate, however, was not based on vital registration data, under the assumption that '[n]o adequate . . . Indian data exist.' The figure was reached indirectly, instead, by extrapolating from the experience of Sri Lanka where marked post-WW2 crude death rate decline had already been assumed largely due to DDT. Major post-war decline in mortality in India was simply assumed to have begun *after* 1951, corresponding to initiation of the residual insecticide spray program in the country.[52]

This latter assumption has since been recognized as inaccurate. Much of the post-WW2 mortality decline in India in fact *preceded* initiation of the DDT spray program in the early 1950s. In Punjab, for example, an abrupt fall in crude death rates took place in the mid-1940s (Figure 7.1),[53] as Dyson and Murphy also show for Maharashtra, Gujarat, and Tamil Nadu, associated more generally, they suggest, with an economic and employment boom in developing countries in the immediate post-war period related to sudden very favourable terms of trade.[54] Admittedly, the Coale-Hoover estimates were not presented as epidemiological in purpose, the goal of their 1958

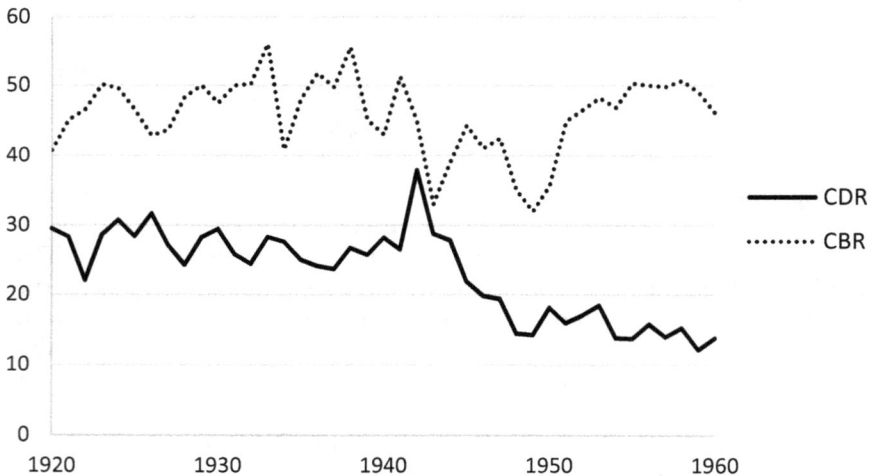

*Figure 7.1* Mean annual crude death rate,* crude birth rate (per 1,000), 11 plains districts,** (East) Punjab, 1920–60.

*Sources*: 1920–1947: *PSCR, PPHA*; 1948–1950: Directorate General of Health Services, *Report for the Quadrennium, 1949–1952*, 28; 1951–1960: *Census of India, 1961*. Punjab. District Handbooks. See S. Zurbrigg, *Epidemic Malaria and Hunger in Colonial Punjab* (London/New Delhi: Routledge, 2019), p. 385.

* Plague deaths omitted. For discussion of the 1948–9 dip in vital rates associated with Partition, see *ibid.*, pp. 386–7.

** Hissar, Rohtak, Gurgaon, Karnal, Amballa, Hoshiarpur, Jullundur, Ludhiana, Ferozepur, Amritsar, Gurdaspur.

report lay instead in conveying the authors' apprehension regarding the economic effects of post-war demographic growth in India. Yet their academic prominence, as in the case of Davis, ensured that their conclusions would be influential.[55] Likewise, the earlier view of Sri Lankan crude death decline as substantially related to malaria control – upon which the estimates of lives saved by DDT-based malaria control in India were based – continues to inform South Asian post-WW2 experience and much contemporary global health analysis as well.[56] In addressing current understanding of modern South Asian malaria mortality history, then, familiarity with malaria control in Sri Lanka is a necessary starting point – if risking some tedium in revisiting earlier debate.

### Post-WW2 mortality decline in Sri Lanka (Ceylon)

In the case of Sri Lanka, the thesis that DDT was responsible for much of the decline in mortality in the immediate post-WW2 period would be questioned by a number of Sri Lankan analysts. In his 1958 *Demography of Ceylon* K.N. Sarkar pointed out that mortality levels on the island were already in decline before initiation of the DDT spray program in mid-1946. Economic development programs along with school feeding and primary health care initiatives were undertaken in the late 1930s and early 1940s, programs that were greatly expanded in the immediate post-WW2 period.[57] S.A. Meegama notes that neonatal tetanus deaths in Colombo had declined by 75 per cent in the early years of the twentieth century and puerperal sepsis deaths by 67 per cent between 1930 and 1939.[58] In 1960, Harald Frederiksen, a program officer with the U.S. Public Health Service and USAID advisor to the National Malaria Eradication Programme in India, concurred with Sarkar, pointing out additional gaps in the Coale-Hoover assessment of DDT's role. In a series of articles[59] Frederiksen showed that the malaria control explanation failed to take into account the timing of DDT spraying in different regions of the country. The major drop in crude death rate in Sri Lanka, he pointed out, occurred very rapidly between 1946 and 1947 across the island. Both the malarious and non-malarious regions experienced similar proportionate declines in mortality between 1945 and 1947 (Table 7.1), although only 28 per cent of the population at that point was covered by the DDT spray program. Moreover, most of the decline in crude death rate occurred in the second half of 1946, the July–December death rate for the country as a whole declining from 21.3 in 1945 to 15.4 in 1946 (Table 7.2), at a time when only 18 per cent of the population was included in the DDT program.[60]

Frederiksen also stressed, as had Sarkar, that death rates were already in decline pre-DDT, and that some of the major stepwise decline post-war likely represented resumption of this earlier trend interrupted by the wartime

*Table 7.1* Death rates (all causes) in the malarious and non-malarious areas of Ceylon [Sri Lanka] during the second semesters, 1944–1948 and 1953

| Second semester | Malarious area (spleen rate > 10%) | Non-malarious area (spleen rate < 10%) | Ceylon |
|---|---|---|---|
| 1944 | 21.0 | 19.2 | 19.9 |
| 1945 | 23.8 | 19.1 | 20.8 |
| 1946 | 17.6 | 14.5 | 15.7 |
| 1947 | 14.6 | 13.7 | 14.0 |
| 1948 | 13.6 | 14.1 | 13.9 |
| 1953 | 10.9 | 11.3 | 11.2 |

*Source*: H. Frederiksen, 'Malaria control and population pressure in Ceylon,' *Public Health Reports*, 75, 10, Oct. 1960, p. 867, Table 4.

*Table 7.2* Percentage of population protected against malaria by residual spraying of insecticides and semestral death rates (all causes), Ceylon, 1944–1953

|  | Semiannual death rates* | | Percent of population protected |
|---|---|---|---|
|  | First semester | Second semester | |
| 1944 | 21.6 | 21.1 | 0 |
| 1945 | 22.6 | 21.3 | 3 |
| 1946 | 25.1 | 15.4 | 18 |
| 1947 | 15.2 | 13.2 | 28 |
| 1948 | 13.5 | 13.2 | 40 |
| 1949 | 13.0 | 12.1 | 36 |
| 1950 | 12.3 | 12.9 | 35 |
| 1951 | 13.1 | 12.7 | 36 |
| 1952 | 12.3 | 11.7 | 38 |
| 1953 | 10.8 | 11.1 | 36 |

*Source*: H. Frederiksen, 'Malaria control and population pressure in Ceylon,' *Public Health Reports*, 75, 10, Oct. 1960, p. 866, Table 2.

exigencies of plummeting rice imports.[61] He went on to identify improvement in a range of economic indicators, among them a substantial rise in personal consumption between 1938 and 1947.[62] Beginning in the final years of WW2, irrigation development and colonization was undertaken in the highly malarious dry zone, prompted by the cut-off of rice imports in late 1942 with the Japanese occupation of Burma.[63] Moreover, in the immediate post-war period food security programs were greatly expanded such that coverage of the wartime program of subsidized rice rations (2 kgs per person per week) was universal by 1948.[64] By that year, 3,500 milk feeding centres were distributing free milk to pregnant women, infants, and preschool children, its beneficial effect reaching 'colonist' families in the highly malarial dry zone in particular.[65] As well, government spending on school meals increased four-fold between 1943 and 1947 from Rs 1.6 to 7.1 million,[66] and rural school enrolment rose to over 870,000 children with the 1945 abolition of school tuition fees.[67]

In other words, far-reaching shifts in food security – and in agricultural employment in the dry malarious zone – took place in the immediate post-war period. Though exact timing, month to month, of coverage of such programs over the 1946–1947 period is unclear, it seems probable that much of their expansion began in 1946 itself. Additionally, as mentioned above, the immediate post-war years saw an economic boom in developing countries, including in Sri Lanka.[68] 'Improvements in the whole range of economic indices,' Frederiksen observed, 'were more or less concurrent with the decline in the death rate.'[69] Nutritional anthropometric data also supports the view of major improvement in post-war food security, the mean weight of school children 6 to 18 years of age increasing by 10 per cent between 1945 and 1950.[70] Government health care spending also increased post-war.[71] However, taking inflation into account, Frederiksen estimated that total health care expenditure in 1947 was still roughly at 1938 levels, suggesting such services were unlikely to have played a major role in the abrupt decline in mortality between 1946 and 1947.[72]

### The Newman assessment

Despite much evidence to suggest alternate explanations for Sri Lankan post-war malaria mortality decline, the DDT thesis has remained prominent in Western academic literature. In the 1963 edition of *Practical Malariology*, for example, Russell would repeat his earlier assertion as to the role of DDT, with no mention of the questions raised in 1960 by Frederiksen in the [U.S.] *Public Health Reports*.[73] In 1965, Peter Newman acknowledged Frederiksen's critique, but argued that there were too many factors at play in the key period of 1946–1947 to allow for a 'disentangling' of determinants of death rate decline. He offered instead an *indirect* method of analysis, one based on pre-DDT spleen rate levels (1938–1941) in relation to 'post-1945' mortality decline in the malarious 'dry zone' and non-malarious 'wet zone' divisions of the island. Regression analysis, he concluded, showed DDT to have contributed 42 per cent of post-war mortality decline nationally.[74]

The Newman analysis was problematic methodologically in a number of ways, in addition to eschewing the opportunity for direct analysis of timing of mortality decline in relation to DDT coverage. The validity of the regression model employed itself was seriously at question where confounding variables clearly were at play, among them major shifts in food security pre- and post-1945 associated with government programs and the post-war economic boom.[75] Moreover, use of spleen rate data as a measure of malaria transmission rates was also questionable, malarial splenic enlargement having long been recognized as influenced by socio-economic factors beyond local malaria transmission levels.[76] Langford rightly observes that 'in some degree improvements in nutrition and general state of health would be expected to reduce spleen rates, and malaria morbidity, and malaria mortality, even if exposure to the risk of malaria remained unchanged.'[77]

It would not be until the early 1990s that the questions raised by Frederiksen with respect to post-war mortality decline in Sri Lanka would be revisited however, this time from the pen of an historical demographer. As Frederiksen had done, C.M. Langford tracked timing of DDT initiation in relation to regional patterns of general and infant mortality decline. Like Sarkar, Langford placed post-war crude death rate decline in the context of longer-term post-1920 patterns of mortality decline in the country. He also attempted to take into account expansion in health, anti-malarial, and school feeding programs over the period from 1930 through to 1954, remarking that 'there was clearly a great deal going on' across the 1936–1949 period in addition to DDT spraying.[78] Even without factoring in post-war economic expansion or most food security and agricultural support measures (for which less specific data was available), Langford concluded that DDT interruption of malaria transmission could explain little of the largest stepwise drop in mortality, that which occurred between 1946 and 1947. At most, DDT interruption of malaria transmission on the island might explain *some* of the more modest *subsequent* decline in crude death rate that occurred between 1948 and 1951 (Langford estimates less than 16 per cent), itself an assessment based upon counterfactual estimates about *potential* increase in malaria mortality in the two subsequent low-rainfall years of 1948–1949 had there been no DDT-spraying, and assuming drought-enhanced transmission on the island.[79] As Langford points out, however, even this post-1947 estimate of DDT impact is open to question for not taking into account very different conditions of food security and quinine access in the later period.[80]

Despite the compelling questions raised by analysts such as Frederiksen, Sarkar, and Langford, the influence of the early literature positing a primary role for DDT in post-WW2 global mortality decline remains strong, with 1950s malaria transmission control continuing to be cited as a major contributor to post-war mortality decline in South Asia and among low-income countries in general.[81]

## Privileging the microbiologic

The indirect and highly tenuous statistical modelling approach employed by Newman to arrive at a microbiological (parasite transmission) explanation of post-war mortality decline in Sri Lanka contrasts starkly with the casual, indeed negligible, treatment accorded by the same author to shifts in food security in post-war Sri Lanka. In this, Newman was not alone. The analytic invisibility of food security can be seen as well in analysis by R.H. Gray who in 1974 reworked the Newman analysis ostensibly to take into account the methodologically confounding variable of 'nutrition' and the question of longer-term mortality trend.[82] Gray acknowledged that possible differences in nutritional status between the malarious and non-malarious regions of the country undermined the validity of the regression model employed by Newman. To rectify the problem, he turned to a 1940–1941 dietary survey which showed, he suggested, that '[i]f anything . . . the endemic areas had marginally better diets' than did the 'wet' non-malarial zone of the island,[83] a conclusion he considered to allow the Newman regression analysis to stand methodologically.

Given the well-recognized limitations of dietary surveys, the choice of the 1941 survey as a means of assessing nutritional status is curious[84] – all the more so given that it was conducted over a single 10-day interval in the post-monsoon agricultural harvest months from late February through March, a period unlikely to capture the seasonal hunger typical of the dry endemic zone where only single harvests per year were then feasible.[85] The choice was that much more puzzling in light of the availability of direct data on nutritional status. A nutritional anthropometry study published in the same journal in 1949, for example, indicated greater nutritional stunting prevalence in 1948 among students from the dry malarial zone relative to the wet zone,[86] a finding consistent with abundant accounts of extreme food insecurity and poverty in much of the dry northern zone of the country.[87] There also was evidence of major post-war improvement in nutritional status apparently in all regions of the country as Frederiksen had earlier pointed out, the Director of Health Services reporting a 10 per cent increase in weight and heights of children between 1945 and 1950.[88]

What is remarkable here is that despite empirical evidence of substantial improvement in post-war food security and nutritional status, neither Newman nor Gray attempted to incorporate these data in their assessment of post-war mortality decline in Sri Lanka.[89] It is difficult to avoid the conclusion that the 1941 dietary survey was employed in the latter's analysis not so much to investigate shifts in hunger, but rather to set aside methodological concerns relating to a confounding influence of food security in the original Newman analysis. Notwithstanding serious limitations to the Newman-Gray analyses, Samuel Preston, a leading U.S. demographer and economist, concluded in 1975 that Frederiksen's 'arguments have been convincingly refuted by Newman.'[90] From there, the Newman analysis has continued to appear in contemporary literature, interpreted as confirming a substantial role for DDT in post-war Sri Lankan mortality decline.[91]

The first half of the twentieth century was a seminal period in the health history of the Sri Lankan people. In the years immediately preceding initiation of the DDT spray program, there were dramatic shifts in food security brought about by social welfare policies, resumption of pre-war levels of foodgrain imports, and the post-war boom in economic growth. These years brought employment growth, food rationing programs, and undoubtedly also subtle but key shifts in conditions of women's work affecting child care and feeding, above all in the dry zone of the country. A major impact of these policies is suggested in improved nutritional anthropometric indices, as noted above. Improvement is seen as well in decline in those causes of infant mortality associated with severe hunger.[92] With the exception of the work of Frederiksen, however, there has been a near-complete absence of investigation of food security trends across the period of post-war Sri Lankan mortality decline in Western demographic and health literature, a neglect that stands in contrast to analysis by Sri Lankan historians.[93]

We have seen the invisibility of human subsistence in malaria control analysis before, in relation to the construction of the Panama Canal. Frank Snowden suggests a similar omission of economic factors in accounts of the WW2 malaria control campaign in Italy.[94] Once the global residual insecticide program had begun, assumptions with respect to mortality impact came to be more or less 'locked in' – slipping into certitude within the broader historiographical domain.[95] Yet even before the era of residual insecticides, an academic privileging of the 'germ' side of the epidemic equation was evident in relation to the 1934–1935 Sri Lankan epidemic, as seen in chapter two. In his analysis of the epidemic presented to the Royal Society of Medicine meeting in November 1935, Briercliffe, chief medical officer of colonial Ceylon, omitted any reference to destitution, though his administration had been fully occupied throughout the epidemic with famine relief efforts in addition to malaria treatment. Interestingly, included in Briercliffe's Royal Society presentation was a photograph of a young child in a state of extreme emaciation (marasmus) with typical signs of skeletal upper arm circumference and hair depigmentation. The photo revealed the classic lower-body swelling ('kwashiorkor') of end-stage starvation, yet was entitled 'Child with post-malarial oedema.'[96] One year later, Lewis Hackett, a leading proponent of vector control with the Rockefeller Foundation, suggested in his prominent text, *Malaria in Europe*, that

> [e]pidemics of any disease seem to develop a sinister character which tempts observers to assume either an unusual susceptibility on the part of the population produced by famine, economic stress etc. . . . We no longer resort to any influence more mysterious than summer heat, an abundance of anopheles, and a few good infectors . . . [that allow] new infection [to] increase by geometrical progression.[97]

Unintentionally perhaps, Hackett here epitomizes the wider epistemic shift where consideration of 'social' factors in epidemic disease causation is now seen as unscientific ('mysterious') and unprofessional.

Clearly, this is not to suggest that malaria transmission in Sri Lanka was innocuous among the well-fed. Malaria's inherent case fatality rate is not negligible, particularly falciparum malaria among the non-immune, above all in regions of intense holoendemic transmission. It is a toll that includes substantial stillbirth risk among pregnant women as well – if here too the historical mortality toll in South Asia appears to have risen markedly under conditions of food crisis. Yet in assessing historical determinants of malaria mortality decline, the question, Frederiksen reminds us, 'is not whether malaria is a potential killer but whether malaria control actually had a major role in the dramatic post-war island-wide reduction in mortality in Ceylon.'[98] Empirical evidence from South Asia suggests it did not. Indeed, post-WW2 experience in Sri Lanka has direct parallels with that in Punjab one decade later where little evidence exists of substantial mortality decline with the 1950s DDT-based interruption of malaria transmission in the state.[99] Nor is the view of malaria as the 'great debilitator' (in the absence of acute hunger-debility) supported by subsequent mortality patterns with the resurgence of malaria transmission from the late 1960s in Sri Lanka or India.[100] It is Frederiksen's larger question that frames the conclusions of this study.

# Notes

1 R. Ross, 'Malaria Prevention at Mian Mir,' *Lancet*, Jul. 3, 1909, 43–45. See S. Zurbrigg, *Epidemic Malaria and Hunger in Colonial Punjab: 'Weakened by Want'* (London and New Delhi: Routledge, 2019), 245. For similar pressures evident in the 1950 debate regarding extension of residual insecticide-based malaria transmission control programs to holoendemic regions in Africa, see WHO Registry files. WHO.2.DC.Mal.2. Africa Reports, 3, as cited in M.J. Dobson, M. Malowany, and R.W. Snow, 'Malaria Control in East Africa: The Kampala Conference and Pare-Taveta Scheme: A Meeting of Common and High Ground,' *Parassitologia*, 42, 149–166, 2000, 157–158.

2 On the food and labour policy changes initiated by Gorgas, see Zurbrigg, *Epidemic Malaria and Hunger*, 230; S.R. Christophers, and C.A. Bentley, *Malaria in the Duars: Being the Second Report to the Advisory Committee Appointed by the Government of India to Conduct an Enquiry regarding Black-water and Other Fevers Prevalent in the Duars* (Simla: Government Monotype Press, 1911), 56–57; P. Hehir, *Malaria in India* (Oxford: Oxford University Press, 1927), 9.

3 'Perhaps after the great demonstrations are over and money begins to fail a little,' Lewis Hackett would surmise regarding potential waning public interest in continued DDT spraying in rural Kanara district, India, 'the control of malaria could be continued with the collateral effect on flies, cockroaches, fleas, lice and all the insects which we have including also some mammals like bats and mice which seem to disappear at the same time'; L. Hackett, *Proceedings of the Fourth International Congresses on Tropical Medicine and Malaria*, Washington, D.C., May 10–18, 1948, vol. 2, 879.

4 W. Bynum, and C. Landry, *The Western Medical Tradition: 1800 to 2000* (Cambridge: Cambridge University Press, 2006), 239.

5 R. Ross, *Memoirs: With a Full Account of the Great Malaria Problem and Its Solution* (London: Murray, 1923), 115. In McLeod's colourful phrasing, the history of tropical medicine is written in 'the language of military and political

conquest; the history of conflict in biblical dimensions, between the heroic endeavours of human beings and the vast microscopic armies and resources of the animal kingdom. Memoirs of tropical doctors are the journals of medical Caesars confronting microbial Gauls'; R. Macleod, and M. Lewis, eds., *Disease, Medicine and Empire: Perspectives on Western medicine and the experience of European expansion* (London: Routledge, 1988), 6.

6　R. Packard, and P. Gadehla, 'A Land Filled with Mosquitoes: Fred L. Soper, the Rockefeller Foundation, and the Anopheles Gambiae Invasion of Brazil,' *Medical Anthropology*, 17, 1994, 215–238, at 233.

7　P. Manson, *Tropical Diseases: A Manual of the Diseases of Warm Climates* (London: Cassell, 1898), xvi.

8　M. Worboys, 'Germs, Malaria and the Invention of Mansonian Tropical Medicine: From "Diseases in the Tropics" to "Tropical Diseases",' in D. Arnold, ed., *Warm Climates in Western Medicine: The Emergence of Tropical Medicine, 1500–1900* (Amsterdam: Redopi, 1996), 181–207 at 195. Arnold notes similar professional opportunities in nutritional science; 'The "Discovery" of Malnutrition and Diet in colonial India,' *Indian Economic and Social History Review*, 31, 1, 1994, 1–26, at 17.

9　G. Harrison, *Mosquitoes, Malaria and Man: A History of the Hostilities since 1880* (New York: E.P. Dutton, 1978), 198, 208; S. Litsios, *The Tomorrow of Malaria* (Wellington, NZ: Pacific Press, 1996), 61. S.P. James and E. Brumpt would both question shifts in vector species and human exposure associated with agriculture modernization as the explanation for the disappearance of malaria in Europe; S.P. James, 'The Disappearance of Malaria from England,' *Proceedings of the Royal Society of Medicine*, 23, 1, Nov. 1929, 71–87; E. Brumpt, 'Anophélisme sans paludisme et régression spontanée du paludisme,' *Ann. Parasit. hum. comp.*, 20, 1944, 67–91.

10　Worboys notes the late nineteenth-century 'relative decline in the influence of epidemiology [that] signaled declining interest in social factors, as disease was constituted in relations between bacteria and individual bodies where personal behaviour, not social structures and social relations, determined the balance of disease and health'; M. Worboys, *Spreading Germs: Disease Theories and Medical Practice in Britain* (Cambridge: Cambridge University Press, 2000), 285.

11　R. Packard, and P.J. Brown, 'Rethinking Health, Development, and Malaria: Historicizing a Cultural Model in International Health,' *Medical Anthropology*, 17, 1997, 181–194, at 191–192.

12　N.H. Swellengrebel, 'Some Aspects of the Malaria Problem in Italy,' in League of Nations Malaria Commission, *Report on its Tour of Investigation in Certain European Countries in 1924* (Geneva: League of Nations, 1925), Annex 11, 168–171, at 171. See ch. 1 at note 44.

13　S. Amrith, 'Political Culture of Health in India: A Historical Perspective,' *Economic and Political Weekly*, Jan. 13, 2007, 114–121.

14　Hackett to Russell, October 18 and November 3, 1924; cited in J. Farley, *To Cast Out Disease: A History of the International Health Division of the Rockefeller Foundation (1913–1951)* (New York: Oxford University Press, 2004), 118.

15　L. Hackett, *Malaria in Europe: An Ecological Study* (London: Oxford University Press, 1937), 320. Prefacing his 1937 text as an effort for 'reconciliation of these two points of view,' Hackett acknowledged the distinction between malaria infection and debilitating disease, yet returned to a singular concern with transmission, concluding, '[t]here has never been any indication that malaria will spontaneously die out under such conditions': returning, in other words, to the view that infection *per se* was the principal problem and its interruption needed to be the goal; ibid., xiv–xvi. Hackett's argument parallels that expressed by Chadwick's sanitarian colleagues, that 'filth was the [factor] most easily remedied'; C. Hamlin, 'Predisposing Causes and Public Health in Early Nineteenth-Century Medical Thought,' *Society for the Social History of Medicine*, 5, 1, Apr. 1992, 43–70, at 66.

16  P. Russell, L.S. West, and R.D. Manwell, *Practical Malariology* (Philadelphia: W.B. Saunders, 1946), 555. Yet, arguably, even here, the socio-economic and basic chemotherapy route for removing or abating the mortality-morbidity burden of malaria was hardly long, as seen in the case of Italy or indeed even Punjab, though such measures were not within the direct power of the consultant vector eradicationist.

17  Litsios notes that 'the Cold War undermined the possibility of addressing politically sensitive issues, such as rural indebtedness and iniquitous land tenure systems'; 'Malaria Control, the Cold War, and the Postwar Reorganization of International Assistance,' *Medical Anthropology*, 17, 1997, 255–278, at 267–271. See also R. Packard, 'Malaria Dreams: Postwar Visions of Health and Development in the Third World,' *Medical Anthropology*, 17, 1997, 279–296; S. Amrith, *Decolonizing International Health: India and Southeast Asia, 1930–65* (Basingstoke: Palgrave Macmillan, 2006), 83–85; J. Siddiqui. *World Health and World Politics: The World Health Organization and the UN System* (London: Hurst, 1995); H. Cleaver, 'Malaria and the Political Economy of Public Health,' *International Journal of Health Services*, 7, 4, 1977, 557–79 at 568–73 [hereafter, *IJHS*]; J. Farley, *Brock Chisholm, the World Health Organization, and the Cold War* (Vancouver: University of British Columbia Press, 2008); J.A. Gillespie, 'Social Medicine, Social Security and International Health, 1940–60,' in *The Politics of the Healthy Life: An International Perspective* (Sheffield: European Association for the History of Medicine and Health, 2002), 219–239.

18  Farley, *To Cast Out Disease*, 296.

19  J. Ettling, *The Germ of Laziness: Rockefeller Philanthropy and Public Health in the New South* (Cambridge, MA: Harvard University Press, 1981), 185. See also, E. Richard Brown, 'Public Health in Imperialism: Early Rockefeller Programs at Home and Abroad,' *American Journal of Public Health*, 66, 9, 1976, 897–903 [hereafter, *AJPH*]; J.C. Goulden, *The Money Givers* (New York: Random House, 1971), ch. 2.

20  Ettling, *Germ of Laziness*, 206–208. Likewise, it is impossible to doubt Paul Russell's belief in the technological approach, if deeply shaped by ideological geopolitical views. His personality was complex: for example, he criticized neo-Malthusian arguments of colleagues who argued against malaria eradication over population 'explosion' concerns. As an ardent eradication proponent, Russell's rejection of that argument was of course logically required. But he went further, to include a relatively sophisticated (in the prevailing Western academic climate) articulation of demographic transition, an exposition on the economic need for children under conditions of poverty and precarious survival; in *Man's Mastery of Malaria*, 254. Russell would also warn against exclusive reliance on insecticides, and even acknowledged in 1936, if obliquely, the importance of drainage as an economic measure. Yet it is difficult to square this with the concerted exclusion of socio-economic perspective in policy formation within the ECM.

21  Over half of all Foundation funding between 1925 and the late 1930s was channelled to yellow fever research and programs; Farley, *To Cast Out Disease*, 88. Arguably Rockefeller Foundation funding of the LNHO reflected a similar

interest in protecting global trade, where a large portion of its work was directed to epidemiological surveillance, and standardization of microbiologic measurements, all congruent with the Rockefeller Foundation germ philosophy but also with rampant U.S. fears of imported microbes. At the first meeting of the trustees of the newly formed Rockefeller Foundation in 1913, concern over immigrant hookworm carriers loomed large: 'Every Indian coolie already in California was a center from which the infection continued to spread throughout the state'; Farley, *To Cast Out Disease*, 4.

22 In 1906, William H. Welch, the first dean of the Johns Hopkins Medical School and its School of Hygiene and Public Health, would praise the facilitating role of medical science in European and American 'efforts to colonize and to reclaim for civilization vast tropical regions'; H.H. Welch, 'The Benefits of the Endowment of Medical Research,' in *Addresses Delivered at the Opening of the Laboratories in New York City, May 11, 1906* (New York: Rockefeller Institute for Medical Research, 1906); as cited in Brown, 'Public Health in Imperialism,' 902.

23 J.S. Simmons, 'Welcoming Address at the Conference on Industry and Tropical Health. Conference Proceedings, Industry and Tropical Health,' *Industry and Tropical Health* 1, 12; as cited in Packard, 'Malaria Dreams,' 282. See also Marcos Cueto, *Cold War, Deadly Fevers: Malaria Eradication in Mexico, 1955–1975* (Washington, D.C.: Woodrow Wilson Centre Press, 2007), 49–69. Rieff notes Andrew S. Natsios, head of USAID and former vice president of World Vision, describing USAID as ' "a key foreign policy instrument . . . an important tool for the President to further America's interests . . . help[ing] nations prepare for participation in the global trading system and become better markets for U.S. exports" '; *A Bed for the Night: Humanitarianism in Crisis* (New York: Simon and Schuster, 2002), 236–237, 120.

24 R. Packard, 'Visions of Postwar Health and Development and Their Impact on Public Health Interventions in the Developing World,' in F. Cooper, and R. Packard, eds., *International Development and the Social Sciences: Essays on the History and Politics of Knowledge* (Berkeley: University of California Press, 1997), 93–115.

25 S. Franco-Agudelo, 'The Rockefeller Foundations' Antimalarial Program in Latin America: Donating or Dominating?,' *IJHS*, 13, 1, 1983, 51–67 at 59–60, at 64. Packard observes 'tropical disease control quickly became viewed as a critical weapon in the war against international Communism. . . . Malaria control programs were defined by the US Special Technical and Economic Missions to Vietnam and Thailand as "impact programs" . . . designed to have a rapid positive effect on local populations in order to build support for local governments and their US supporters'; 'Malaria Dreams,' 282–283.

26 P.F. Russell, *Man's Mastery of Malaria* (London: Oxford University Press, 1955), 221. Russell recounts the strategic origins of U.S. malaria control programs in 1940 in 18 Latin American countries, prompted by concerns for ensuring 'strategic materials'; ibid., 222–227. A summary account of the economic and military benefits accruing to the United States with global malaria control, including elimination of a $175 million annual 'malaria tax' on resource imports (malaria-related increased production costs) from developing countries, is given in P.F Russell, 'A Lively Corpse,' *Tropical Medicine News*, Jun. 5, 1948, 25.

27 Cleaver, 'Malaria and the Political Economy of Public Health.' Roger Jeffrey has estimated that, in the period 1950–1959, foreign aid to India accounted for 14 per cent of the total expenditure on health. 'Of this the UN (WHO and UNICEF) . . . accounted for only 15 per cent, most of the remainder coming from U.S. bilateral aid to India, channeled through the Public Law 480 programme'; *The Politics of Health in India*, (Berkeley: University of California Press, 1988), 102.

28 D.K. Viswanathan, *The Conquest of Malaria in India: An Indo-American Co-operative Effort* (Madras: Law Institute Press, 1958), 3–4, 58. See also K. Mankodi, 'Political and Economic Roots of Disease: Malaria in Rajasthan,' *Economic and Political Weekly*, Jan. 27, 1996, PE42–48; D. Kinkela, *DDT and the American Century: Global Health, Environmental Politics, and the Pesticide That Changed the World* (Chapel Hill: University of North Carolina Press, 2011). Packard cites early 1950s Iran as 'caught in a serious political upheaval' involving the 1953 U.S.-assisted overthrow of the Mossadegh government, with a 1956 International Development Advisory Board report suggesting that ' "the malaria component of the U.S. technical assistance program . . . play[ed] an important role in supporting our diplomatic representations with a concrete manifestation of our sincerity and mutual interest" '; 'Visions of Postwar Health,' 98–99.

29 Amrith, 'Political Culture of Health in India,' 118. For a similar pattern in Latin America, see M. Cueto, 'The Cycles of Eradication: The Rockefeller Foundation and Latin American Public Health, 1918–1940,' in P. Weindling, *International Health Organisations and Movements, 1918–1939* (Cambridge: Cambridge University Press, 1995), 222–243, at 228.

30 A. Hooton, Major IMS, Agency Surgeon, Kathiawar, letter to the *Indian Medical Gazette*, April 24, 1909, in *Transactions of the Bombay Medical Congress*, 93. See Zurbrigg, *Epidemic Malaria and Hunger*, 264–265.

31 Ibid., 225–226, 265.

32 Hamlin, *Public Health and Social Justice in the Age of Chadwick* (Cambridge: Cambridge University Press, 1998), 338.

33 Ibid., 157.

34 C. Hamlin, 'Could You Starve to Death in England in 1839? The Chadwick-Farr Controversy and the Loss of the "Social" in Public Health,' *AJPH*, 85, 6, Jun. 1995, 856–866.

35 'Dominated solely by the actuarial problems of pecuniary profit and loss, Chadwick laid no claims to universal humanitarianism but frankly admitted his narrow interests in keeping the poor rates down'; S.E. Finer, *The Life and Times of Sir Edwin Chadwick* (New York: Barnes and Noble, 1952), 157.

36 Margaret Jones recounts how reluctance on the part of the new indigenous government in Sri Lanka in the early 1930s to pursue aggressive weekly oiling of municipal cesspools and stocking wells with larvivorous fish had 'enabled hostile commentators at the metropolitan centre to place responsibility for the loss of life in 1934–35 at the feet of the new government . . . elected three years before'; *Health Policy in Britain's Model Colony: Ceylon, 1900–1948* (New Delhi: Orient Longman, 2004), 187. Rieff observes a modern parallel, the 'humanitarian' content of development assistance 'serv[ing] to immunize the public against any political questioning'; *A Bed for the Night*, 170.

37 Hamlin, 'Public Health and Social Justice,' 289 [emphasis added].

38 Rieff observes in relation to recent USAID military-aid in Afghanistan that '[t]he mainline relief agencies depend largely on young people who work on short contracts . . . and quickly get back to start real careers'; *A Bed for the Night*, 236–237, 120.

39 S.P. James, Presidential Address, 'Advances in Knowledge of Malaria Since the War,' *Transactions of the Royal Society of Tropical Medicine and Hygiene*, 31, 3, Nov. 1937, 263–280, at 276.

40 Harrison, *Mosquitoes, Malaria and Man*, 140. There were of course instances where technical assistance was appropriate. Amrith for example describes a technical assistance agreement between the GOI, WHO and UNICEF signed in

July 1951 for construction of a penicillin factory near Pune, production beginning in 1955; *Decolonizing International Health*, 105.

41 'The Rockefeller Foundation phased out its International Health Division in 1951, merging it with the medical sciences program'; P. Weindling, 'American Foundations and the Internationalizing of Public Health,' in S. Gross Solomon, L. Murand, and P. Zylberman, eds., *Shifting Boundaries in Public Health: Europe in the Twentieth Century* (Rochester: University of Rochester Press, 2008), 63–85, at 79. A June 1951 Rockefeller Foundation report concluded: 'The problem of food has become one of the world's most acute and pressing problems; and . . . is the cause of much of the world's present tension and unrest. . . . Agitators from Communist countries are making the most of the situation. The time is now ripe, in places possibly over-ripe, for sharing some of our technical knowledge with these people. Appropriate action now may help them to attain by evolution the improvements, including those in agriculture, which otherwise may have to come by revolution'; 'The World Food Problem, Agriculture, and the Rockefeller Foundation,' by Advisory Committee for Agricultural Activities, June 21, 1951, RG 3, series 915, box 3, folder 23, Rockefeller Foundation Archives; as cited in J.H. Perkins, *Geopolitics and the Green Revolution: Wheat, Genes, and the Cold War* (New York: Oxford University Press, 1997), 138–139. Perkins concludes '[t]his specific report was instrumental in leading the Rockefeller Foundation to start its Indian Agricultural Program. . . . American plant-breeding science thus became part of the cold war's defense of capitalist political economies,' although the Rockefeller Foundation was already engaged in funding Borlaug's hybrid grain research by the early 1940s; ibid.,107. For a detailed account of the Foundation's influence in population analysis in India, see M. Rao, *From Population Control to Reproductive Health: Malthusian Arithmetic* (New Delhi: Sage, 2004), 27, 106–111.

42 A century earlier the vice-chairman of the Cockermouth [Poor Law] Union lamented, Hamlin recounts, that '[t]he people themselves are inert. . . . Their thoughts are engrossed by the great business of finding daily food; and they will not listen to any lectures upon the theory of infection, or the connexion [sic] between dirt and disease'; *Public Health and Social Justice*, 204.

43 Farley observes that it was only in 1926, following failure to eradicate hookworm infection in the U.S. South and after international malaria control activities were well underway, that a statistician was appointed to the IHB to begin analysis of projects' effectiveness, to dubious account; *To Cast Out Disease*, 112–113, 120, 176.

44 See above, ch. 4, note 4.

45 With the claims of the sanitationist portrayed as simple common sense, Hamlin observes, 'their confirmation by independent inquirers has not seemed particularly problematic to historians'; *Public Health and Social Justice*, 220, 160–161.

46 'Virtually nowhere,' Packard observes, 'was research conducted to investigate local conditions, or to study in a scientific manner the relative effectiveness of various approaches. The "R" word was not to be spoken and research activities were certainly not funded'; 'Malaria dreams,' 290.

47 K. Davis, 'The Population Specter: Rapidly Declining Death Rate in Densely Population Countries: The Amazing Decline of Mortality in Underdeveloped Areas,' *American Economic Review*, 46, 2, 1956, 305–318, at 311. Davis's source for his DDT conclusion was H. Cullumbine, 'An Analysis of the Vital Statistics of Ceylon,' *Ceylon Journal of Medical Science*, Dec. 1950, 134–135; possibly also, E.J. Pampana, who by 1951 had concluded: 'Il semble donc évident que cette baisse doit être en grande partie mise au crédit du DDT,' in 'Lutte

antipaludique par les insecticides à action rémanents: résultats des campagnes antipaludiques,' *Bull. Org. Mond. Santé*, 3, 557–619, at 592. In neither article was analysis of timing and location of mortality decline in relation to DDT spraying offered.

48 Davis, 'The Population Specter,' 312; also, Pampana, 'Lutte antipaludique,' 600.

49 P.F. Russell, *Man's Mastery of Malaria* (London: Oxford University Press, 1955), 167, 244. Early on, G. Macdonald offered a similar interpretation: 'A similar reduction [with malaria control], from 31.8 to 15.4 per 1000, has been seen in the notorious North Central Province of Ceylon, which has for long been one of the most malarious parts of that country'; 'Community Aspects of Immunity to Malaria,' *British Medical Bulletin*, 8, 1951, 33–36, reprinted in L. Bruce-Chwatt, and V.J. Glanville, eds., *Dynamics of Tropical Diseases: The Late George Macdonald* (London: Oxford University Press, 1973), 77–84, at 84.

50 F.J. Dy, 'Present Status of Malaria Control in Asia,' *Bulletin of the WHO*, 11, 1954, 725–763, at 726, 736. This interpretation is puzzling given that the full complement of Sri Lankan mortality data had been sent, Frederiksen relates, to WHO officials in Bangkok for the 1953 conference and 1954 Taipei conference; H. Frederiksen, 'Malaria Control and Population Pressure in Ceylon,' *Public Health Reports*, 75, 10, Oct. 1960, 865–868. See also 'First Asian Malaria Conference in September 1953,' *Chronicle of the WHO*, 8, 4, Apr. 1954, 117–123, at 120.

51 A.J. Coale, and E.M. Hoover, *Population Growth and Economic Development in Low Income Countries: A Case Study of India's Prospects* (Princeton: Princeton University Press, 1958), 62–67. A subsequent analysis of the 1950s Indian malaria eradication program (MEP) was limited to assessing the 'costs and benefits' of eradication versus simply ongoing control; E.J. Cohn, 'Assessing the Costs and Benefits of Anti-Malarial Programs: The Indian Experience,' *AJPH*, 63, 12, Dec. 1973, 1086–1096, at 1095.

52 Coale, and Hoover, *Population Growth and Economic Development*, 14–15, 62, 65. The 2 million figure is also J.A. Sinton's estimate in the mid-1930s; in 'What malaria costs India, nationally, socially and economically,' *Records of the Malaria Survey of India*, 5, 3, Sept. 1935, 223–264, at 256, and that cited by Paul Russell in 1941; 'Some Social Obstacles to Malaria Control,' *Indian Medical Gazette*, Nov. 1941, 681–690. One-quarter of all fever deaths, it appears, was assumed due to malaria, an estimate first offered in the pre-1909 period. On this, see Zurbrigg, *Epidemic Malaria and Hunger*, 102.

53 For discussion of possible factors contributing to this marked step-wise decline, see Zurbrigg, *Epidemic Malaria and Hunger*, ch. 12.

54 T. Dyson and M. Murphy, 'Macro-level Study of Socioeconomic Development and Mortality: Adequacy of Indicators and Methods of Statistical Analysis,' in J. Cleland, and A. Hill, eds., *The Health Transition: Methods and Measures*. Health Transition Series No. 3 (Canberra: Australian National University, 1991), 147–164, at 153. For analysis of economic and food security conditions in post-WW2 Punjab, see Zurbrigg, *Epidemic Malaria and Hunger*, 389–394.

55 See, e.g., R.P Sinha, *Food in India: An Analysis of the Prospects for Self-Sufficiency by 1975–76* (Delhi: Oxford University Press, 1961), 39.

56 Harrison, *Mosquitoes, Malaria and Man*, 229; S. Anand, and R. Kanbur, 'Public Policy and Basic Needs Provision: Intervention and Achievement in Sri Lanka,' in J. Drèze, and A. Sen, eds., *The Political Economy of Hunger* (Oxford: Clarendon, 1991), vol. 3, 59–92 at 63–64; L.T. Ruzicka, and H. Hansluwka, 'Mortality in Selected Countries of South and East Asia,' in WHO, ed., *Mortality in South and East Asia: A Review of Changing Trends and Patterns, 1950–1975* (Manila:

World Health Organization), 1982, 83–155, at 123, in WHO, *Mortality in South and East Asia: A Review of Changing Trends and Patterns, 1950–1975* (Manila: World Health Organization, 1982); D.F.S. Fernando, 'Health Statistics in Sri Lanka, 1921–80,' in S.B. Halstead, et al., eds., *Good Health at Low Cost* (New York: Rockefeller Foundation, 1985), 85; P. Jha, and A. Mills, *Improving Health Outcomes of the Poor: The Report of the Working Group 5 of the Commission on Macroeconomics and Health* (Geneva: World Health Organization, 2002), 38; M. Worboys, 'Colonial Medicine,' in R. Cooter, and J. Pickstone, eds. *Medicine in the Twentieth Century* (Amsterdam: Harwood Academic Publ., 2000), 79; R. Packard, *The Making of a Tropical Disease* (Baltimore: Johns Hopkins University Press, 2007), 146.

57  K.N. Sarkar, *The Demography of Ceylon* (Colombo: Govt Press, 1958), at 123.

58  S.A. Meegama, 'The Decline in Maternal and Infant Mortality and its relation to Malaria Eradication,' *Population Studies*, 23, 2, 1969, 289–302. Together, if such efforts were extended widely beyond the urban population through the 1940s they potentially could have reduced infant mortality rate by as much as 40 per 1,000 live births, assuming near-universal mortality among those infants without access to breastfeeding in cases of maternal deaths.

59  H. Frederiksen, 'Malaria Control and Population Pressure in Ceylon,' *Public Health Reports*, 75, 10, Oct. 1960, 865–868; H. Frederiksen, 'Determinants and Consequences of Mortality Trends in Ceylon, *Public Health Reports*, 76, 8, Aug. 1961, 659–663; H. Frederiksen, 'Economic and Demographic Consequences of Malaria Control in Ceylon,' *Indian Journal of Malariology*, 16, 4, Dec. 1962, 370–391; H. Frederiksen, 'Dynamic Equilibrium of Economic and Demographic Transition,' *Economic Development and Cultural Change*, 14, 1, Oct. 1965, 316–322; H. Frederiksen, Book Review of P. Newman, '*Malaria Eradication and Population Growth 1965*,' *American Journal of Tropical Medicine and Hygiene*, 15, 2, 1966, 262–264; H. Frederiksen, 'Determinants and Consequences of Mortality and Fertility Trends,' *Public Health Reports*, 81, 8, Aug. 1966, 715–727; H. Frederiksen, 'Malaria Eradication and the Fall of Mortality: A Note,' *Population Studies*, 24, 1, Mar. 1970, 111–113.

60  Frederiksen, 'Malaria Control and Population Pressure,' at 866, Table 2. Wernsdorfer also supported Frederiksen's analysis, noting that '[i]n the non-malarious areas the average [death rate] decrease was 30.6%, in the malarious areas 33.5%. This difference is statistically significant (p < 0.001) but in absolute terms it would account for only 784 lives saved from malaria during the second semester of 1953, representing some 1.7% of deaths from all causes and certainly not enough to explain the major drop in mortality rates'; 'Social and Economic Aspects,' 1434, in W.H. Wernsdorfer, and I.A. McGregor, eds., *Malaria: Principles and Practice of Malariology* (Edinburgh: Churchill Livingstone, 1988), vol. 2, 913–998.

61  Frederiksen, 'Determinants and Consequences of Mortality Trends in Ceylon,' 659. Per capita food imports, primarily rice, declined by 25 per cent in 1942–1943 relative to pre-war levels following the 1942 Japanese occupation of Burma, triggering hyperinflation similar to that in Bengal; Frederiksen, 'Economic and Demographic Consequences,' 380, 383. Meyer suggests the 1934–1935 malaria epidemic marked a turning point in accountable governance in Sri Lanka; E. Meyer, 'L'Épidémie de malaria de 1934–1935 à Sri-Lanka: Fluctuations économiques et fluctuations climatiques,' *Cultures et Développement*, 14, 2–3, 1982, 183–226, at 186; 14, 4, 589–638, at 629–633.

62  Frederiksen, 'Determinants and Consequences of Mortality Trends,' 661–662, Table 5.

63 With marked decline in rice imports in 1942, government '[i]nvestment on peasant colonisation schemes in the dry zone was increased, and the range of free services given by government to the colonists expanded well beyond what had been envisaged in 1939'; K.M. De Silva, *A History of Sri Lanka* (Delhi: Oxford University Press, 1981), 472. As in Punjab a war-economy boom was felt in Sri Lanka 'with Sri Lanka the main source of natural rubber for the Allied powers after the Japanese overran Malaya and the Dutch East Indies,' and Sri Lanka established as the South East Asia Command with its network of bases on the island; ibid., 470–471. Severe drought and harvest failure in 1945–1946, however, triggered a 'sharp rise in the death rate from starvation, malnutrition and malaria'; S.A. Meegama, 'Malaria Eradication and its Effect on Mortality Levels,' *Population Studies* 21, 3, Nov. 1967, 207–237, at 217.

64 De Silva, *A History of Sri Lanka*, 470–472; W.A.A.S. Peiris, *Socio-Economic Development and Fertility Decline in Sri Lanka* (New York: United Nations, Dept. International Economic and Social Affairs, 1986), 57–58. On food rationing in Sri Lanka, see P. Isenman, 'Basic Needs: The Case of Sri Lanka,' *World Development*, 8, 1980, 237–258.

65 Imports of milk and milk foods into Ceylon rose exponentially from 2,184,000 lbs in 1942 to 8,112,000 in 1945, then to 28,880,000 lbs by 1947; Meegama, 'Malaria Eradication and its Effect on Mortality Levels,' 213, 222.

66 C. Langford, 'Reasons for the Decline in Mortality in Sri Lanka Immediately after the Second World War: A Re-Examination of the Evidence,' *Health Transition Review*, 6, 1993, 3–23, at 15.

67 De Silva, *A History of Sri Lanka*, 198, 475.

68 Dyson and Murray, 'Macro-level study of socioeconomic development and mortality.'

69 Frederiksen, 'Economic and demographic consequences,' 386. Frederiksen was not criticizing the program itself. As USAID consultant, by the mid-1960s he was actively involved with the National Malaria Eradication Programme in India and applauded both the reduced morbidity from the disease and increase in dry zone acreage under cultivation; 'Economic and demographic consequences,' 391. Indeed, a major concern for him, Litsios points out, was to refute the pessimism emerging from Western analysts who, under a neomalthusian perspective, questioned DDT programs as precipitating a population explosion that would 'overwhelm resulting economic gains'; S. Litsios, 'Malaria Control and Future of International Public Health,' in E. Casman, H. Dowlatabadi, eds., *The Contextual Determinants of Malaria* (Washington, D.C.: Resources for the Future, 2002), 292–328 at 316.

70 Frederiksen, 'Determinants and Consequences of Mortality Trends,' 661.

71 Health expenditures increased from Rs 12.9 million in 1939 to 37.2 million in 1947, by 1952 reaching 82.5 million; Langford, 'Reasons for the decline in mortality in Sri Lanka,' 15.

72 Frederiksen, 'Mortality Rates and Economic Development,' 17; Frederiksen, 'Determinants and Consequences of Mortality Trends,' 661–662.

73 P. Russell, L.S. West, R.D. Manwell, and G. Macdonald, *Practical Malariology* (London: Oxford University Press, 1963), 501. One decade later, this view would appear in an official Sri Lankan government report; *The Population of Sri Lanka* (Colombo: Dept of Census and Statistics, 1974), 5.

74 P. Newman, *Malaria Eradication and Population Growth with Special Reference to Ceylon and British Guiana*, Bureau of Public Health Economics, Research Series No. 10, School of Public Health (Ann Arbor: University of Michigan, 1965), 157; P. Newman, 'Malaria Control and Population Growth,' *Journal of Development Studies*, 6, 2, Jan. 1970, 133–158; P. Newman, 'Malaria

Eradication and Its Effects on Mortality Levels: A Comment,' *Population Studies*, 23, 2, 1969, 285–288; P. Newman, 'Malaria and Mortality,' *Journal of the American Statistical Association* 72, 358, 1977, 257–263. Newman, Frederiksen observed, 'prefers a more elaborate and circumstantial method . . . [one that] fails to quantify the extension of insecticides in time and place . . . [and] overlooks or ignores this opportunity to directly compare the reductions in mortality in areas with malaria and with spraying of insecticides, and in areas without malaria and without spraying of insecticides . . . substitut[ing] hypothetical extrapolation of the regression technique for empirical observation of the [mortality] results of the natural experiment'; Frederiksen, 'Book Review of P. Newman' [*Malaria Eradication and Population Growth*, 1965], 262–264; Frederiksen, 'Malaria Eradication and the Fall of Mortality,' 111–13).

75 Dyson and Murray, 'Macro-Level Study of Socioeconomic Development,' 147–164.
76 See Zurbrigg, *Epidemic Malaria and Hunger*, 101, 191–192; *Report on the Sanitary Administration of the Punjab*, 1908, 14.
77 Langford, 'Reasons for the Decline,' 18.
78 Ibid., 14.
79 As suggested by Newman, 'Malaria Control and Population Growth,' 157.
80 Langford, 'Reasons for the Decline,' 21–22. Moreover, a significant 'pre-emptive' role for DDT post-1947 is questionable, resting as it does on the assumption that epidemic mortality was driven primarily by malaria transmission levels. Major drought in 1938 as severe as that in 1948 (79.0 inches rainfall cf a mean of 99 inches) triggered increased malaria transmission, a high vector infection (sporozoite) rate (4.97 per cent), and a four-fold rise in 1939 dispensary fever cases; S. Rajendram, and S.H. Jayewickreme, 'Malaria in Ceylon,' *Indian Journal of Malariology*, 5, 1, Pt. 1, Mar. 1951, 1–73, at 57, 29, 67, 59. Yet 1939 mortality increased only marginally to 21.8 per 1,000 compared to 21.0 the year before; Frederiksen, 'Malaria Control and Population Pressure,' 866. Margaret Jones also notes the limited mortality outcome in 1939; *Health Policy in Britain's Model Colony*, 203–204.
81 See above, note 57.
82 R.H. Gray, 'The Decline of Mortality in Ceylon and the Demographic Effects of Malaria Control,' *Population Studies*, 28, 2, Jul. 1974, 205–229.
83 Gray, 'Decline of Mortality in Ceylon,' Table 11, 219; citing L. Nicholls, and A. Nimalasuriya, 'Rural Dietary Surveys in Ceylon,' *Ceylon Journal of Science* (D), V, Pt. D, Nov. 12, 1941, 59–110.
84 League of Nations, 'The Most Suitable Methods of Detecting Malnutrition due to the Economic Depression, Conference Held at Berlin from December 5th to 7th, 1932,' *Quarterly Bulletin of the Health Organisation*, 2, 1, Mar. 1933, 116–129.
85 Gray's interpretation of the Nicholls study itself is questionable. The eight highly malarious 'dry zone' study villages show caloric consumption to be slightly lower, not 'marginally better,' than that in the wet-zone villages. Average daily calorie consumption of the eight dry zone villages, listed as nos. 2–5 and 10–13, is recorded as 2,390 compared to a mean of 2,461 calories per day in the remaining five southwest wet-zone survey villages; in Nicholls and Nimalasuriya, 'Rural Dietary Surveys in Ceylon,' 63. Bibile and colleagues observed that 'in south-east Uva province . . . peasants consume three meals a day during the harvest, ie. from March onwards . . . [and in] August onwards, the number of meals become two and sometimes one for a day. The traders and landed proprietors have a regular supply of food throughout the years'; S.W. Bibile, H. Cullumbine, R.S. Watson,

and T. Wickremananake, 'A Nutritional Survey of Various Ceylon Communities,' *Ceylon Journal of Medical Science* (D), VI, Pt. 1, Mar. 21, 1949, 54.

86  H. Cullumbine, 'The Influence of Environment on Certain Anthropomorphic Characters,' *Ceylon Journal of Medical Science* (D), 6, 3, (1949), 164–170, at 171, Table 3. Gray was aware of this later study and cited its anthropometric findings, yet concluded that 'on balance . . . disparities in diet could not account for the mortality differences between zone of malaria prevalence before 1945'; Gray, 'Decline of Mortality in Ceylon,' 220.

87  The climatically precarious agricultural economy in the dry malarial zone was marked by 'hungry seasons . . . [m]alnutrition, and even starvation'; conditions Meegama described as 'inherent in the type of cultivation forced by circumstances on those people.' He pointed to 'innumerable references' in the annual colonial administrative reports to 'famine conditions and distress in this region' compared to the 'agriculturally prosperous' wet zone with its more secure agriculture and diversified economy, hence 'stable supply of food'; Meegama, 'Malaria Eradication and its Effect on Mortality Levels,' 211. See also above, ch. 2, at notes 13 and 46.

88  *Administrative Reports of the Director of Health Services, Ceylon,* no date; cited in Frederiksen, 'Determinants and Consequences of Mortality Trends in Ceylon,' 661.

89  Nor was there any attempt, as Brown points out, to incorporate any of the available literature on changing economic conditions in the dry zone, such as a 1952 International Bank for Reconstruction and Development report [*The Economic Development of Ceylon* (Baltimore: Johns Hopkins Press, 1952)]; P.J. Brown, 'Socioeconomic and Demographic Effects of Malaria Eradication,' *Social Science Medicine*, 1986, 852–853. Curiously, Brown also comes to accept the Gray analysis.

90  S. Preston, 'The Changing Relationship between Mortality and Level of Economic Development,' *Population Studies*, 29, 2, July 1975, 231–248, at 239; S. Preston, 'Causes and Consequences of Mortality Declines in Less Developed Countries during the Twentieth Century,' in R.A. Easterlin, ed., *Population and Economic Change in Developing Countries* (Chicago: University of Chicago Press, 1980), 296, 313. This, though in his own analysis Preston was unable to establish a statistical relationship between life expectancy increase and pre-DDT malaria endemicity; 'Causes and Consequences,' 311–312.

91  See, e.g., L. Molineaux, 'The Epidemiology of Human Malaria as an Explanation of its Distribution, Including Implications for Its Control,' in Wernsdorfer and McGregor, eds., *Malaria: Principles and Practice*, 974–976; R. Cassen, *India: Population, Economy, Society* (London: Macmillan, 1978), 86; R. Carter, and K.N. Mendis, 'Evolutionary and Historical Aspects of the Burden Of Malaria,' *Clinical Microbiology Reviews,* Oct. 2002, 564–594, at 584.

92  Among the four leading causes of infant mortality in Sri Lanka between 1935 and 1948, three were associated with undernourishment: 'debility'; 'rata' (a local term for a skin disease condition associated with malnutrition); and 'prematurity' (a term applied to low birth weight newborns, often associated with intrauterine undernourishment). Both 'debility' and 'rata' are recorded showing marked decline between the periods 1935–1939, 1944–1946 and 1948; in Sarkar, *The Demography of Ceylon*, 161. The fourth major cause of infant mortality listed, 'convulsions,' also shows major decline, a diagnosis that Nicholls suggested applies to '[m]any of the children who die within a week of birth appear[ing] to be of low vitality'; in 'A Nutritional Survey of the Poorer Classes in Ceylon,' *Ceylon Journal of Science.* (D), IV, Pt. 1, Apr. 30, 1936, 1–70, at 51–52. It is unlikely that many convulsion deaths were malarial, the large majority (71 per cent) occurring under one month of age, half within one week of birth; 'A Nutritional Survey,' 52.

93 'These [wartime] food subsidies . . . were continued thereafter to become one of the island's social welfare services'; De Silva, *A History of Sri Lanka*, 476. Both Frederiksen and Langford are acknowledged in Packard's important critique of the MBD thesis as questioning the DDT explanation of post-WW2 Ceylon mortality decline, but the actual content of the latter's analyses unfortunately is left unarticulated; R. Packard, ' "Roll Back Malaria"? Reassessing the Economic Burden of Malaria,' *Population and Development Review*, 35, 1, Mar. 2009, 53–87, at 66.

94 F. Snowden, *The Conquest of Malaria: Italy, 1900–1962* (New Haven: Yale University Press, 2006), 219–220.

95 William McNeill's reading is perhaps the most emphatic: 'The sudden lifting of the malarial burden brought by liberal use of DDT in the years immediately after World War II was one of the most dramatic and abrupt health changes ever experienced by humankind'; *Plagues and People* (Garden City, NY: Anchor Press, 1976), 249. See also, P. Kennedy, *Preparing for the Twenty-first Century* (New York: Random House, 1993), 25; A. Hardy, and E.M. Tansey, 'Medical Enterprise and Global Response, 1945–2000,' in W. Bynum, et al., *The Western Medical Tradition* (Cambridge: Cambridge University Press, 2006), 472; R. Fogel, *The Fourth Great Awakening* (Chicago: University of Chicago Press, 1999), 46; A.K. Bagchi, *The Political Economy of Underdevelopment* (Cambridge: Cambridge University Press, 1982), 204.

96 R. Briercliffe, and W. Dalrymple-Champneys, 'Discussion on the Malaria Epidemic in Ceylon 1934–1935,' *Proceedings of the Royal Society of Medicine*, 29, 1936, 537–562, at 554, Fig. 16. The severe edema in the child's lower extremities may have been exacerbated by malaria-induced anemia, but the state of extreme undernourishment evident in the severe muscle mass loss and sparse, depigmented hair indicates underlying severe undernourishment.

97 Hackett, *Malaria in Europe*, 227.

98 Frederiksen, 'Malaria Eradication and the Fall of Mortality,' 113. In 1970 Frederiksen noted that despite 'the dramatic and massive resurgence of malaria in Ceylon,' by early 1968 reaching a million cases, '[r]esident and visiting observers from the host government, the World Health Organization, the U.S. Public Health Service and the Population Council have so far not noted any significant increase in mortality since the start of the malaria epidemic'; ibid.

99 On this, see Zurbrigg, *Epidemic Malaria and Hunger*, ch. 12, analysis that encompasses the eastern half of the colonial province of Punjab making up the post-1947 Indian state of Punjab.

100 Ibid. See also, Wernsdorfer, 'Social and Economic Aspects of Malaria,' in Wernsdorfer and McGregor, eds., *Malaria: Principles and Practice*, 1421–1472, at 1435. Limited impact of malaria transmission resumption on general death rate levels has often been attributed to improved access to treatment; D. Bradley, 'Malarial Old Infections, Changing Epidemiology,' *Health Transition Review*, 2, Suppl. 1992, 137–153. But for much of rural 1950s India, assured access to anti-malarials appears unlikely; Zurbrigg, *Epidemic Malaria and Hunger*, 387.

# 8

# WHAT WAS LOST

When I teach the social impact of technology, I do not find it difficult to make it clear to engineers that technology has a social impact; however, it is almost impossible for me to make it clear to them that *they* are being impacted.

—— Ursula Franklin, 'Educating Engineers for the
Modern World,' in *Ursula Franklin Speaks:
Thoughts and Afterthoughts, 1986–2012* (Montreal:
McGill-Queen's University Press, 2014), p. 155

A new scientific truth does not triumph by convincing its opponents and making them see the light, but rather because its opponents eventually die, and a new generation grows up that is familiar with it.

—— Max Planck, *Scientific Autobiography and
Other Papers*, trans. F. Gaynor (New York
Philosophical Society, 1949), pp. 33–34

What was lost in understanding of human health with the nineteenth-century ascendance of sanitationist epidemic theory and a laboratory-based medicine was not just a single factor in infective disease causation. Set aside amidst the enthusiasm for applying the new microbiological insights of germ transmission were the broader discerning powers of observation of an earlier era. In the annals of modern medical and public health history, early twentieth-century figures in colonial India such as S.R. Christophers and C.A. Bentley had their nineteenth-century European counterparts in W.P. Alison, Rudolf Virchow, and Louis-René Villermé. The most prominent amongst them have not been forgotten. But posterity has often remembered their work selectively for their microbiologic or statistical contributions; less for their broader epidemiologic insights to which that expertise led them. In his 1840 descriptions of typhus fever amongst the Scottish poor, Alison's carefully detailed observations predicted with near-clairvoyant accuracy the characteristics of spontaneous recrudescent typhus under conditions of

229

human destitution, a phenomenon that would be unravelled scientifically only a century later as Brill-Zinsser disease.[1] These were powers of observation that extended beyond infection transmission alone, encompassing that 'tapestry of social relations'[2] within which the specific disease epidemiology was set, and discerning key relationships from this broader context. 'It is not asserted,' Alison wrote in his treatise on typhus ('fever') and poverty in Scotland

> that destitution is a cause adequate to the *production* of fever (although in some circumstances I believe it may become such); nor that it is the *sole* cause of its extension. What we are sure of is, that it is a cause of the *rapid diffusion* of contagious fever, and one of such peculiar power and efficacy, that its existence may always be presumed, when we see fever prevailing in a large community to an unusual extent. The manner in which deficient nourishment, want of employment, and privations of all kinds, and the consequent mental depression favour the diffusion of fever, may be matters of dispute; but that they have that effect in a much greater degree than any cause external to the human body itself, is a fact confirmed by the experience of all physicians who have seen much of the disease.[3]

It was the 'peculiar power and efficacy' of destitution (hunger-induced immune-suppression and 'mental depression') that a handful of the early malaria researchers in the Indian Medical Service also were recognizing and attempting to assess in teasing apart the interaction of biological and socio-economic factors underlying highly lethal malaria in India. Though more constrained perhaps by imperial allegiances than was Alison, their intellectual facility allowed them to consider and comprehend relationships transcending the specific confines of the sanitary paradigm of germ transmission. That they employed their scientific talents enthusiastically in the service of the British imperial state cannot be doubted. It could well be argued they could have done more, and that in their politically privileged positions, the obligation to do so was there. But that is a different historical question. Here what is considered is simply the significance of that broader understanding, and its common fate: how such epidemiological insights and experience were overshadowed and effectively set aside. 'The role of predisposition was not something that could be disproved,' Hamlin observes in the post-1842 context of industrializing England, 'but it could be ignored.'[4]

These larger insights stand in stark contrast to the vision of public health conjured in the nineteenth-century daily tasks of sanitary engineering, a vision increasingly narrowed to the elimination of environmental 'dirt' or 'moisture.' In his re-examination of the Chadwickian legend, Hamlin anticipates something of the interpretative power of the sanitationist model evident in the accounts of W.J. Gilbert, an Assistant Poor Law Commissioner selected by Chadwick to co-compile testimony on urban filth and 'bad air' (mal-aria). 'The diseases arising from malaria,' Gilbert would lament on the first page of the Local Reports (England and Wales) from which Chadwick selectively synthesized the Sanitary Report of 1842, are ascribed to various causes, 'heredity or personal infection, to low or unsuitable diet, hard work, exposure to cold, and other causes; but whenever such a regularly recurring complaint is found, almost invariably there is some open drain, some stagnant pool.'[5] Here, miasma-engendering filth functions as the default causal explanation of disease: ubiquitous, and in its invisible mechanism of 'noxious vapours,' impossible to disprove. The frailty of the logic is transparent. 'Dirt' not only trumps diet (hunger), but it does so even where its presence is simply a theoretic *possibility*. Indeed, it was precisely the invisibility of the miasmic threat that endowed sanitarianism with its power and corresponding sense of professional obligation.

A parallel shift to the privileging of microbiologic factors external to the human host in explanations of epidemic behaviour can be traced equally clearly in the late colonial South Asian malaria literature, in Major A. Hooton's absorption with anopheline vectors in the Kathiar Agency of Gujarat, as seen above in chapter seven.[6] The invisible, but ever-present potential threat of infected mosquitoes would soon be accompanied by its counterpart, the twentieth-century risk of 'hidden (micronutrient) hunger.' It is seen as well in Passmore and Sommerville's 1940 paper where Christophers's 1911 'scarcity' conclusions regarding malaria lethality are set aside on the basis of their laboratory work on simian malaria, work that addressed micronutrient-deficient dietaries rather than caloric insufficiency (hunger).[7] 'Mere association,' they argued in relation to the 1911 report, 'cannot be taken as proof' of a causal relationship.[8] Despite the manifest analytic limitations of the 1940 study, Paul Russell would make similar arguments in his 1946 text, *Practical Malariology*, citing the Passmore-Sommerville article. 'A good deal has been said about famine as a causative factor in regional epidemics, . . . [but] no proof of a causal relationship has been found,' he argued. '[F]requently the same climatic factor which brought about famine also made conditions favorable for the breeding of vector mosquitoes.'[9] Here, the 'exciting' or 'precipitating' cause – entomological conditions – of malaria epidemicity was accorded preferential explanatory power over 'predisposing' factors and selectively relieved of the burden of proof in the process, what Hamlin describes in nineteenth-century sanitationist argument as 'the arbitrary elevation of one set of correlations to the status of *the cause*.'[10] To qualify as scientific, the epidemiological observations as contained in earlier studies such as *Malaria in the Punjab* now required experimental (microbiologic) validation, where the sufficiency of vector and related immunological aspects in explaining epidemic mortality patterns, however uncorroborated by epidemiological evidence, did not.

Had Russell been asked directly for his assessment of malaria mortality in the absence of destitution, he might well have replied that the *amount* of mortality was immaterial. It was enough that there was *any* mortality (which there was) and *any* economic debility associated with infection (which again there unquestionably was), whether or not either became dramatically magnified under conditions of acute hunger (which they did). And as a vector sanitationist or medical clinician, he was right. Yet in the context of health policy decision-making, the amount of mortality *did matter*. As it matters also to health historiography.

This 'gravitational' pull to factors external to the human host in epidemic causation was not new. But it was becoming that much more exclusivist within the confines of industrializing Europe. In his efforts to document the class differentials in mortality he saw in early nineteenth-century Paris, the French hygienist, Villermé, would lament that '[w]e far too often attribute . . . the very different life expectancies of the masses of individuals who make up each nation, to difference in climate.'[11] One century later, Ackerknecht would point to 'the extraordinary brilliancy of the bacteriological era' that has come to 'obscur[e] . . . everything lying behind it in the field.'[12] In relation to the World Health Organization's Malaria Eradication Program, Packard similarly describes 'a compelling logic' to the idea of eradication of the plasmodial parasite that

> continually draws one into the narrow medical, technical and organizational factors that shaped the program. . . . [O]ne needs to continually work against the logic and resist its pull. For it is a logic that isolated the history of malaria eradication from the world in which it occurred, a logic that excluded from vision a wide range of social, economic, and political forces that were operating during this period.[13]

What drives this 'extraordinary brilliancy' and privileged status? Beyond the undisputed effectiveness of microbiologic techniques in specific instances, explanations of epidemic behaviour narrowed to germ-transmission are deemed more credible because microbes are identifiable and in theory at least amenable to controlled experiment, hence grounded by scientific proof. Hunger, in contrast, is viewed as not admitting of scientific analysis, under the assumption perhaps that it is not possible to control for myriad confounding social dimensions ('complexities'). This privileging, one can suggest, turns in part on the conflation of scientific and microbiologic. Microbial (also, micronutrient) explanations of ill-health are preferentially 'scientific' because they are reproducible in laboratory conditions, the bedrock of scientific investigation. Human destitution triggered by crop failure, work injury, or death of a primary wage-earner, for self-evident ethical reasons, generally is not. The microbiologic is academically 'safe,' by comparison.[14] Interestingly, in their 1909 paper on the 'Human Factor,' Christophers and Bentley themselves hint at this dichotomy, referring to observations on economic conditions as 'study whose object is not in one sense scientific research but simply the getting of information absolutely necessary to action.'[15] Here, wage levels, grain prices, destitution, physiological poverty (macrobiological conditions) comprise 'information,' while parasite rates and entomological observations constitute scientific research.[16]

The consequences of the selective microbiologic focus for historical epidemic enquiry have been many. One example in relation to malaria is seen in Macdonald's mathematical modelling of malaria transmission, work in which host recovery rate was assigned a constant value, presumed unmeasurable and unsuitable for statistical analysis and prediction. In the process, however, the immense range in lethality (case fatality rate) of malarial infection was effectively removed from the epidemic equation, as we have seen: and along with it, a dimension central to understanding much endemic disease mortality in history, and the larger question of secular trends in human life expectancy, in turn.[17] Quantifiability in this sense thus tends to shape what data qualify as scientifically useful, but also what questions are asked, and by whom investigated. Weindling points to the dilemma, observing in the context of the International Labour Organisation's early work on health and economics, that 'in seeking to justify its reformist demands in the universalist terms of science, [the organisation] *had to* devolve initiatives to scientific experts whose empirically based approaches were necessarily limited to what could be proven in the laboratory.'[18]

In relation to mid-twentieth-century South Asian epidemiological thought, a particularly transparent window on the impact of the biomedical model's 'brilliancy' can be seen in the official report on the 1943 Bengal famine. In the deliberations of Famine Commission members regarding the causes of epidemic mortality, a range of entomological and parasitic factors were considered in seeking to explain the enormous malaria mortality witnessed. Various vector explanations outlined in the earlier 1940 Passmore-Sommerville paper were discussed at some length.[19] Unable to identify ecological changes capable of affecting malaria transmission rates across Bengal, the Commission turned to the recent 'influx of refugees from Burma [Myanmar]' as creating conditions 'propitious for the dissemination of unfamiliar strains' of malaria parasites, 'exotic strains' to which the population would have had little previously acquired specific immunity. This, too, was an unlikely explanation, it ultimately was acknowledged, leading members to 'tentatively express . . . that the high mortality from malaria can be largely accounted for without pre-supposing any change in the virulence of the infecting organism.'[20]

Remarkably, this statement effectively brought the committee's report to a close. It was followed by a simple paraphrasing of a Croonian Lecture recently given before the Royal Society, a quote inserted, it seems, as a concluding statement to the medical portion of the famine Inquiry report. The Topley paper, the 1945 Commission members urged, 'brings out the complexity of the problem' of epidemic causation in relation to famine. Clarity was often elusive due to

> [o]ur present lack of knowledge of all the factors concerned in the rise and fall of epidemics and their interaction. . . . It may be difficult to account satisfactorily for the cause and course of epidemics even in a well-fed static human population, even indeed, in a closed colony of experimental animals. To do so in the case of a socially disorganized famine-stricken population is an impossible task.[21]

A definitive explanation of the 1943–1944 Bengal famine's soaring malaria mortality, the medical enquiry report appears to suggest, was as yet out of reach where an expanding list of potential microbiological factors could not expressly be ruled out.

What is striking in the 1945 Famine Commission's closing statement on Bengal famine mortality is the degree of circumspection, a hesitancy in marked contrast to the conclusions of earlier observers such as W.R. Cornish and A.P. MacDonnell who linked malaria lethality in the late nineteenth-century famines in British India indisputably to human starvation.[22] On the one hand, the 1945 enquiry commissioners clearly understood at a common-sense level that starvation was the overriding driver of lethality in Bengal in 1943–1944, indeed at one point acknowledging Christophers's 1911 Punjab conclusions. On the other hand, such a relationship could now only be viewed as, at best, 'tentative,' with both the micronutrient nutritional research and 1940 Passmore-Sommerville paper before them – the latter quoted at length – and a growing range of entomological theses also as explanatory possibilities.[23] It is as if Commission members were throwing up their hands in the face of such microbiologic 'complexity.' But for some perhaps also finding comfort in its academic safety.

One can suggest this was scientism at its most paralyzing, a forfeiting of the basic capacity to weigh relative roles. But it was more than this, too, because in the malaria literature such a tentativeness was often unequally applied. As in the case of Ceylon, the microbial-immunological argument often was privileged, less subject to interpretative caution, indeed, requiring at times no empirical evidence at all. A similar example of microbiologic privileging can be seen three decades later at an international famine and nutrition symposium. In a paper addressing 'different degrees of starvation,' W.R. Aykroyd, leading medical contributor to the 1945 Bengal Famine Commission report, would suggest that the common association between famine and disease 'is in the main social rather than physiological, i.e., it is due to the disruption of society, facilitating the spread of epidemic disease, rather than lowered bodily resistance to invading organisms.'[24]

## Consequences of the germ paradigm's 'brilliancy'

A similar tendency to gravitate to microbiologic explanations of epidemic behaviour can be traced running through recent South Asian epidemic and demographic historiography. Researchers of epidemic and mortality decline history generally acknowledge the findings of prominent nutritionists such as Nevin Scrimshaw that undernourishment compromises immune capacity, and thus recovery, for many common (endemic) infections.[25] But if recognized in theory, understanding of the large range in lethality of many infective diseases often fails to be incorporated in assessing relative roles for microbe transmission, public health interventions, and staple-food security in historical mortality decline. It is often assumed, for example, that interrupting transmission of one particular pathogen will effect a decline in mortality levels equivalent to those deaths triggered by such infection preceding the transmission 'intervention.' This may be the case for inherently virulent infections such as smallpox; but not necessarily for the leading historical triggers of death such as malaria, tuberculosis, typhus, the diarrhea-pneumonia complex, and others where undernourishment and acute hunger have played a prominent predisposing role in their lethality, and continue to do so among impoverished populations. This of course raises the issue of 'competing risk.' As explored in relation to the 1950s DDT-based malaria control program, the overall impact of the abrupt interruption in malaria transmission on general mortality levels in (East) Punjab state appears to have been very limited.[26] The most likely explanation is that many of the deaths averted by the DDT program were simply postponed to subsequent seasons: those children most vulnerable to dying of malaria by virtue of undernourishment remaining vulnerable to other common endemic infections at other times of the year.[27]

Conceptual consequences of the germ theory's brilliancy for epidemic historiography lie at other levels as well. In employing the tools and microbiologic insights of the expanding medical subdisciplines for understanding human health history (secular trends in life expectancy), only infrequently have historians addressed the interpretive constraints so posed. The dilemma for them is considerable because the range of possible microbiological factors – and hence the number of potentially relevant medical subdisciplines – involved in any particular epidemic event or time-trend is essentially unlimited. The onus is there to take them sufficiently into account, to 'cover all biomedical bases,' or at least to attempt to do so. This has meant that in the face of complex technical questions, the historian often defers to the medical literature, hesitating to ask for scientific 'proof,' or to pose self-evident questions. Here, Hamlin, in citing Gilbert's example of 'some open drain,' remarks that 'we do not read other areas of social science so naively.'[28]

The interpretive difficulty lies in the ease with which microbiological findings come to be accorded explanatory power for epidemiological phenomena in advance of being tested adequately, or at times at all. In the case of malaria, entomological hypotheses such as 'vector deviation' continue to be cited as likely contributing explanations of epidemic outbreaks – in this case, famine-induced livestock mortality posited as resulting in a shift in mosquito feeding from cattle to humans – though unaccompanied by substantive empirical examination.[29] The difficulty lies not in the citing of potentially relevant biological phenomena; but rather in doing so in the absence of accompanying effort to weigh their contribution in relation to other factors. Any possibility of a microbiologic explanation – or simply its possibility – suffices often to sideline adequate assessment of hunger.

In recent accounts, for example, of the emergence of an 'exalted' form of malaria ('Burdwan fever') in the 'dying river' tracts of nineteenth-century western Bengal, potential entomological effects of interrupted inundation irrigation are generally cited alongside the economic effects of embankments in lowering soil productivity.[30] '[A]nother consequence of the declining [inundation] flows through the western arms of the Ganges delta,' Marshall observes, was that 'as the rivers became more stagnant, malaria-bearing mosquitoes bred more freely.'[31] In this, the author is taking into account 1940s studies that suggested a link between lower water-table levels in the embankment-affected tracts and a more conducive habitat for the main malaria vector in the region, *An. philippinensis*, ecological changes that may well have enhanced malaria transmission levels.[32] Here, again, the interpretative difficulty arises where the citing of a microbiological aspect distracts from, or arrests, deliberation regarding relative roles: *viz.*, consideration of broader context that could shed light on the likely contribution of each.[33] In the case of Burdwan fever, a broader epidemiological perspective could include post-1920 decline in mortality levels in the region;[34] and as well, the experience of epidemic malaria during the 1943–44 Bengal famine. In the latter case, as explored in chapter three,[35] malaria lethality soared as the leading cause of mortality across the course of the famine although ecological conditions (including subsoil water-table levels) remained unchanged – a heightened malaria mortality that was sharply circumscribed to the period of epidemic starvation. In other words, the famine was a dramatic demonstration of the power of human famishment to alter the lethality of malarial infection.[36] Of course, access to such broader context is not always so readily at hand. Nonetheless, acknowledgement of the need for a weighing of relative import remains.

Similar interpretive difficulties can be seen in relation to analysis of the massive canal irrigation projects in colonial Punjab. Interpretation of their 'malariogenic' consequences has often focused on vector-transmission parameters, overshadowing the economic impacts of blocked surface drainage and waterlogging.[37] This has meant it has been difficult to place the specific, and very real, deleterious effects in the context of mortality trends over time: an impasse that in turn has impeded integration of the region's 'public health' history into the rest of South Asian history.

Faced with the seeming incongruity of continuing malaria transmission but declining epidemic and general mortality after 1920, historians of South Asian epidemic history have turned at times to alternate microbiological hypotheses, positing a general rise in acquired immunity levels in the population[38] – a thesis unsupported empirically, and itself a function of vector transmission.[39] Macdonald earlier, as we have seen, also turned to an immunologic hypothesis of malaria epidemicity, if in a somewhat different framework: in this case, suggesting year-to-year fluctuation in numbers of non-immunes in the Punjab population to explain the region's epidemic malaria history. Default reliance on acquired immunity hypotheses is of course a much broader phenomenon within epidemic historiography:[40] a reflection of the continuing epistemic power of the germ-transmission paradigm, but arguably also an expression of the underlying absence of an adequate epidemiological approach to hunger in historical analysis.

## From too obvious to invisible

This study has sought to trace the decline in Western medical understanding of hunger in human health and epidemic history. What was once obvious, even 'truistic,'[41] by the mid-twentieth century now verged on the invisible: the history of mortality decline, aside from famine control, was now understood primarily in terms of the control of pathogen transmission and chemotherapeutics. In one sense, the historical relationship between hunger and infective disease lethality was *too* obvious, often failing to merit discussion within medical texts. In the 1894 edition of the *Indian Manual of Hygiene*, for example, a single reference acknowledged that '[i]n a country like India, the influence of rainfall upon General Health and well being of the community is very marked.' But the consequences of 'failure of the crop' were deemed 'too well known to need any further explanation.'[42] Hamlin also reminds us that the ancient Hippocratic treatises addressed the medical diseases of individuals, whereas those of society associated with crop failure were not the domain, or within the capacity, of the physician.

> Knowing that . . . a harvest had failed might allow one to anticipate disaster but rarely allowed one to prevent it. Indeed, such events marked the limits of a medicine based on individualized dietetics. Powerless to . . . guarantee the crops, Hippocratic writers . . . focused instead on what they could do.[43]

In the case of South Asia, hunger runs through the colonial records, but largely obliquely. During the famine-related malaria epidemic of 1878, the Sanitary Inspector for Jullunder city noted, for example, that 'food tickets' distributed by the municipal committee 'as recommended by the Native Doctors . . . [had] done great good,' while the insufficiency of such funds also was acknowledged.[44] Three decades later, hunger would weave inferentially through the deliberations of the 1909 Imperial Malaria Conference held at Simla, well beyond the 'scarcity' conclusions of Christophers's Punjab presentation. When a malaria 'cess' was proposed for funding anti-malaria work, it was opposed by one of the few 'Native' delegates. Taxing the poor for whom resistance to malaria was already low could not be justified, Mr. Kishori Lal Goswami, Member of the Bengal Provincial Legislative Council, argued: 'poverty was accountable for malaria, poverty reduced the people's power of resistance, and if further taxation was to be imposed that resistance would be further reduced.'[45] He was not challenged, and the proposed tax, it appears, was quietly abandoned.

This broader, seemingly self-evident, understanding of disease lethality as shaped by the subsistence conditions of the human host was not limited to South Asian experience. The relationship continued to be reappear episodically in Britain into the early twentieth century. In the 1902 annual oration to the Medical Society of London, S. Mackenzie described the role of poverty in tuberculosis as 'a powerful predisponent,' adding,

> I remember many years ago, before the discovery of the bacillus, someone pressing the late Dr. H.G. Sutton to define what tubercle *really* was. He replied, 'Tubercle is making shirts at 5s. a week.'[46]

But if the disease and destitution relationship was a commonplace, hunger was also deeply incriminating, as seen in Edwin Chadwick's efforts to remove starvation as a cause of death category from vital registration reports.[47] Where obvious, hunger was often veiled linguistically. The various epidemic 'fevers' (often typhus) seen typically among the livelihood-desperate were grouped, for example, under the nineteenth-century English category of 'crowd diseases,' the term connoting contagion as the central dynamic underlying their epidemic manifestation, less so starvation.

In nineteenth-century colonial India as well, starvation deaths were rarely registered as such, but rather slotted under categories of 'old age' or 'fever' by low-level functionaries, often for 'fear of getting into trouble with the authorities.'[48] The commonly documented 'exalted' form of malaria evident on colonial construction sites would be interpreted in miasmic terms of 'turning up the soil,' the indentured and often times semi-starving migrant labourers who did the 'turning,' left out of sight.[49] At the same time, the heinous methods resorted to by the state to control the desperate actions of the famished went largely unrecorded. Only a single reference to whipping – a measure employed to discourage deliberate courting of imprisonment to access food – appears in the voluminous nineteenth-century British

India famine commissioner reports, an inadvertent remark by a district official that found its way into the Punjab provincial report on the 1899–1900 famine.[50]

Where specific measures to alleviate hunger appear in the colonial sanitary and malaria records, they too were phrased in oblique terms. In Christophers's case, policies to prevent famine and the notorious associated malaria epidemics were referred to as 'general sanitary reforms';[51] flood-related food relief in Punjab, simply as 'other ameliorative measures.'[52] At the 1909 malaria conference, 'great privation and hardship' was openly acknowledged to underlie the 'very fatal' form of epidemic malaria. But such transparency was the exception,[53] prompted, as I have suggested elsewhere, by even greater 'obloquy' directed to the British Raj by prominent figures publicly excoriating the government for its reluctance to embrace vector eradication as a central malaria control policy.[54]

In historical records generally, reticence to record the human agony of famishment prevails, as 'that of which one cannot speak.' One small glimpse of the extremes of starvation misery appears in Aykroyd's 1974 *Conquest of Famine*. 'Cannibalism occurred' during the 1846–1847 Irish famine, 'as it does in many major famines,' he acknowledged, 'but it was apparently confined to a few people driven mad by suffering. The [Quaker] Friends had to give up buying cheap sausages when some were found to contain human flesh.'[55] Such stark accounts however are rare. As Millman and Kates have pithily observed, '[t]he history of hunger is for the most part unwritten. The hungry rarely write history, and historians are rarely hungry.'[56]

From being once 'too obvious,' hunger within professional circles by the early twentieth century had swung to its socially 'hidden' form, increasingly viewed in the micronutrient domain as largely a qualitative problem. 'One of the most difficult problems facing the investigator,' scientists with the All-India Institute of Hygiene and Public Health lamented in 1949, 'is to determine the nutritional status of an individual without carrying out a series of elaborate biochemical tests which are beyond the realm of practicability in a survey . . . unless unmistakable signs of vitamin deficiency are present.'[57] Increasingly interpreted now as an educational problem, hunger in turn came to be shorn of its ethical and emotive implications.

At the methodological level, reliance on aggregate economic measures to assess 'nutritional status' within mortality decline analysis has further contributed to hunger's invisibility by obscuring differential access to food within populations. When it became evident in the mid-twentieth century that national Gross Domestic Product data poorly predicted life expectancy across the world,[58] 'nutrition' itself, along with the index, was sidelined as a substantial factor in post-WW2 mortality decline, and the inherent inadequacies of aggregate indices such as GDP as a measure of hunger within societies were overlooked. Within Western medical fora, the questions raised by Frederiksen in the 1960s in relation to post-WW2 Sri Lankan post-war mortality decline were simply set aside as 'not . . . realistic.'[59]

> [T]he falls in mortality in the developing countries have been so sharp, and the rise in living standards so gradual – indeed in some there has been no rise at all – that on this score alone it is difficult to accept his hypothesis. . . . We may therefore conclude that medical measures of one kind or another are responsible for the fall in mortality.[60]

Here, a role for food security in rising life expectancy was not just invisible, but verging on the inconceivable, with mortality decline credited instead to medical measures 'of one kind or another.'

Within Western academic thought, macroeconomic indices have continued to be employed as indicators of nutritional status in health analysis, despite conveying little about distribution of food within societies, shifts in security of staple food access, or the myriad constraints to access presented by prevailing conditions of work.[61] Moreover, the language employed in recent epidemic historiography has added a further veil, with aspects of food insecurity commonly grouped under the rubric of 'social' factors, leading to attributions of dysfunctional cultural or behavioural practices.[62] Equally problematic has been the increasing use of the term 'environmental' to encompass both subsistence insecurity (economic conditions) and exposure to infection,[63] terminology generally directing attention to the latter – conditions external to the human host related to infection transmission.

Quantitative hunger – not enough to eat – would begin to be reclaimed in clinical medicine in the 1960s and early 1970s through nutritional anthropometry, where childhood undernourishment was rendered obvious as cumulative faltering growth on paediatric weight ('road-to-health') charts,[64] most prominently in low-income populations. Hunger's impact on immune capacity and the lethality of many infective diseases was also confirmed in this period,[65] if analysis of broader socio-economic determinants was often limited.[66] Ensuing historical nutritional anthropometry research also began to reclaim visibility of 'chronic' hunger at this time by tracing secular trends in human stature as a marker of cumulative endemic undernourishment.[67] It was in this period as well that recognition of the immense variation in lethality (case fatality rate) of infective diseases re-emerged in analysis of mortality decline in nineteenth-century Britain in the work of Thomas McKeown.[68] Perceived in some instances however as a dismissal of public health efforts to control infection transmission,[69] the key issue of shifts in the lethality of endemic infections tended to recede once again in epidemic and public health historiographic analysis.[70]

## 'Good Health at Low Cost'

One example of waning visibility of subsistence (in)security in contemporary health history analysis can be seen in the 1985 document *Good Health at Low Cost* [*GHLC*].[71] Addressing the dramatic post-WW2 rise in child survival rates and life expectancy recorded in the low-income (GDP) 'developing' countries of Sri Lanka, China, and Kerala state in India,[72] the *GHLC* report identified four main contributing factors: 'education for all'; public health measures (immunization, protected water supplies and sanitation, vector control); accessible primary health care; and 'adequate caloric intake by all.'[73] Of the four, much of the conference report however came to focus on the first three factors: primary health care, public health programs, and female literacy. Aggregate *per capita* foodgrain figures and trends for each population were reported,[74] along with a brief review of the 'linkages' between nutritional status and mortality risk.[75] But shifts in food access *within* the case-study populations and specific economic reforms – such as rural land reforms, public distribution programs, and minimum wage legislation – and their consequences for access made up relatively little of the 248-page report.[76] Surprisingly as well, little attempt was made to assess *timing* of the various programs in relation to observed mortality trends.

In light of the document's considerable subsequent influence,[77] several questions unaddressed in the 1985 report are considered here.

### China as case study

In regard to China, mortality decline appears to have been most rapid at the beginning of the 1950–1980 case study period, that is, between the years 1950 and 1957.[78] In the absence of country-wide vital registration before 1955, estimates of mortality levels in the immediate pre-1950 period have generally relied upon local surveys conducted in the pre-revolution period. Those data considered approximately representative of national (*viz.*, largely rural) conditions come from a 1929–1931 study conducted in 16 provinces in rural areas not directly affected by then-prevailing warfare.[79] Adjusted for under-registration, the 1929–1931 data have suggested a rural crude death rate of 41.5 per 1,000 population, with life expectancy estimated at 24.2 years.[80] Such conditions, Judith Banister has suggested, likely continued through the 1930s and 1940s: 'In 1950, warfare had just ceased and recovery from the ravages was just beginning.'[81] The crude death rate in 1949 for China as a whole she estimated as 38 per 1,000 population, indicating life expectancy likely below 30 years.[82]

By 1957, national life expectancy had almost doubled to 50 years.[83] By the early 1970s, a further 13 years in average life span had been gained.[84] Together, these figures translate into hundreds of millions of deaths averted, the population increasing from 542 million at the end of 1949 to 830 million in 1970.

What explains this rapid rise in survival rates? Certainly, the return of peace, of rudimentary administrative capacity, and of a civilian economy, played a major role, conditions directly affecting livelihood and food security. A number of national disease control campaigns also were initiated in the early 1950s. Among them, smallpox was effectively eradicated by 1957 through universal vaccination.[85] As well, an anti-syphilis campaign saw the entire adult population of Shanghai, for example, tested and treatment provided for positive cases, a government-funded program that extended substantially also to village level.[86] These two diseases together however appear to have accounted for only a small portion, possibly 8 per cent, of total preventable mortality in the pre-1950 period.[87] Other programs, such as the Patriotic Health Campaigns were considerably less effective in controlling transmission of major parasitic infections such as malaria and schistosomiasis in these early years.[88] Major improvements in water and sanitation infrastructure in the initial two decades also appear to have been limited, the prevalence of intestinal parasitic infections remaining high through to the early 1980s.[89] Primary education was massively expanded post-1950, but it is unlikely increased child literacy could explain a significant portion of the initial rapid decline in mortality. Basic rural health care services, moreover, largely awaited initiation of the barefoot doctor program in 1968–1969 and its expansion in the 1970s,[90] at a point in other words when a good deal of the 1950–1980 gains in life expectancy nationally had already taken place.[91]

Measles immunization began in 1965, and expanded childhood immunization campaigns in the later 1960s and early 1970s.[92] Yet well before, a major drop in the lethality of common endemic infections in the country appears already to have taken place. Tuberculosis was a leading cause of mortality in pre-1950 China, estimates suggesting 200–300 deaths annually per 100,000 population.[93] By 1957 the tuberculosis death rate in major cities was reported as 54.6 per 100,000 population, declining further to 36.2 six years later.[94] Improved access to treatment through concerted efforts to identify cases undoubtedly contributed.[95] Yet levels of access to effective treatment beyond the urban centres is unclear, with specialist tuberculosis personnel numbering only 4 per million population in 1960.[96] Moreover, even in the major urban centres tuberculosis transmission rates, based on Mantoux testing, appear to have remained high across the 1950s.[97] A similar decline also appears to have occurred in the lethality of measles, a major contributor to pre-1950 childhood mortality. The national case fatality rate was estimated to be 8.6 per cent in 1950; six years later a figure of 1.6 per cent was reported. A similar proportionate decline was recorded in Beijing.[98]

The sources and representativeness of the above few mortality data are unclear, making definitive conclusions on lethality trends for many endemic diseases yet out of reach. Improved access to preventive or curative care may well explain some decline in tuberculosis mortality, particularly in urban areas. Health care services, however, are unlikely explanations for mortality decline in the case of measles: a near-universal childhood viral infection for which immunization or effective treatment, at the time, had yet to be developed.

The decline in death rates in post-1950 China clearly merits far more detailed study, certainly more than is offered here. One development, however, that suggests a major role for improved food security in declining infective disease lethality is the dramatic improvement documented in child nutritional status. Between 1951–1958 and 1979, the mean height of boys 12 years of age had increased by 8.4 centimetres; mean weight, by 4.2 kilograms, with comparable increases for girls.[99] These figures reflect to a large extent conditions of child feeding and care in early childhood and *in utero*, and thus conditions preceding each of these two nutritional survey periods, *viz.*, the 1940s decade, and the mid- and later 1960s. This degree of improved child nourishment after 1949 would have been accompanied by a major increase in general immune-competence in the population.[100]

The magnitude and rapidity of nutritional improvement and rise in life expectancy in China is historically unprecedented, an increase in human survival that took over a century to achieve in far smaller populations in nineteenth- and early twentieth-century Europe. In addition to the cessation of military invasion and civil warfare by 1949, the rise corresponds temporally to initiation of major food security programs. Between 1950 and 1952, an estimated 30 to 45 per cent of China's arable land was redistributed, bringing about an immediate narrowing of rural wealth and livelihood disparity, and was accompanied by a 25 per cent increase in crop output by 1958.[101] In urban areas, by 1955 a food ration system guaranteed access to subsidized staple foodgrains, the 'iron rice-bowl,' that provided 1,800–2,600 kcal daily per adult.[102] No formal rationing system was established for the almost 90 per cent of the population in rural China, but a system of grain transfers from surplus to deficit areas was established to maintain 'a floor level of grain consumption.'[103]

Mortality decline would be reversed, tragically, with frank famine conditions in 1960 that saw life expectancy fall that year to 1930s levels:[104] an inverse example – quite possibly largely preventable – of the mortality-hunger link. The earlier trend soon resumed, however, with life expectancy reaching an estimated 61 years by 1969.[105]

The composition of the diet in China between 1950 and 1970 remained essentially unchanged from its traditional content: based almost entirely on traditional staple foodgrains and tubers.[106] But it was much more secure, and sufficient, it appears, to satisfy hunger for many. Few aspects, however, of the food security programs established in these initial years are traced in the *GHLC* report.[107]

Considerable undernourishment still remained in China in 1975, affecting 23 per cent of young suburban children; and one-third of the population still lived in absolute poverty, levels that were far higher in the poorest western and southwestern provinces of the country.[108] Thus further improvement in child and adult nourishment nationally likely continued to contribute to ongoing decline in mortality levels in the post-1975 period, life expectancy reaching 71 years in 1999–2000.[109]

## Kerala state

Infant mortality in the southwestern Indian state of Kerala fell rapidly from 120 deaths per 1,000 live births in the 1950s to 39.1 by 1981, and further to 15 by 1990.[110] The 1960s and 1970s was a period of major economic reforms, policies that included modest land reforms, security of tenancy legislation, a rural Public Distribution System (PDS or 'fair price shops') program, minimum wage legislation, and in the 1970s agricultural labourer pensions.[111] These reforms were accompanied by important expansion of rural health care services[112] and primary education, overlap that makes assessment of relative roles in mortality decline in the state more challenging.

Once again, however, trends in childhood nutritional status shed important light. Despite below-average mean per capita calorie intake for Kerala state as a whole compared to all-India figures, prevalence of severe malnutrition among young children (weight less than 60 per cent normal) in Kerala by the 1970s was recorded already below levels in other states, at 10.2 per cent. By the 1980s, reported severe malnutrition prevalence was down to 2.0 per cent.[113] The significance of this decline lies in the five- to 10-fold greater mortality risk for severely underweight children relative to normal growth, or even to lesser degrees of undernourishment.[114] By 1976 as well, the height of rural school boys 6 years of age in the state had increased by 4.9 cm relative to 1963.[115] In contrast to this improvement in child stature, there is little evidence that sanitation and protected water supply improved substantially. As in China, intestinal parasitic infection rates remained extremely high as late as the early 1980s.[116]

Curiously, data on trends in prevalence of severe undernourishment in young children are not included in the Kerala case study analysis, nor those on increased child stature. Moreover, little exploration of the potential impact of the economic reforms for food security was offered.[117] Instead, based upon aggregate (state-level) per capita caloric consumption figures and Gini coefficients, the case study at one point concluded that 'nutritional differences cannot explain the lower mortality rate in Kerala' relative to other Indian states.[118]

## Tamil Nadu

Twenty-five years later, a further series of case studies was undertaken as a follow-up to the original 1985 *Good Health at Low Cost* report. In this case, the focus was directed even more specifically to 'health systems': preventive and curative care health services.[119] Among the cases included in the 2011 report was that of the south Indian state of Tamil Nadu, neighbouring to Kerala. Between 1983 and 2005, infant mortality had declined from 100 deaths per 1,000 live births to 35 across the state, a period that saw expansion of rural primary health care services through 'village health nurses' and a thorough overhaul of the rural supply of essential drugs and laboratory services – both extremely welcome initiatives.[120] Once again, however, little information was provided on the timing of these programs in relation to the trajectory of child mortality decline. But unmentioned also were major rural food security programs launched in the state in the 1980s and early 1990s.

Initiated in the wake of the 1985 state election, a Public Distribution System ('fair price shops') guaranteed rural access to 20 kgs of rice per village household each month at controlled and subsidized prices. Its timing appears to have corresponded to the initial major drop in infant mortality to 65 per 1,000 live born by 1991, following a 1970s decade of stagnating rates.[121] And as in Kerala, this drop was associated with a major decline in the prevalence of severe undernourishment in young children: from 13.9 per cent in 1983–1984 to 4.2 per cent by 1988–1990[122] – data that also do not appear in the case study analysis.[123] Subsequently, 25,000 village creches were established for children 0 to 3 years of age, as well as maternity benefits of Rs 300 for 'nutritional support.[124]

## View from a southern Tamil Nadu village

In light of the limited attention directed to basic subsistence issues in the two *GHLC* documents, one glimpse of how the new food security programs in Tamil Nadu state were perceived at village level is offered here. When asked by the author in early 1997 how child health conditions in the southeastern district of Ramanathapuram had changed from 17 years earlier, Rakku, traditional midwife of Puliyur village, turned to a small box on the shelf of her thatched one-room home. Taking out her household ration card, she pointed to the family's rice allotments, marked in monthly instalments. Then she gestured to the local 'fair price' shop at the village's edge and explained how she would 'sell' her sugar and kerosene ration to 'big' (landowning) households during periods of scarce daily wage employment, the modest earnings helping her to purchase *ragi*, a local staple millet, to bridge seasonal livelihood gaps. She went on to describe the more recent establishment of a child care centre where women could leave their infants and toddlers for care during field labour through the day.[125]

Beyond the impact, momentous enough, of stable foodgrain prices across the agricultural year, and their modest subsidy through the ration shop, what the midwife described might be considered a type of 'micro-credit' benefit of the PDS program – if unintended perhaps by administrators. Its impact went beyond the direct nourishing of young children. In a small but concrete way, the PDS program appears to have effected a shift in relations of dependency within the village: the ration card replacing to some extent the traditional role of the village landlord-moneylender, a function now in her own possession (if in her husband's name) and that of other landless, illiterate *dalit* women.[126]

The realities of hand-to-mouth subsistence, understood intimately by the women of Puliyur village, are captured poorly, one can suggest, in aggregate econometric analyses. Even less so are the constraints of time that subsistence realities ordain for the feeding of their young children, including those *in utero* – above all, the necessary frequency of 'meals-per-day' required by infants and toddlers. Such constraints, and gaps, remain largely unrecorded, and invisible. Likewise, too, it seems, their beginning alleviation, and the shift in female empowerment that even modest food security policies instantiate.

Discussion of women's 'empowerment' can at times be left at a somewhat abstract level, interpreted primarily in terms of access to health care services. Such services are of course fundamentally important also for these women and their children. But there can often be limited acknowledgement of the importance of minimum food and employment security in allowing women to access that care without jeopardizing the survival of other children and the larger household. Similarly, minimally sufficient time and work flexibility for women to attend to child feeding and care during episodes of diarrhea and other common childhood infections is crucial for ensuring recovery and lessening nutrient drain.[127]

The further removed by class, caste, and personal experience analysis is from the subsistence lives of such women, the less comprehensible, it seems, insufficient and insecure daily subsistence can become. There is some irony in this. For in disciplines outside medical and health historiography, the consequences of food insecurity on mortality are more evident. A central methodological tool in historical demographic research, for example, involves examining mortality patterns in response to foodgrain price levels ('price shocks') as an indicator, if crude, of shifts in access to staple food.[128] In a different domain, the importance of food security was a founding premise of the International Labour Organisation in 1919: an understanding that '[p]ay and social security benefits were the keys to good health.'[129] Two decades later, the hunger-epidemic relationship remained strategically self-evident within the halls of post-WW2 Western geopolitical power, as we have seen, giving rise to the 1942 Hot Springs food conference and subsequent establishment of UNRRA and the FAO.[130]

Yet in modern epidemic historiography such understanding has waned. Disease epidemics are more comprehensible, and visible, than are epidemics of hunger, or for that matter, is endemic hunger. 'It is striking,' Michel Garenne and colleagues have observed of the 1987–1989 malaria epidemic in

Antananarivo, Madagascar, 'that malaria came back at about the same time' as food shortage and soaring prices. 'Perhaps more striking still,' they add,

> the malaria epidemic, which killed about 700 people in the city in three years, has been well documented and studied. Indeed, several scientific publications and many articles in local and international newspapers have appeared on the subject. However, the more silent food shortage which killed perhaps 11 times more people has been ignored.[131]

'News coverage and scientific publications,' they suggest, 'do not always follow a demographic logic. . . . Diseases or causes of death which for some reasons are considered to be shameful tend to be ignored.'[132] The *GHLC* and Antananarivo analyses are but two among many examples of a receding visibility of subsistence (in)security in contemporary health, and health history, analysis, and of the limitations this poses for interpreting historical, and recent modern, experience of mortality decline.[133]

It bears restating perhaps that the attempt in this study to reclaim human subsistence in health historiography is not a dismissal of the value of modern medical and public health techniques or safe water supply. Each of the health care programs detailed in the *GHLC* case studies is indisputably important for saving lives. Anti-natal tetanus toxoid and anti-diphtherial/pertussis immunization, two examples among many, are true 'wonder' techniques in the ease of their administration and the numbers of newborns and young children saved – deaths for which 'daily bread' in such cases could offer limited or negligible protection. So also is emergency obstetrical care, and assured access to a range of basic drugs. A right to all is fundamental. Indeed, the importance of assured access to such preventive and curative services is far greater for those who can least afford livelihood losses associated with even brief periods of physical incapacity.

Nor is attention to human subsistence a denial of public health 'agency' such as the efforts of those who struggled for reforms in housing and water supply in early twentieth-century Beijing or in the slums of nineteenth-century industrializing Britain. The importance of a strong public health system in addressing continuing disease outbreaks and the emergence of new ones is of eminent importance, as evidenced with recent HIV, Ebola, SARS, and most recently, Zika epidemics. But public 'agency' clearly was not limited to germ-transmission control interventions in the case study countries above, nor indeed in Britain a century earlier where historic shifts in conditions of work and livelihood security ultimately took place through the efforts of the emerging trade unions and labour-oriented political movements in achieving economic and social welfare legislation.[134]

Ultimately, measures of disease control cannot substitute for subsistence security because hunger undermines survival chances not for a single infective disease, but for a host of common endemic infections. Those children most at risk of succumbing to a specific infection such as measles or pneumonia by virtue of undernourishment-compromised immune capacity are more vulnerable to a range of other endemic infections at other times of the year – including those microbes represented in the catch-all 'pulmonary-diarrhea complex' category, still responsible for up to one-third of all preventable childhood deaths in the modern non-industrial world:[135] in the words of the 1878 Punjab Sanitary Commissioner, 'distress for food . . . render[ing] them incapable of resisting the assaults of any disease going.'[136] At another level, when analysis is directed principally to technical interventions to specific diseases one can suggest there is often limited comprehension of the magnitude of prevented deaths that underlie secular trends in life expectancy for entire populations – indeed, of even a few years' increase.

It is not a matter, then, of choosing between health care systems and food security, but of addressing both. Yet the relative sidelining of food security policies in recent analysis of the modern mortality decline suggests instead a fundamental loss in understanding of the central role of staple-food security in 'good health,' and of the importance of conditions of women's work upon which child nourishment depends.[137] These are issues that take on even wider contemporary significance with the challenges already unfolding with global climate destabilization. In this context, perhaps one of the more important insights from the 1985 *GHLC* report is the finding that the composition of the diet for all three Asian populations studied had remained essentially unchanged from its traditional content across the period of dramatically rising life expectancy: which is to say, staple food made up almost entirely of traditional foodgrains and tubers.[138] Nothing fancy, in other words: sufficient daily 'bread.'

## A larger significance to South Asian malaria history

One example of the importance of staple-food security can be seen, inversely, in the 1950s experience in Punjab[139] where abrupt interruption in malaria transmission appears to have had only a marginal effect, at most, on general mortality levels – suggesting, in other words, that post-1920 decline in acute hunger accounted for most of the reduction in the region's historical malaria mortality burden, though much 'chronic' undernourishment remained.[140] Across the final years of the nineteenth-century, there was increasing awareness in British India of malaria as the leading 'vehicle' by which acute hunger markedly magnified death rates from autumnal malaria infection. During this period and into the early twentieth century, epidemiological analysis transcended the conceptual constraints of sanitationist epidemic theory of the British metropole, where epidemic causality had increasingly been reduced to 'exciting' or 'precipitating' factors. First queried by W.R. Cornish in his painstaking account of famine mortality in the 1876–1877 Madras famine, those reductive conceptual constraints were formally challenged two decades later in the pages of the 1901 Famine Commission Report.[141] Moreover, for reasons that included looming imperial exigencies, this understanding of the hunger-epidemic malaria relationship was soon extended beyond episodic famine (epidemic acute starvation), to include the general 'difficulties under which the people . . . get their food supply . . . throughout the year.' In the wake of the 1918 influenza epidemic, the Madras Corporation in its 1919 annual report stressed the 'potent influence' of economic conditions upon the death rates of the population.

> Supplies may exist and still be beyond the purchasing power of many members of the population . . . the excessive mortality accompanying the diminution of the means of support though not caused by actual starvation is brought about by disease. The working of this factor so easily perceived when people are dying of starvation is often overlooked when a population is decimated by disease.[142]

Such non-famine conditions of economic stress S.R. Christophers would refer to as 'private hardship': acute hunger triggered by injury, debility, or individual loss of employment or of a household wage-earner; but also manifested in 'hunger seasons,' regular intervals where little agricultural employment was available and increasingly unremunerative work was resorted to in an effort to stave off frank starvation.[143]

Already, at the third annual meeting of the General Malaria Committee in 1912, Bentley stressed the distinction between infection and disease, and pointedly challenged the view 'that our knowledge of malaria . . . [based upon] blood examination, spleen counting, . . . dissection of anopheles, and the mapping out of [vector] breeding places . . . is now so complete that it can be reduced to mathematical formulae.'

> [A]lthough the brilliant discoveries of Laveran and Ross have extended our knowledge of the parasitology of malaria . . . we are still ignorant of many of the factors responsible for the occurrence of malaria *disease*, more especially when it appears in epidemic form among populations like those to be met with in India; and there are reasons for believing that until our conception of infectious diseases in general and malaria in particular undergoes a radical change, these gaps in our knowledge may not only remain unfilled but actually pass *unrecognized*.[144]

The 'radical' change envisioned by Bentley entailed recognition of the immense variation in clinical morbidity and mortality historically observed for common endemic infections under conditions of hunger-induced suppression of immune capacity. In a very concrete sense, a small handful of malaria researchers in early twentieth-century South Asia had found themselves undertaking an epidemiology of what W.P. Alison in Scotland articulated almost a century earlier as the 'grand level of Poverty itself.'[145]

Bentley's fears, and Forster's a decade later, that comprehension of the role of hunger in epidemic and endemic mortality patterns in British India was being lost would prove well founded. In the case of malaria, the three decades 1920–1950 were a key period of contestation in Western infectious disease thought in which acknowledgement of the distinction between infection and morbid disease was in marked retreat in international fora – which is to say, at a point in time when subsistence precarity yet remained a central dimension of public health in much of the then malaria-endemic world.

In December 1949, with growing Western optimism for residual insecticide-based malaria eradication, V. Venkat Rao would survey malaria control efforts in India and conclude with a prophetic warning that '[t]he human factor involved in epidemic malaria has not perhaps received the emphasis that it deserves.'[146] His reference was possibly the last to a concept which had centrally informed malaria research and analysis three decades before, in that 'golden age' of malaria research.[147] That it could fade so thoroughly, and so rapidly, from medical and intellectual discourse – though the practical reality of hunger remained pervasive in the society in which he worked – speaks to how many fundamental concepts relating to disease and social conditions had already been set aside. Ironically, across this period of conceptual demise, a demonstrable 'success' in one area of malaria control was unfolding quietly in the background: the near elimination after 1920 of the once 'fulminant' malaria epidemics of northwest India, unfolding without external philanthropic expertise, without vector sanitation, or indeed without any perceptible decline in malaria transmission rates among the rural population. But rather with the politically imperative control of epidemic acute hunger. Yet this quiet pre-DDT success would fail to be reflected in the new, post-WW2 World Health Organization, as the region's exactingly documented historical experience was set aside.

The demise in understanding of the role of destitution in South Asian malaria history – and its inverse, the triumph of the 'malaria as block to development' thesis – stemmed from a confluence of forces: academic, professional, technological, and geopolitical, with antecedents that predated the 1908 Punjab epidemic. In one sense, 'malariology' as a discipline could no longer 'see' or know what was missing because, for new entrants to the profession, elemental concepts and the very language of human hunger were gone. Relatively few medical figures were left in modern tropical medicine institutes who had extensive field experience of malaria in relation to acute hunger, or the broader professional stature, to be in a position to argue successfully those insights.

Now in his mid-70s, Christophers did not attend the 1948 Washington Malaria Congress. Though he would be formally lauded *in absentia* for his life-time malaria research by congress attendees,[148] economic dimensions to malaria formed no part of the proceedings. At the very end of the twentieth century, *An Illustrated History of Malaria* would commemorate the great medical figures who contributed historically to the elucidation of malaria science. Among the 129 photographic portraits and 346 names included in the text's index, S. Rickard Christophers was missing.[149]

What happened a century earlier in the lead-up to and formulation of the 1842 Sanitary Report, Hamlin suggests, was 'not a beginning, but the kind of revolutionary change that obliterates an earlier landscape,' one where a broader predispositionist understanding of disease came to be 'intentionally effaced from professional memory.'[150] With scarcely less efficiency, and possibly no less intentionality on the part of key figures, a similar effacing was re-enacted a century later with the relinquishing of earlier research and understanding of the 'Human Factor' in malaria. In the process, historical common experience, and arguably common sense itself, was set aside. Binding together the two (public) health histories was the Chadwickian sanitationist legacy in which the very language of hunger had been erased.

## Notes

1 See ch. 4, note 4.
2 C. Hamlin, *Public Health and Social Justice in the Age of Chadwick* (Cambridge: Cambridge University Press, 1998), 289.
3 W.P. Alison, *Observations on the Management of the Poor in Scotland, and Its Effects on the Health of Great Towns*, 2d ed. (Edinburgh: Blackwood, 1840), 10–11. For a comprehensive overview of Alison's work as professor of medicine at Edinburgh University and Edwin Chadwick's 'nemesis,' see C. Hamlin, 'William Pulteney Alison, the Scottish Philosophy, and the Making of a Political Medicine,' *Journal of the History of Medicine and Allied Sciences*, 61, 2, 2006, 144–186.
4 C. Hamlin 'Predisposing Causes and Public Health in Early Nineteenth-Century Medical Thought,' *Society for the Social History of Medicine*, 5, 1, Apr. 1992, 43–70.
5 Hamlin, *Public Health and Social Justice*, 195–196.
6 See ch. 7, at notes 30 to 36; also, S. Zurbrigg, *Epidemic Malaria and Hunger in Colonial Punjab* (London and New Delhi: Routledge, 2019), 264–265.
7 R. Passmore and T. Sommerville, 'An investigation of the effect of diet on the course of experimental malaria in monkeys,' *Journal of the Malaria Institute of India*, 3, 4, Dec. 1940, 447–455, 448 [hereafter, *JMII*].
8 In the specific case of epidemics among labour camps '[i]t seems more probable,' they concluded, that 'labour forces are exposed to infection with strains of malaria parasites to which they have previously had no opportunity of acquiring immunity'; ibid.
9 P. Russell, L.S. West, R.D. Manwell, *Practical Malariology* (Philadelphia: W.B. Saunders, 1946), 374. As had Ross in his criticism of the work at Mian Mir, Russell would fault Christophers for 'largely ignor[ing]' the anopheline factor in

the 1911 Punjab study, arguing that 'methods for measuring anopheline density have never been satisfactory'; ibid., 376.

10 Hamlin, *Public Health and Social Justice*, 196 [emphasis in original].

11 E. Ackerknecht, 'Hygiene in France, 1815–1848,' *Bulletin of the History of Medicine*, 22, 1948, 117–155, at 141. For an overview of the work of Louis René Villermé, see N. Krieger, *Epidemiology and the People's Health* (Oxford: Oxford University Press, 2014), 78–80.

12 Ackerknecht, 'Hygiene in France,' 144.

13 R.M. Packard, 'Malaria Dreams: Postwar Visions of Health and Development in the Third World,' *Medical Anthropology*, 17, 1997, 279–296, at 280.

14 Noting Gill's reference to famine as a contributing factor in the 1934–1935 Ceylon epidemic, Lewis Hackett responded: 'What is lacking to this case is any sound evidence, other than influential opinion, that it is true.' In acknowledging host factors, he argued, 'we are no longer on solid ground. We have cut loose from our experimental data and become engaged at once in a battle of opinion.'; L. Hackett, *Malaria in Europe* (Oxford: Oxford University Press, 1937), 263, 261.

15 S.P. James, S.R. Christophers, 'Malaria in India: What the State can do to prevent it?' *Lancet*, 26 Jun. 1909, 1860–1862, at 1862.

16 Of course hunger too could also be observed and investigated 'scientifically' under controlled conditions, as S.P. Ramakrishnan would pursue; S. Zurbrigg, 'Did starvation protect from malaria?: Distinguishing between severity and lethality of infectious disease in colonial India,' *Social Science History*, 21, 1, 1997, 27–58.

17 It would be this question that framed Thomas McKeown's 1970s analysis of mortality decline from infective disease in Britain: 'The virulence of an organism is not . . . a distinct character like its size or shape; it is an expression of an interaction between a particular organism and a particular host'; T. McKeown, *The Modern Rise of Population* (London: Edward Arnold, 1976), 73. For further discussion in relation to colonial Punjab epi-/endemic mortality history, see Zurbrigg, *Epidemic Malaria and Hunger*, 406–409.

18 P. Weindling, 'Social medicine at the League of Nations Health Organisation and the International Labour Office compared,' in P. Weindling, ed. *International Health Organisations and Movements, 1918–1939* (New York: Cambridge University Press, 1995), 134–153. [emphasis added]).

19 Famine Inquiry Commission, *Report on Bengal* (New Delhi: Government of India Press, 1945), 116–123.

20 Ibid.

21 W.W.C. Topley, 'The biology of epidemics,' Croonian Lecture, *Proceedings of the Royal Society of London. Series B, Biological Sciences*, 130, 861, May 8, 1942, 337–359.

22 W.R. Cornish, *Report of the Sanitary Commissioner for Madras for 1877* (Madras: Government Central Branch Press, 1877), 11, 142, xxviii [hereafter, *MSCR*]; A.P. MacDonnell, *Report of the Indian Famine Commission 1901* (Calcutta: Government Printing Office, 1901), 2, 61–62. For details, see Zurbrigg, *Epidemic Malaria and Hunger*, 187, 329.

23 *Report on Bengal*, 121.

24 W.R. Aykroyd, 'Definition of Different Degrees of Starvation,' in G. Blix, Y. Hofvander, B. Vahlquist, eds. *Famine: A Symposium dealing with Nutrition and Relief Operations in Times of Disaster* (Uppsala: Swedish Nutrition Foundation, 1971), 17–24. Dissension among 1945 Famine Commission members as to the role of starvation in epidemic mortality may explain the vacillation in

emphasis, with Indian members perhaps stressing testimony from earlier famine commission reports, and Aykroyd, judging from later statements, veering to the microbial: some form of 'consensus' ultimately reached by deferring to Topley's 'complexity.' In a subsequent overview of the Bengal famine, Aykroyd would also refer to the '[r]efugees from Burma [who] poured into Bengal through Assam and Chittagong, bringing with them a virulent form of malaria'; *The Conquest of Famine* (London: Chatto & Windus, 1974), 72.

25 N.S. Scrimshaw, C.E. Taylor, J.E. Gordon, *Interactions of Nutrition and Infection* (Geneva: World Health Organization, 1968); N.S. Scrimshaw, 'The Phenomenon of Famine,' *American Review of Nutrition*, 7, 1987, 1–21.

26 Zurbrigg, *Epidemic Malaria and Hunger*, ch. 12.

27 Ibid., 384, 281. Moreover, hunger itself likely has played a substantial role secondarily in maintaining transmission of major infective diseases such as tuberculosis; and certainly in the severity of others, as suggested by Punjab malaria history in relation to dose of infection; ibid., ch. 5.

28 Hamlin, 'Social Justice and Public Health,' 11.

29 See, e.g., E. Whitcombe, 'Famine Mortality,' *Economic and Political Weekly*, 28, 1993, 1169–1179; B. Mohanty, 'Case Study of the Indian Famines of 1896–97 and 1899–1900,' in S.N. Singh, et al., eds., *Population Transition in India*, v. 2 (Delhi: B.R. Publishing, 1989), 371–379.

30 P.J. Marshall, *Bengal: The British Bridgehead: Eastern India 1740–1838* (Cambridge: Cambridge University Press, 1987); I. Klein, 'Population Growth and Mortality in British India Part I: The Climacteric of Death,' *Indian Economic and Social History Review*, 26, 4, 1989, 387–403 [hereafter, *IESHR*].

31 Marshall, *Bengal: British Bridgehead*, 4–5, 20.

32 M.O.T. Iyengar, 'Studies on Malaria in the Deltaic Regions of Bengal,' *JMII*, Dec. 1942, 435–446.

33 Klein considers both, but ultimately argues the impact of increased vectors 'far outpaced any agricultural decline from soil decay'; 'Development and death: Reinterpreting malaria, economics and ecology in British India,' *IESHR*, 38, 2, 2001, 147–179. Yet the effect of interrupted inundation flows on cropping frequency would have been immediate, as Bentley conveyed; C.A. Bentley, 'Some economic aspects of Bengal malaria,' *IMG*, Sept. 1922, 321–326; Bentley, *Malaria and Agriculture in Bengal. How to reduce malaria in Bengal by irrigation* (Calcutta: Bengal Govt Press, 1925). For recent Burdwan fever analysis, see ch. 1, note 56.

34 Zurbrigg, *Epidemic Malaria and Hunger*, 273–276.

35 See also, Zurbrigg, 'Did Starvation Protect from Malaria?'

36 A. Sen, *Poverty and Famines: An Essay on Entitlement and Deprivation* (Oxford: Oxford University Press, 1981); A. Maharatna, *The Demography of Famines: An Indian Historical Perspective* (Delhi: Oxford University Press, 1996).

37 E. Whitcombe, 'The Environmental Costs of Irrigation in British India: Waterlogging, Salinity, Malaria,' in D. Arnold, R. Guha, eds., *Nature, Culture, Imperialism: Essays on the Environmental History of South Asia* (Delhi: Oxford University Press, 1995), 237–259; K. Wakimura, 'Epidemic malaria and "Colonial Development": Reconsidering the Cases of Northern and Western India,' Economic History Congress XIII, Buenos Aires, Argentina, July 2002, mimeo.

38 The apparent paradox has redirected interpretation of South Asian mortality decline away from 'nutritional' explanations to instead immunological hypotheses; Klein, 'Population Growth and Mortality in British India,' 392, 403; I. Klein, 'Population Growth and Mortality in British India Part II: The Demographic Revolution,' *IESHR*, 27, 1, 1990, 33–63, at 60; Klein, 'Development

and Death,' at 177–179. In contrast, others have pointed to initial shifts in food security to explain beginning decline in mortality post-1920; S. Guha, 'Mortality Decline in Early Twentieth Century India: A Preliminary Enquiry,' *IESHR, 28,* 4, 1991, 371–387; C. Guilmoto, 'Towards a New Demographic Equilibrium: The Inception of Demographic Transition South India,' *IESHR, 28,* 3, 1992, 247–289.

39 Zurbrigg, *Epidemic Malaria and Hunger,* chs. 2, 4.

40 See, e.g., W.H. McNeill, *Plagues and Peoples* (New York: Anchor Books, 1976), 116.

41 'Malthus saw no need to appeal to learned medicine to support these claims,' Hamlin points out, 'for nothing he said about disease was controversial. It seemed obvious, even truistic, that disease was deadlier to the weak than to the strong'; Hamlin, *Public Health and Social Justice,* 26.

42 Surgeon-Captain H.E. Grant, *The Indian Manual of Hygiene being King's Madras Manual,* rev. ed., (Madras: Higginbotham & Co., 1894), 326.

43 C. Hamlin, *More Than Hot: A Short History of Fever* (Baltimore: Johns Hopkins University Press, 2014), 61–62.

44 *Report on the Sanitary Administration of the Punjab* (Lahore: Medical Department, Punjab), 1878, 67.

45 GOI, *Proceedings of the Imperial Malaria Conference held at Simla in October 1909* (Simla: Government Central Branch Press, 1910), 103 [hereafter Simla Conf.].

46 S. Mackenzie, 'The Powers of Natural Resistance, or the Personal Factor in Disease of Microbic Origin,' The Annual Oration, May 26, 1902, *Transactions of the Medical Society of London, 25,* 302–318, at 312.

47 C. Hamlin, 'Could you starve to death in England in 1839? The Chadwick-Farr controversy and the loss of the "social" in public health,' *American Journal of Public Health, 85,* 6, Jun. 1995, 856–866.

48 W.R. Cornish, MSCR 1877, 147.

49 P. Manson, *Tropical Diseases: A Manual of the Diseases of Warm Climates* (London: Cassell and Co., 1898), 98. On this and the larger issue of malaria and 'tropical aggregation of labour,' see Zurbrigg, *Epidemic Malaria and Hunger,* 228–231.

50 *Famine Commission Report* (Punjab), 1900, Vol. I, 35. See Zurbrigg, *Epidemic Malaria and Hunger,* 347; D. Arnold, 'Looting, grain riots and government policy in South India 1918,' *Past and Present,* no. 84, 1979, 111–145; D. Arnold, 'Social Crisis and Epidemic Disease in the Famines of Nineteenth-century India,' *Social History of Medicine,* 6, 3, Dec. 1993, 385–404, at 396.

51 See also, ch. 4, at note 52. Cornish, who attempted to tally 1876–1877 Madras famine starvation-induced deaths, was very much the exception, sufficiently senior, experienced, and administratively and intellectually above reproach; MSCR, 1876–1877.

52 Simla Conf., 43; P. Hehir, *Malaria in India* (London: Humphrey Milford, 1927), 442.

53 Simla Conf., 5.

54 See, Zurbrigg, *Epidemic Malaria and Hunger,* chs. 7, 8.

55 Aykroyd, *Conquest of Famine,* 93.

56 S. Millman, R.W. Kates, 'Toward Understanding Hunger,' in L.F. Newman, et al., eds., *Hunger in History: Food Shortage, Poverty, and Deprivation* (Oxford: Basil Blackwell, 1990), 3–24, at 22.

57 R.B. Lal, S.C. Seal, *General Rural Health Survey, Singur Health Centre, 1944,* (Calcutta: GOI Press, 1949), 118.

58  A.J. Coale, E.M. Hoover, *Population Growth and Economic Development in Low Income Countries: A Case Study of India's Prospects* (Princeton: Princeton University Press, 1958), 62–67; S. Preston, 'Causes and Consequences of Mortality Declines in Less Developed Countries during the Twentieth-century,' in R.A. Easterlin, ed., *Population and Economic Change in Developing Countries* (Chicago: University of Chicago Press, 1980), 296, 313.

59  T.W. Meade, 'Medicine and population,' *Public Health*, 82, 3, 1968, 100–110. For a similar assessment, see, Editorial, 'Malaria and the Population Explosion,' *Lancet*, Apr. 27, 1968, 899–900.

60  Meade, 'Medicine and population.' In addition to GDP figures, Frederiksen referred to the public distribution system and agricultural development programs.

61  Important exceptions are studies that investigate caloric consumption by income-deciles, a rare example of which is seen in the 1937 rural Madras study discussed in ch. 3 at note 78; W.R. Aykroyd, B.G. Krishnan, 'Diets surveys in south Indian villages,' *Indian Journal of Medical Research*, 24, 3, Jan. 1937, 667–688.

62  That the poor continued to work despite illness is cited for its effect on infection dissemination; less for the looming hunger that drove the sick to work, often to death; A. Hardy, *The Epidemic Streets: Infectious Disease and the Rise of Preventive Medicine, 1856–1900* (Oxford: Clarendon Press, 1993), 270–271.

63  S. Szreter, *Health and Wealth: Studies in History and Polity* (Rochester: University of Rochester Press, 2005), 313–328. McKeown, *Modern Rise of Population*, 156, 159. Curiously, McKeown also grouped 'improvement in diet' under the umbrella term of 'environmental' factors, along with 'conditions of exposure to disease'; 'Medicine and world population,' *Journal of Chronic Diseases*, 18, 1965, 1067–1077.

64  D. Morley, *Paediatric Priorities in the Developing World* (London: Butterworth-Heinemann, 1973).

65  R. Martorell, T.J. Ho, 'Malnutrition, morbidity and mortality.' In H. Mosley, L. Chen, eds., *Child Survival: Strategies for Research*, Supplement to vol. 10, *Population and Development Review*, 1984, 49–68; Scrimshaw and Gordon, *Interactions of Nutrition and Infection*.

66  An important exception is seen in the work of R. Chambers, R. Longhurst, A. Pacey, eds., *Seasonal Dimensions to Rural Poverty* (London: Frances Pinter, Institute of Development Studies, 1981), 164, 167, 174.

67  For a comprehensive overview of this work, see R. Floud, R. Fogel, B. Harris, Sok Chul Hong, eds., *The Changing Body: Health, Nutrition, and Human Development in the Western World since 1700* (Cambridge: Cambridge University Press, 2011). It is unclear however to what extent adult stature also captures prevalence of acute hunger (semi- or frank starvation), given the much greater associated mortality. For discussion of this distinction and likely implications for interpreting trends in nutritional stunting in South Asia, see Zurbrigg, *Epidemic Malaria and Hunger*, 25–32, 354, 410.

68  McKeown, *Modern Rise of Population*; McKeown, *The Role of Medicine*. In part, lack of clarity regarding the meaning of 'nutritional improvement' left his argument readily open to rebuttal on the basis of little demonstrable *qualitative* (micronutrient) improvement in the late nineteenth- and early twentieth-century period of initial rising life expectancy.

69  S. Szreter, 'The importance of social intervention in Britain's mortality decline,' *Social History of Medicine*, 1, 1, 1988, 1–37.

70  Moreover, geographic and institutional distance from the dominant epistemic community often was too great to counter dominant germ-transmission

paradigms in mortality decline analysis. Egyptian demographers 'profoundly disagreed' with U.S. economists, for example, regarding timing of post-WW2 crude death rate decline in Egypt, finding most decline occurred in the immediate post-war years, thus pre-dating the country's DDT malaria control program, rather than in the 1950s as the latter argued. Their views, however, were apparently disregarded; T. Dyson and M. Murphy, 'Macro-Level Study of Socioeconomic Development and Mortality: Adequacy of Indicators and Methods of Statistical Analysis,' in J. Cleland, A. Hill, eds., *The Health Transition: Methods and Measures* (Canberra: Australian National University, 1991), Health Transition Series No. 3, 147–164, at 149. On the marked mid-1940s drop in mortality levels in Punjab associated with food rationing and a post-war economic boom, see, Zurbrigg, *Epidemic Malaria and Hunger*, 392–393.

71 S.B. Halstead, J.A. Walsh, K.S. Warren, *Good Health at Low Cost* (New York: Rockefeller Foundation, 1985) [hereafter, *GHLC*].

72 A fourth case study was Costa Rica, if somewhat less representative as a very low-income country.

73 *GHLC*, 246.

74 *GHLC*, 200–213.

75 Ibid., 200; R. Martorell, R. Sharma, 'Trends in Nutrition, Food Supply and Infant Mortality Rates,' *GHLC*, 200–213.

76 Food subsidies were listed in tabular form (203, 177), with a passing reference to land reform (204, 62, 64). But brevity allowed little discussion of their potential impact, or timing in relation to mortality decline. One contributor emphasized that 'the rapid growth of the national economy . . . [in China was] certainly the material basis of the continuously progressing health status of the people,' but again without specific policy or timing details; ibid., 35.

77 'What matters most [in achieving high life expectancy] is that people come to understand disease risks, and how to manage them. . . . Low-income countries found low-cost ways to control these diseases, relying more heavily on educating people to do things for themselves and less on public financing, expert intervention, medical technology, or hospitals'; J.C. Riley, *Low Income, Social Growth, and Good Health: A History of Twelve Countries* (Berkeley: University of California Press, 2008), 5–7, 159.

78 J. Banister, *China's Changing Population* (Stanford: Stanford University Press, 1987), 83; J. Banister, K. Hill, 'Mortality in China 1964–2000,' *Population Studies*, 58, 1, 2004, 55–75 at 55, reported 20 per 1,000 to 10.2 per 1,000 by 1958.

79 F.W. Notestein and Chi-ming Chiao, 'Population,' in J.L Buck, ed., *Land Utilization in China* (Chicago: University of Chicago Press, 1937), vol. 1, 358–399. For a summary, see Banister; *China's Changing Population*, 79, Table 4.2.

80 G. Barclay, A. Coale, M. Stoto, J. Trussell, 'A reassessment of the Demography of Traditional Rural China,' *Population Studies*, 42, 4, 1976, 605–635, at 608, 621.

81 Death rates (per 100,000) in Beijing for the 1937–1945 period also show no decline relative to earlier decades; Campbell, 'Mortality Change,' 236, Table 11.3.

82 J. Banister, 'Population Policy and Trends in China, 1978–83,' *The China Quarterly*, 100, Dec. 1984, 717–741, at 740.; Banister, *China's Changing Population*, 80. It is possible that rates of survival had improved somewhat prior to 1949 in Communist-held areas through land distribution measures; Liping Bu, *Public Health and the Modernization of China, 1865–2015* (London: Routledge, 2017), 192, 197–198.

83 Banister, *China's Changing Population*, 116. See also, J. Banister, S.H. Preston, 'Mortality in China,' *Population and Development Review*, 7, 1, 1981, 98–110 at 107–108.

84 Banister and Preston, 'Mortality in China,' 104.
85 Banister *China's Changing Population*, 55; J. Salaff, 'Mortality decline in the People's Republic of China and the United States,' *Population Studies*, 27, 1973, 551–576 at 566.
86 Banister, *China's Changing Population*, 53–54; Salaff, 'Mortality decline,' 563.
87 Smallpox in 1929–1931 reportedly contributed 7.7 per cent of total deaths; Notestein and Chiao (1937) mortality survey, 393; cited in J. Banister, *China's Changing Population*, 51. Syphilis mortality is generally a later consequence of the infection, thus lives saved due to treatment likely contributed only a small proportion to the overall decline. Neonatal tetanus was also targeted in the 1950s, mortality in Beijing declining from 7.2 deaths per 1,000 live births in 1941 to 0.7 in 1957 with the shift to hospital deliveries (Salaff, 'Mortality decline,' 566), though rural decline through rudimentary village midwife training is unclear. Priority was given to development of 2,379 Maternal and Child Health (MCH) stations by 1952 (World Bank, *China: The Health Sector*, Washington, D.C., 1984, 14), yet each was responsible for a population of 250,000. Moreover even had rural neonatal tetanus rates declined as fast as urban, the contribution to infant and overall mortality decline would have been small.
88 Much has been written about the national 'patriotic' vector control campaigns also initiated in the early 1950s. Their impact on *transmission* of endemic infections such as malaria and schistosomiasis however has been questioned; C. Campbell, 'Mortality Change and the Epidemiological Transition in Beijing, 1644–1990,' in Ts'ui-jung Liu, et al., eds., *Asian Population History* (Oxford: Oxford University Press, 2001), 221–269, at 237–238; Salaff, 'Mortality Decline,' 567; Banister, *China's Changing Population*, 57–58. Farley points out the extreme difficulties of controlling the snail vector of schistosomiasis; *Bilharzia: A History of Imperial Tropical Medicine* (Cambridge: Cambridge University Press, 1991), 284–285.
89 As of 1982, only half the urban population had access to piped water; in rural areas, 6 per cent, with another 34 per cent benefitting from 'improved wells.' As late as 1981, dysentery remained 'the most commonly reported communicable disease in China,' with 'great deficiencies' remaining; GHLC, 192, 193; Banister, *China's Changing Population*, 64–66.
90 D. Zhang, P. Unschuld, 'China's barefoot doctor: Past, present, and future,' *Lancet*. 372 (9653), 2008, 1865–1867; J. McConnell, 'Barefoot No More,' *Lancet*, 341 (8855), 1993, 1275.
91 Estimated life expectancy in 1980 was 65 years; Banister, 'Population Policy and Trends,' 740–741.
92 Campbell, 'Mortality Change,' 239.
93 GHLC, 15. Notestein and Chiao, 'Population,' cited in Banister, *China's Changing Population*, 51; E.L. Opie, 'Tuberculosis of first infection in adults from rural districts of China,' *Chinese Medical Journal*, 56, 3, 1939, 216–224; Bu, *Public Health and the Modernization of China*, 257.
94 GHLC, 16.
95 Tuberculosis hospitals increased from 13 to 48 between 1949 and 1957; Campbell, 'Mortality Change,' 233.
96 Ibid., 233. Much TB-control effort in the 1950s was directed to BCG production and vaccination, the effectiveness of which has since been shown, however, to be very limited in preventing pulmonary TB; the single exception being the uncommon meningeal form in children; Centers for Disease Control, *Morbidity and Mortality Weekly Report*, Apr. 26, 1996.
97 Salaff, 'Mortality decline,' 569.
98 Ibid., 566; Banister, *China's Changing Population*, 56.

99  By comparison, the 'lack of any significant change in nutritional status during 1915–25 to 1951–58 is quite striking'; D.T. Jamison, A. Piazza, 'China's Food and Nutrition Planning,' in J.P. Gittinger, J. Leslie, C. Hoisington, *Food Policy: Integrating Supply, Distribution, and Consumption* (Baltimore: Johns Hopkins Press, 1987), 467–484, at 479; A. Piazza, *Food Consumption and Nutritional Status in the PRC* (Boulder: Westview Press, 1986), 140–141, 154–155. This improvement is all the more significant because the children represented in the earlier 1915–1925 survey figures were school children likely from the least poor subgroups, those attending school. No major differences in stunting prevalence were observed between males and females in 1979; but significant regional and urban (2.6%): rural (12.7%) differences remained; ibid., 481.

100  The leading causes of death in pre-1949 Beijing (respiratory and gastrointestinal diseases, and tuberculosis) (Campbell, 'Mortality Change,' 235–236) are all strongly linked to undernourishment. Reported incidence of low birth weight (birth weight < 2.5 kg) in Shanghai also apparently declined from 6.3 per cent in 1936–1940 to 3.2 per cent in 1950–1955; Salaff, 'Mortality decline,' 574.

101  Jamison and Piazza, 'China's Food and Nutrition,' 477, 470, 472, Table 36.2.

102  Elizabeth Croll, *The Family Rice Bowl: Food and the Domestic Economy* (London: UNRISD/Zed Press, 1983), 113.

103  Jamison and Piazza, 'China's Food and Nutrition,' 470.

104  Banister, 'Population Policy, 740.

105  Ibid., 741.

106  *GHLC*, 209.

107  Passing reference to 'improvement in nutrition' in China appears in a very detailed account of the country's health care system (*GHLC*, 24), but the reader is directed elsewhere for data. The one case study where food security programs were considered in somewhat more detail was Sri Lanka; *GHLC*, 114.

108  World Bank, *China: The Health Sector*, 174; Banister, 'Mortality in China,' 65.

109  Banister and Hill, 'Mortality in China 1964–2000, 69.

110  *GHLC*, 41, 40–45; P.G.K. Panikar, and C.R. Soman, *Health Status of Kerala: Paradox of Economic Backwardness and Health Development* (Trivandrum: Center for Development Studies, 1984), 24. By 1990, infant mortality had fallen to 15 deaths per 1,000 live births; S. Irudaya Rajan and P. Mohanachandran, 'Estimating Infant Mortality in Kerala,' *Economic and Political Weekly*, vol. 34, no. 12 (Mar. 20–26, 1999), 713–716.

111  *GHLC*, 64.

112  The number of primary health centres in Kerala doubled in the 1960s, as did rural dispensaries a decade later.

113  National Nutrition Monitoring Bureau (NNMB), *Report of Repeat Surveys: 1988–90* (Hyderabad: National Institute of Nutrition, Hyderabad, 1991), 55, Table 9.1. There are limitations to the earlier NNMB survey data; but the trendline of decline in severe malnutrition prevalence in Kerala is consistent from the late 1970s, and corresponds to trends in child stature over the same period.

114  R. Martorell, and T.J. Ho, 'Malnutrition, morbidity, and mortality,' *Population and Development Review Suppl.*, 10, 1984, 49–68; J.C. Waterlow, et al., *Protein-energy Malnutrition* (London: Edward Arnold, 1992), 336, Fig. 18.4.

115  Panikar and Soman, *Health Status of Kerala*, 28. Between 1961–1962 and 1983, calorie intake in Kerala increased by 40 per cent; B.G. Kumar, 'Quality of Life and Nutritional Status: A reconsideration of some puzzles from Kerala,' in P. Bardhan, M. Datta-Chaudhuri, and T.N. Krishnan, eds., *Development and Change: Essays in Honour of K.N. Raj* (Bombay: Oxford University Press,

1993), 318–340, at 321. For assessment of the impact of the PDS program on low-income household food consumption, see e.g., S.K. Kumar, 'Impact of Subsidized Rice on Food Consumption and Nutrition in Kerala,' International Food Policy Research Institute, Research Report, no. 5, Jan. 1979.

116 Panikar and Soman, *Health Status of Kerala* 74–75. Over 90 per cent of school girls in 1980 were found with intestinal nematode infections, and over 70 per cent with ascariasis. Moreover, infant and child mortality rates were similar in households with pipe water source compared to wells; also with flush toilet, latrine, or neither; *GHLC*, 193, 194.

117 For example, in a single stroke the PDS program substantially mitigated seasonal foodgrain price swings ('hunger seasons'), and security of dwelling (ownership of housing plots) arguably would have helped empower the landless 30 per cent of households to insist on newly legislated minimum wage levels.

118 *GHLC*, 63, 73. To be fair, reliable data from initial 1970s NNMB survey work may not have been available to analysts in the early 1980s, although it appears data on child stature was. Based solely upon aggregate calorie availability, Kerala continues to be seen as one with malnutrition levels 'among the highest in India'; D. Lal, *The Hindu Equilibrium* (Oxford: Clarendon Press, Oxford, 2005), 323.

119 D. Balabanova, M. McKee, A. Mills, eds., *'Good Health at Low Cost': Twenty Years On* (London: London School of Hygiene and Tropical Medicine, 2011) [hereafter, *GHLC-25*]. The 2011 report's overview of 'lessons gained' from the earlier 1985 *GHLC* analysis pointed again, in the case of China, to the control of communicable disease transmission and to barefoot doctors; with food security policies unmentioned; ibid., 2–3, 236.

120 *GHLC-25*, 172, 176–177. Most recently 24-hour emergency medical services has been extended through a growing network of rural health centres; ibid., 188.

121 *GHLC-25*, 166, Fig. 6.2.

122 *Report of the NNMB-NNSO Linked Survey, 1983–84*, National Institute of Nutrition: Hyderabad, Table 20; *Report of the First Repeat Rural Surveys* [1988–90], National Institute of Nutrition: Hyderabad, 55. Though the 1988–1990 NNMB survey reports 'very little change in average income status' in the state, average *calorie* intake among children 1–3 years was found to have increased by 9 per cent and among 4–6 year-olds by almost 13 per cent; NNMB 1988–90, 12, 18, 47.

123 The Tamil Nadu report mentions increased industrial and transportation development across the state, as well as passing reference to the Noon Meal Scheme for school children, but with little exploration of the impact on food security or timing in relation to infant mortality decline; *GHLC-25*, 184–185. Most recently, the PDS has expanded to include wheat flour and lentils; www.tncsc.tn.gov.in/PDS.html; and Tamil Nadu has successfully implemented the National Rural Employment Guarantee program; J. Drèze, A. Sen, *An Uncertain Glory: India and its Contradictions* (Princeton: Princeton University Press, 2013), 168–176.

124 R. Chhabra, 'Reaping rewards of social development,' *People and the Planet*, 3, 3, 1994, 16–20.

125 Personal interview, February 1997.

126 'We have seen the close links between seasonality, poverty and dependence. If counter-seasonal programmes can enable the poorer rural people to gain more adequate flows of food and income and to become less vulnerable and less dependent, they may then be more able and ready to assert themselves. More

food and better health may provide the physical and psychological preconditions for political organization and pressure to achieve reforms'; R. Chambers, S. Maxwell, 'Practical Solutions,' in Chambers, Longhurst and Pacey, eds., *Seasonal Dimensions to Rural Poverty*, 226–240, at 238.

127 Studies in contemporary West African agricultural populations vividly document pronounced rainy-season weight loss and infant/toddler failure to grow; M.G.M Rowlands, et al., 'Seasonality and the Growth of Infants in a Gambian Village,' in Chambers, Longhurst and Pacey, eds., *Seasonal Dimensions to Rural Poverty*, 164–174. See also, A.M.K. Chowdhury, S.L. Huffman, and L.C. Chen, 'Agriculture and Nutrition in Matlab Thana, Bangladesh,' ibid., 52–66.

128 See, e.g., Allen, R.C., T. Bengtsson, and M. Dribe, eds., *Living Standards in the Past: New Perspectives on Well-Being in Asia and Europe* (Oxford: Oxford University Press, 2005).

129 P. Weindling, 'Social medicine at the League of Nations Health Organisation and the International Labour Office compared,' in Weindling, *International Health Organisations*, 139.

130 See above, ch. 6 at notes 91–95. See also, J.H. Perkins, *Geopolitics and the Green Revolution: Wheat, Genes, and the Cold War* (New York: Oxford University Press, 1997), 128.

131 M. Garenne, D. Waltisperger, P. Cantrelle, O. Ralijona, 'The Demographic Impact of a Mild Famine in an African City: The Case of Antananarivo, 1985–87,' in T. Dyson, C. Ó Gráda, eds., *Famine Demography: Perspectives from the Past and Present* (Oxford: Oxford University Press, 2002), 204–217.

132 Ibid.

133 In a 2015 analysis of post-1949 mortality decline in China, food security policies were hardly mentioned. Nor were child nutrition indices reported. 'Nutrition' was addressed solely in terms of *per capita* provincial grain production, price trends, and an undefined 'campaign against malnutrition' in four western provinces, possibly a local selenium micronutrient deficiency program (Table 2); the authors concluding that 'increases in educational attainment and public health campaigns jointly explain 50–70 per cent of the dramatic reductions in infant and under-five mortality between 1950 and 1980'; K.S. Babiarz, et al., 'An Exploration of China's mortality decline under Mao: A provincial analysis, 1950–80,' *Population Studies (Camb)*, 69, 1, 2015, 39–56. Interestingly, almost four decades ago, Chambers and colleagues observed, '[t]he very high life expectancies and low fertility of Sri Lanka and Kerala are usually attributed to education, health services, and late marriage. It is at least possible that a major factor is the exceptional food security of poor families in those two regions'; Chambers, et al., eds., *Seasonal Dimensions to Rural Poverty*, 231.

134 For a glimpse of the political impact of such efforts on hours and conditions of work both in Britain and British India, see ch. 1, at notes 30–36.

135 C.L. Fischer-Walker, et al., 'Global burden of childhood pneumonia and diarrhea,' *Lancet*, 381 (9875), 2013, 1405–1416.

136 *Punjab Sanitary Commission Report*, 1878, 28–29.

137 The question of the 'nutrition drain' associated with recurrent infections, and related impact of clean water and sewerage infrastructure interventions, can be seen also within a wider additional context that encompasses subsistence (in) security: the constraints of time available for nourishing young children through the frequent infections of childhood. In this sense, the time- and energy-sparing impact of ready access to safe water is likely also to encompass a 'nutritional' element.

138 *GHLC*, 209. Moreover, decline in mortality levels was at least as great in the Asian case study countries where staple foods were primarily grains and tubers, as in Cuba and Costa Rica where the traditional diet included considerable amounts of food of animal origin.

139 Zurbrigg, *Epidemic Malaria and Hunger*, ch. 12.

140 Ibid., 384.

141 See above, note 22.

142 *Annual Report of the Madras Corporation, Health Dept*, 1919, 2.

143 S.R. Christophers, 'Endemic and Epidemic Prevalence,' in M.F. Boyd, ed., *Malariology* (Philadelphia: W.B. Saunders, 1949), 698–721, at 715. For a contemporary portrait of seasonal hunger by women landless labourers in Midnapore district, West Bengal, see N. Mukherjee, A. Mukherjee, 'Rural Women and Food Insecurity: What a Food Calendar Reveals,' *Economic and Political Weekly*, Mar. 12, 1994, 597–599. See also note 127.

144 C.A. Bentley, 'A New Conception Regarding Malaria,' *Proceedings, 3rd Meeting of the General Malaria Committee, Nov. 18–20, 1912, held at Madras* (Simla: Govt. Monotype Press, 1913), 61–84 [emphasis added].

145 W.P Alison, *Observations on the Management of the Poor in Scotland*, x. I am indebted to Christopher Hamlin for insights into the significance of Alison's work.

146 V. Venkat Rao, 'A critical review of malaria control measures in India,' *IJM*, 3, 4, Dec. 1949, 313–326, at 324.

147 Three years later, the Director of the Malaria Institute would highlight Christophers's 'famous memoir,' *Malaria in the Punjab*, that 'has remained an authoritative report on the subject' of malaria, yet refer to its economic conclusions only obliquely: 'In places like the Punjab . . . there is no well marked innate immunity and there are periodic severe or fulminating epidemics . . . the result, *under certain circumstances*, of exceptionally heavy rainfall accompanied by river flooding, usually following one or more years of comparative drought'; Jaswant Singh, 'Malaria and its Control in India,' *Perspectives in Public Health*, 72, 1952, 515–525, 515–516 [emphasis added].

148 In presenting the Laveran Prize to H.E. Shortt at the 1948 International Malaria Congress in Washington, N.H. Swellengrebel referred to Shortt's work (identifying the long-missing exoerythrocytic stage of development of the malaria parasite in humans) as 'a builder of bridges spanning chasms of ignorance . . . like that other constructor of foundations, the man we admire so much, Sir Rickard Christophers. . . . I want your name coupled with his.' He added, '[s]ome of our friends from India and Pakistan called Sir Rickard their father. In time to come they may call *you* by that name'; 'Presentation of the Laveran Prize to Prof. Henry E. Shortt by Prof N.H. Swellengrebel,' *Proceedings of the Fourth International Congress on Tropical Medicine and Malaria*, 19–20.

149 C.M. Poser, Geo. W. Bruyn, *An Illustrated History of Malaria* (New York: Parthenon Publ., 1999). In a remarkable parallel, Hamlin notes how 'Alison is oddly absent from big-picture histories of public health'; 'William Pulteney Alison, the Scottish Philosophy,' at note 1.

150 'Public Health and Social Justice,' 18.

# Appendix I

# MALARIA TRANSMISSION
# IN PUNJAB

Malaria is caused by a single-cell protozoan parasite (*Plasmodium*), its transmission involving a complex life cycle with two stages of development. The first stage takes place in humans who form the 'reservoir' of infection; and the second occurs in particular species of *Anopheles* mosquitoes. Transmission of malaria to the human host occurs through the bite of an infected female mosquito, its blood meal being required for egg production. Parasites ('sporozoites') are transmitted along with the insect's saliva that acts as an anticoagulant, and are rapidly sequestered in the liver of the human host. After one to two weeks, large numbers of 'merozoites' are released into the blood stream and infect red blood cells. Characteristic symptoms of episodic fever and chills begin to appear as successive batches of the parasite break down red blood cells, are released into the circulation, and infect further blood cells. Subsequently some merozoites differentiate into male and female gametocytes, at which point the human host becomes infective to further feeding mosquitoes, initiating the second ('extrinsic') phase of the parasite's life cycle. With fertilization of the male and female gametes inside the insect gut, sporozoites develop in the stomach wall, multiply, and migrate to the mosquito's salivary glands where the cycle begins again.

Successful completion of the *Plasmodium* life cycle thus requires two blood meals by the vector mosquito a minimum of 10 days apart, an interval allowing sufficient time for development of the parasite inside the insect. Thus, transmission hinges upon anopheline lifespan, determined by both temperature and atmospheric humidity. Under ideal conditions (28°C. and 60–80 per cent humidity), a single reproductive cycle for the P. *falciparum* parasite requires 30 to 35 days.

Subtropical in latitude but nestled within the Asian continental landmass, the Punjab plains are subject to enormous extremes in temperature and atmospheric humidity. With the exception of the Himalayan hill tracts, annual rainfall is low. Thus for most of the year, low humidity reduces anopheline lifespan well below that required for development of the parasite. With the summer monsoon rains, however, the fine clay soil is quickly saturated, causing further rainfall to collect in countless pools suitable for larval development. Atmospheric humidity levels rise dramatically, and in turn mosquito longevity, such that malaria infection rates can increase exponentially from extremely low pre-monsoon levels to near universal prevalence in the space of three reproductive cycles. With cessation of the rains in mid- or late September, malaria transmission falls off quickly.

The two main malaria species transmitted in Punjab were *P. vivax* ('benign tertian') and *P. falciparum* ('malignant' or 'sub-tertian' malaria), the latter associated with greater morbidity and mortality related to proportionately greater parasitization of red blood cells. In the Punjab plains, the autumn rise in malarial fever typically appeared in late August, initially consisting of vivax infection. In non-drought years, falciparum cases followed within 2 to 4 weeks, largely replacing vivax transmission by early October, its later timing related to the longer period (10 to 14 days) required for the appearance of gametocytes in the human host.

# Appendix II

# AN EPIDEMIOLOGICAL APPROACH TO HUNGER IN HISTORY[1]

To trace the uncoupling of disease and destitution in modern epidemic theory requires the reclaiming of fundamental concepts of human subsistence. Here a tentative epidemiological framework is offered. Three dimensions to hunger considered in this study involve: degree or severity of food (calorie) insufficiency; duration; and prevalence (proportion of a population affected at a given time). If self-evident, these differing aspects can be obscured in modern usage of the terms 'malnutrition,' 'undernutrition,' or 'undernourishment.'

Hunger involves a range of caloric levels of food consumption on a continuum of insufficiency: from slight and moderate inadequacy, at one end of the spectrum, to nothing at all to eat, on the other. In very basic terms, this encompasses two states: 'not enough' to eat (undernourishment), and 'not nearly enough' (semi- or frank starvation). The two can be distinguished, again in very general terms, in relation to basal metabolic rate, that level of energy required for all internal metabolic and physiological functions in a state of complete rest. In this study, 'acute' hunger refers to caloric intake below basal metabolic rate, a level where weight loss is continuous and life cannot be supported beyond the short term. In contrast, undernourishment (often termed 'chronic' hunger) refers to food intake above basal metabolic requirement but below that required to fully meet all *external* energy demands ('normal' activity, and physical labour) as well as growth demands (in children and in pregnant or breastfeeding women).

In both cases, duration largely determines general mortality risk, related to direct effects on immunological capacity (immunosuppression).[2] The mortality risk with undernourishment (chronic hunger), though also elevated, is less than absolute and less immediate compared to that for acute hunger (the term 'chronic' reflects this lower lethality, allowing for a longer duration unremedied). Some physiological 'adaptation' to undernourishment is often possible through reduced physical activity (energy expenditure), or additionally in children, a reduction in physical growth rate (stunting). Both such states of 'adaptation,' however, entail immunological and cognitive

264

costs depending on extent of calorie deficit, as well as likely impairment of (future) work capacity.

While the link between immune-suppression and both undernourishment and semi-/frank starvation is clear, this relationship very likely encompasses immune-suppression effects beyond those directly due to calorie insufficiency. A related component, if largely unmeasurable, derives from the immune-suppression effects of extreme psychological stress associated with food insecurity and acute hunger: the despair and human degradation accompanying inability to protect oneself and family members, above all, one's children. Such despair was routinely expressed in the desperate resort to offering children into servitude for the price of their being fed, or the agony of watching them die in the streets and roadways absent of succour.[3] Separating the two sources of immune-suppression associated with acute hunger is an impossible – one might suggest, unnecessary – task. In this study, both are assumed to be at play.

In young children, cumulative undernourishment is identified clinically by 'stunting' (low height-for-age), and acute hunger, by 'wasting' (low weight-for-height) or emaciation. Both can be evident in the same child as levels of food inadequacy fluctuate over time. In all states of caloric inadequacy, the added energy drain of concurrent infections further reduces the *net* calories physiologically available.

Prevalence of acute and chronic hunger cannot be traced in historical research with the precision expected in modern clinical research. Nevertheless, with a clearer conceptualization of hunger, historical markers can be identified from a range of archival sources. The two general categories of hunger, acute and chronic, can be identified in South Asian historical records, for example, in references to numbers of meals per day consumed: two meals a day generally considered 'enough to satisfy hunger.' The categories of zero, one, and two meals per day encompass, albeit in very general form, the two central aspects of hunger in human history: on the one hand, reflecting (in)sufficiency of levels of food (caloric) intake, and on the other, (ir)regularity of access to food, that is, the frequency with which subgroups of a population slip below one square meal into semi- or frank starvation (acute hunger). If one could graphically sketch acute and chronic hunger through history, one would be tracing, in effect, the relative prevalence in a population of persons with access to two square meals per day, one, or none over time – the term 'prevalence' here being used in its epidemiological sense of frequency, duration, and social extent.

Such a schematic framework requires qualification to take into account the exceptional needs, for example, of infants and young children who require far more than two meals a day because of their extremely high relative food requirements for growth, and their small stomach size. It is here, of course, where conditions of work for women, productive and reproductive, play such a large historical role. Attention has been directed recently to the nutritional drain of repeated infections, again of special relevance to young children. The concept of 'net' nutrition takes into account the potential additional impact on food sufficiency of transient illness-induced anorexia and added nutrient losses associated, in particular, with diarrheal episodes. In addition to questions of water supply, 'net nutrition' thus also reflects conditions of work: time and energy available to feed and care for young children to compensate for such recurring nutrient losses.

Further, such a schema allows consideration of acute hunger well beyond episodic 'famine' (epidemic acute hunger). Indeed, endemic acute hunger plays possibly a greater role in health history than its epidemic form, encompassing regular 'hunger seasons,' intervals in the agricultural year where little employment is available and increasingly unremunerative work is resorted to in an effort to stave off frank starvation. Studies in contemporary agricultural populations document pronounced rainy-season weight loss and infant/toddler failure to grow, related to women's extreme time constraints and depleted food stores.[4] Undernourishment is 'visible' as well, if indirectly, in conditions of work. Most obvious, historically, are wage levels insufficient to meet even minimal calorie requirement; but also intensity and hours of work, constraints that often bore disastrous consequences for nourishing young children and constitute a large, if generally unwritten, chapter of endemic hunger history.

The conceptual distinction between acute and chronic hunger is important for historical analysis for several reasons. The most obvious relates to mortality risk, as indicated above. Another is methodological: the means by which the two states of hunger can be identified from historical records, and potentially measured, often differ. Historical changes in mean physical stature in a population, for example, are likely to reflect change in general levels of (under)nourishment over time more reliably than acute hunger,[5] whereas short-term fluctuations in foodgrain prices probably signal greater relative increases in acute hunger compared to chronic.

The significance of this distinction is evident in the case of South Asia. Recent nutritional anthropometric research for the colonial period suggests little increase in mean stature,[6] and indeed, possibly slight decline in height amongst the poorer and most food-insecure subgroups across the colonial period.[7] This lack of improvement in adult stature appears paradoxical in light of the beginning increase in life expectancy across the final three decades of British rule from very low levels pre-1920. Yet seen from the context of both *gaps* in food access as well as *levels* of food intake, this pattern is perhaps less surprising. More effective famine (acute hunger) control after 1901 likely meant proportionately greater improvement in survival chances among the most poor and chronically undernourished, resulting possibly in a net increase in nutritionally stunted individuals after 1920 within the post-famine population. Seemingly opposite trends – decreasing or stagnant mean stature levels and rising life expectancy – may not necessarily be inconsistent, then, with improving food security, when the distinction between acute and chronic hunger is taken into account.

Finally, the conceptual distinction between acute and chronic hunger is particularly important in health and epidemic history because of potential differences in interaction between specific infectious diseases and type of hunger. In South Asia, the case fatality rate for malaria, for example, appears to have been heightened in particular by acute hunger and less so by lesser degrees of hunger (undernourishment).[8]

## Notes

1 For further discussion, see S. Zurbrigg, *Epidemic Malaria and Hunger: In Colonial Punjab: 'Weakened by Want'* (London and New Delhi: Routledge, 2019), 28–32.

2 'Many of the body's generalized defenses against infectious disease,' Nevin Scrimshaw details, 'are reduced by relatively mild degrees of nutritional deficiency. These include, among others, cell-mediated immunity, phagocyte function, complement function, and delayed cutaneous hypersensitivity. . . . With the more severe deficiencies of famine [acute hunger], specific humoral antibody defenses [macromolecules such as antibodies circulating in the bloodstream and tissues] and capacity to produce phagocytes are also weakened'; 'The Phenomenon of Famine,' *American Review of Nutrition*, 7, 1987, 1–121.

3 P.B. Mukharji addresses such mental misery, in 'Verncularizing Political Medicine: Locating the Medical betwixt the Literal and the Literary in Two Texts on the Burdwan Fever, Bengal c. 1870s,' in R. Deb Roy, and G.N.A. Attewell, eds., *Locating the Medical: Explorations in South Asian History* (New Delhi: Oxford University Press, 2018), 235–263.

4 For further discussion, see Zurbrigg, *Epidemic Malaria and Hunger*, 410–412.

5 See for example, R. Floud, 'The Heights of Europeans since 1750: A New Source for European Economic History,' in J. Komlos, ed., *Stature, Living Standards, and Economic Development: Essays in Anthropometric History* (Chicago: University of Chicago Press, 1994), 12.

6 A.V. Guntupalli, and J. Baten, 'The Development and Inequality of Heights in North, West, and East India 1915–1944,' *Explorations in Economic History*, 43, 2006, 578–608.

7 L. Brennan, J. McDonald, and R. Shlomowitz, 'Long-Term Change in Indian Health,' *South Asia: Journal of South Asian Studies*, 26, 1, 2003, 51–69; Guntupalli and Baten, 'Inequality of Heights,' 592.

8 Zurbrigg, *Epidemic Malaria and Hunger*.

# BIBLIOGRAPHY

Acharya, K.C.S., *Food Security System of India: Evolution of the Buffer Stocking Policy and its Evaluation*, New Delhi: Concept Publ., 1983.

Ackerknecht, E., 'Hygiene in France, 1815–1848,' *Bulletin of the History of Medicine*, 22, 1948, 117–155.

Acton, H.W., 'An investigation into the Causation of Lathyrism in Man,' *Indian Medical Gazette*, Jul. 1922, 241–247.

Adyanthaya, N.K., *Report on the Enquiry into the Family Budgets of Industrial Workers in Madras city, 1935–1936*, Madras: Superintendent, Govt. Press, 1940.

Agnihotri, I., 'Ecology, Land Use and Colonisation: The Canal Colonies of Punjab,' *Indian Economic and Social History Review*, 33, 1, 1996, 37–58.

Alison, W.P., *Observations on the Management of the Poor in Scotland, and Its Effects on the Health of Great Towns*, 2nd ed., Edinburgh: Blackwood, 1840.

Allen, R.C., T. Bengtsson, and M. Dribe, eds., *Living Standards in the Past: New Perspectives on Well-Being in Asia and Europe*, Oxford: Oxford University Press, 2005.

Amrith, S., *Decolonizing International Health: India and Southeast Asia, 1930–65*, Basingstoke: Palgrave Macmillan, 2006.

———, 'Political Culture of Health in India: A Historical Perspective,' *Economic and Political Weekly*, Jan. 13, 2007, 114–121.

Anand, S., and R. Kanbur. 'Public Policy and Basic Needs Provision: Intervention and Achievement in Sri Lanka,' in J. Drèze, and A. Sen, eds., *The Political Economy of Hunger*, vol. 3, Oxford: Clarendon, 1991, 59–92.

Anderson, M., 'India, 1858–1930: The Illusion of Free Labour,' in D. Hay, and P. Craven, eds., *Masters, Servants and Magistrates in Britain and the Empire, 1562–1955*, Chapel Hill and London: University of North Carolina Press, 2004.

Anon [Editorial], 'An Imperial School of Hygiene,' *Lancet*, Mar. 4, 1922, 441.

———, 'Public Health and Medical Research in India,' *British Medical Journal*, Apr. 14, 1923, 640.

———, 'On the Seven Scourges of India,' *Indian Medical Gazette*, Jul. 1924, 351–355.

———, ['from a special correspondent] 'The Need for a Public Health Policy for India,' *Indian Medical Gazette*, Oct. 1927, 575–582.

———, 'Malaria and the Population Explosion,' *Lancet*, Apr. 27, 1968, 899–900.

Arnold, D., 'Dacoity and Rural Crime in Madras, 1860–1940,' *Journal of Peasant Studies*, 7, 2, 1979, 140–167.

————, 'Looting, Grain Riots and Government Policy in South India 1918, *Past and Present*, no. 84, 1979, 111–145.

————, 'Famine in Peasant Consciousness and Peasant Action: Madras 1876–78,' in R. Guha, ed., *Subaltern Studies III: Writings on South Asian History and Society*, Delhi: Oxford University Press, 1984, 62–115.

————, *Colonizing the Body: State Medicine and Epidemic Disease in Nineteenth-Century India*, Berkeley: University of California Press, 1993.

————, 'Social Crisis and Epidemic Disease in the Famines of the Nineteenth-Century India,' *Social History of Medicine*, 6, 3, Dec. 1993, 385–404.

————, 'Colonial Medicine in Transition: Medical Research in India, 1910–47,' *South Asia Research*, 14, 1, 1994, 10–35.

————, 'Crisis and Contradiction in India's Public Health History,' in D. Porter, ed., *The History of Public Health and the Modern State*, Amsterdam: Rodopi, 1994, 335–355.

————, 'The "Discovery" of Malnutrition and Diet in Colonial India,' *Indian Economic and Social History Review*, 31, 1, 1994, 1–26.

————, *Warm Climates in Western Medicine: The Emergence of Tropical Medicine, 1500–1900*, Amsterdam: Rodopi, 1996.

————, 'British India and the "Beriberi Problem," 1798–1942,' *Medical History*, 54, 2010, 295–314.

Aykroyd, W.R., 'Diet in Relation to Small Incomes,' *Quarterly Bulletin of the Health Organisation of the League of Nations*, 2, 1933, 130–153.

————, 'The Problem of Malnutrition in India,' *Current Science*, 4, 2, Aug. 1935, 75–77.

————, *Human Nutrition and Diet*, London: Thorton Butterworth, 1937.

————, 'Economic Aspects of the Problem of Nutrition in India,' *Indian Journal of Social Work*, 2, 3, Dec. 1941, 269–282.

————, *Nutrition*, Oxford Pamphlets on Indian Affairs, No. 21, Bombay: Humphrey Milford, Oxford University Press, 1944.

————, *Diet Surveys in India*, Cawnpore: The Job Press, 1948.

————, 'International Health – A Retrospective Memoir,' *Perspectives in Biology and Medicine*, 11, 2, 1968, 273–285.

————, *Conquest of Deficiency Diseases*, Geneva: World Health Organization, 1970.

————, 'Definition of Different Degrees of Starvation,' in G. Blix, Y. Hofvander, and B. Vahlquist, eds., *Famine: A Symposium dealing with Nutrition and Relief Operations in Times of Disaster*, Uppsala: Swedish Nutrition Foundation, 1971.

————, The *Conquest of Famine*, London: Chatto & Windus, 1974.

Aykroyd, W.R., and B.G. Krishnan, 'Diets Surveys in South Indian Villages,' *Indian Journal of Medical Research*, 24, 3, Jan. 1937, 667–688.

————, 'The Effect of Skimmed Milk, Soya Bean, and Other Foods in Supplementing Typical Indian Diets,' *Indian Journal of Medical Research*, 24, 1937, 1093–1115.

Babiarz, K.S., et al., 'An Exploration of China's Mortality Decline under Mao: A Provincial Analysis, 1950–80,' *Population Studies (Camb)*, 69, 1, 2015, 39–56.

Bagchi, A.K., *The Political Economy of Underdevelopment*, Cambridge: Cambridge University Press, 1982.

Baker, W.E., T.E. Dempster, and H. Yule, *Report of a Committee Assembled to Report on the Causes of the Unhealthiness Which has Existed at Kurnaul*, 1847;

in Collected Memoranda on the Subject of Malaria, *Records of the Malaria Survey of India*, 1, 2, Mar. 1930, 1–68.

Balabanova, D., M. McKee, and A. Mills, eds., *'Good Health at Low Cost': Twenty Years On*, London: London School of Hygiene and Tropical Medicine, 2011.

Balfour, A., and H.H. Scott, *Health Problems of the Empire*, London: W. Collins Sons & Co., 1924.

Balfour, M., and S.K. Talpade, 'Maternity Conditions of Women Mill-Workers in India,' *Indian Medical Gazette*, May 30, 1930, 241–249.

———, 'Maternity Conditions and Anaemia in the Assam Tea-gardens,' *Journal of the Association of Medical Women in India*, vol. 24, 1936.

Bandyopadhyay, P., *Indian Famine and Agrarian Problems: A Policy Study on the Administration of Lord George Hamilton, Secretary of State for India, 1895–1903*, Calcutta: Star Publs., 1987.

Banerjee, H., *Agrarian Society of the Punjab, 1849–1901*, New Delhi: Manohar, 1982.

Banister, J., 'Population Policy and Trends in China, 1978–83,' *The China Quarterly*, 100, Dec. 1984, 717–741.

———, *China's Changing Population*, Stanford: Stanford University Press, 1987.

Banister, J., and K. Hill, 'Mortality in China 1964–2000,' *Population* Studies, 58, 1, 2004, 55–75.

Banister, J., and S.H. Preston, 'Mortality in China,' *Population and Development Review*, 7, 1, 1981, 98–110.

Barclay, G., A. Coale, M. Stoto, and J. Trussell, 'A Reassessment of the Demography of Traditional Rural China,' *Population Studies*, 42, 4, 1976, 605–635.

Baron, C., and C. Hamlin, 'Malaria and the Decline of Ancient Greece: Revisiting the Jones Hypothesis in an Era of Interdisciplinarity,' *Minerva*, 52, 2015, 327–358.

Behal, R.P., *Wage Structure and Labour: Assam Valley Tea Plantations, 1900–1947*, New Delhi: V.V. Giri National Labour Institute, 2003.

———, 'Power Structure, Discipline, and Labour in Assam Tea Plantations under Colonial Rule,' *International Review of Social History*, 51, 2006, Supplement, 143–172.

Behal, R.P., and P. Mohapatra, 'Tea and Money versus Human Life: The Rise and Fall of the Indenture System in the Assam Tea Plantations 1840–1908,' *Journal of Peasant Studies*, 19, 3/4, 1992, 142–172.

Bentley, C.A., *Report of an Investigation into the Causes of Malaria in Bombay*, Bombay: Miscellaneous Official Publications, 1911.

———, 'A New Conception Regarding Malaria,' 3rd Meeting of the General Malaria Committee, Nov. 18–20, 1912, held at Madras, Simla: Govt Press, 1913, 61–84.

———, 'Dr. Bentley on Amelioration of Malaria by Irrigation,' *Indian Medical Record*, Feb. 1922, 41–43.

———, 'Some Economic Aspects of Bengal Malaria,' *Indian Medical Gazette*, Sept. 1922, 321–326.

———, *Malaria and Agriculture in Bengal. How to Reduce Malaria in Bengal by Irrigation*, Calcutta: Bengal Govt Press, 1925.

———, Testimony. *Royal Commission on Agriculture in India*, vol. IV, London: HMSO, 1928, Bengal Evidence, 240–247.

Bhatia, B.M., *Famines in India*, Bombay: Asia Publ. House, 1963.

———, 'Famine and Agricultural Labour in India,' *Indian Journal of Industrial Relations*, 10, 1975, 575–594.

Bhombore, S.R., C. Brooke Worth, and K.S. Nanjundiah, 'A Survey of the Economic Status of Villagers in a Malarious Irrigated Tract in Mysore State, India, before and after D.D.T. Residual Insecticidal Spraying,' *Indian Journal of Malariology*, 6, 4, Dec. 1952, 355–366.

Birn, A.-E., 'Backstage: The Relationship between the Rockefeller Foundation and the World Health Organization, Part I: 1940s-1960s,' *Public Health*, 128, 2014, 129–140.

———, 'Philanthrocapitalism, Past and Present: The Rockefeller Foundation, the Gates Foundation, and the Setting(s) of the International/Global Health Agenda,' *Hypothesis*, 1, 12, 2014, 1–27.

Birn, A.-E., and A. Solórzano, 'The Hook of Hookworm: Public Health and Politics of Eradication in Mexico,' in A. Cunningham, and B. Andrews, eds., *Western Medicine as Contested Knowledge*, Manchester: Manchester University Press, 1997, 147–171.

Birn, A.-E., Y. Pillay, and T.H. Holtz, *Textbook of Global Health*, 4th ed., Oxford: Oxford University Press, 2017.

Biswas, A., 'The Decay of Irrigation and Cropping in West Bengal, 1850–1925,' in B. Chattopadhyay, and P. Spitz, eds., *Food Systems and Society in Eastern India*, Geneva: United Nations Research Institute for Social Development, 1987, 85–131.

Blaxter, K.L., ed., *Nutritional Adaptation in Man*, London: John Libbey, 1985, 13–30.

Boon, T., 'Agreement and Disagreement in the Making of *World of Plenty*,' in D.F. Smith, ed., *Nutrition in Britain: Science, Scientists and Politics in the Twentieth Century*, London: Routledge, 1997.

Boserup, E., *The Conditions of Agricultural Growth*, Chicago: Aldine, 1965.

———, 'The Primary Sector in African Development,' in M. Lundahl, ed., *The Primary Sector in African Development*, London: Croom Helm, 1985, 43–55.

Bouma, M.J., and H. van der Kaay, 'The El Niño Southern Oscillation and the Historical Malaria Epidemics on the Indian Subcontinent and Sri Lanka: An Early Warning System for Future Epidemics?' *Tropical Medicine and International Health*, 1, 1, Feb. 1996, 86–96.

Boyd, M.F., ed., *Malariology: A Comprehensive Survey of All Aspects of This Group of Diseases from a Global Standpoint*, Philadelphia: W.B. Saunders, 1949.

Brennan, L., J. McDonald, and R. Shlomowitz, 'Long-Term Change in Indian Health,' *South Asia: Journal of South Asian Studies*, n.s., 26, 1, 2003, 51–69.

Briercliffe, R., *The Ceylon Malaria Epidemic, 1934–35. Report by the Director of Medical and Sanitary Service*, Colombo: Ceylon Govt Press, Sept. 1935.

Briercliffe, R., and W. Dalrymple-Champneys, 'Discussion on the Malaria Epidemic in Ceylon, 1934–35,' *Proceedings of the Royal Society of Medicine*, 29, 1936, 537–562.

Brooke, M.M., 'Effect of Dietary Changes upon Avian Malaria,' *American Journal of Hygiene*, 41, 1945, 81–108.

Brown, E.R., 'Public Health in Imperialism: Early Rockefeller Programs at Home and Abroad,' *American Journal of Public Health*, 66, 9, 1976, 897–903.

Brown, P.J., 'Socioeconomic and Demographic Effects of Malaria Eradication,' *Social Science Medicine*, 1986, 852–853.

———, 'Malaria, *Miseria*, and Underpopulation in Sardinia: The "Malaria Blocks Development" Cultural Model,' *Medical Anthropology*, 17, 1997, 239–254.

Brumpt, E., 'Anophélisme sans paludisme et régression spontanée du paludisme,' *Ann. Parasit. hum. comp.*, 20, 1944, 67–91.

Brunton, D., and Review of C. Hamlin, 'Public Health and Social Justice,' *Journal of the Society of the Social History of Medicine*, 13, 1, Apr. 2000, 173–174.

Bu, L., *Public Health and the Modernization of China, 1865–2015*, London: Routledge, 2017.

Burnet, E., W.R. Aykroyd, 'Nutrition and Public Health,' *Quarterly Bulletin of the Health Organisation of the League of Nations*, 4, 2, Jun. 1935, 323–474.

Buxton, P.A., 'The Effect of Climatic Conditions upon Population of Insects,' *Transactions of the Royal Society of Tropical Medicine and Hygiene*, 28, 4, 1933, 325–256.

Bynum, W.F., 'Nosology,' in W. Bynum, and R. Porter, *Companion Encyclopedia of the History of Medicine*, London: Routledge, 1993, 335–356.

———, 'An Experiment that Failed: Malaria Control at Mian Mir,' *Parassitologia*, 36, 1–2, 1994, 107–120.

———, 'Malaria in Inter-war British India,' *Parassitologia*, 42, 1–2, 2000, 25–31.

Bynum, W.F., and C. Landry, *The Western Medical Tradition: 1800 to 2000*, Cambridge: Cambridge University Press, 2006.

Campbell, C., 'Mortality Change and the Epidemiological Transition in Beijing, 1644–1990,' in Ts'ui-jung Liu, et al., eds., *Asian Population History*, Oxford: Oxford University Press, 2001, 221–269.

Carpenter, K.J., *Protein and Energy: A Study of Changing Ideas in Nutrition*, Cambridge: Cambridge University Press, 1994.

———, 'A Short History of Nutritional Science: Part 4 (1945–1985),' *Journal of Nutrition*, 133, 2003, 3331–3342.

Carter, H.F., 'Report on Malaria and Anopheline Mosquitoes in Ceylon.' Sessional Paper VII., Colombo: Ceylon Govt Press, 1927.

Carter, H.F., and W.P. Jacocks, 'Observations on the Transmission of Malaria by Anopheline Mosquitoes in Ceylon,' *Ceylon Journal of Science*, Section D, 2, Pt. 2, 1929, 67–86.

———, 'Observations on the Transmission of Malaria by Anopheline Mosquitoes in Ceylon,' *Ceylon Journal of Science*, 2, Pt. 4, 1930.

Carter, R., and K.N. Mendis, 'Evolutionary and Historical Aspects of the Burden of Malaria,' *Clinical Microbiology Reviews*, Oct. 2002, 564–594.

Cassen, R., *India: Population, Economy, Society*, London: Macmillan, 1978.

Catanach, I., 'Plague and the Tensions of Empire: India, 1896–1918,' in D. Arnold, ed., *Imperial Medicine and Indigenous Societies*, Manchester: Manchester University Press, 1988, 149–171.

Celli, A., 'The Restriction of Malaria in Italy,' *Transactions of the Fifteenth International Congress on Hygiene and Demography, Washington, September 23–28, 1912* (Washington, D.C., 1913), 516–531.

Chakrabarti, P., *Bacteriology in British India: Laboratory Medicine and the Tropics*, Rochester: University of Rochester Press, 2012.

Chakrabarty, D., 'Conditions for Knowledge of Working-Class Conditions: Employers, Government and the Jute Workers of Calcutta, 1890–1940,' in R. Guha, ed. *Subaltern Studies II, Writings on South Asian History and Society*, Delhi: Oxford University Press, 1983, 259–310.

Chambers, R., and S. Maxwell, 'Practical Solutions,' in R. Chambers, R. Longhurst, and A. Pacey, eds., *Seasonal Dimensions to Rural Poverty*, London: Frances Pinter Publ., 1981, 226–240.

Chambers, R., R. Longhurst, and A. Pacey, eds., *Seasonal Dimensions to Rural Poverty*, London: Frances Pinter Publ., 1981.

Chandavarkar, R., 'Plague Panic and Epidemic Politics in India, 1896–1914,' in T. Ranger, and P. Slack, eds., *Epidemics and Ideas*, Cambridge: Cambridge University Press, 1992, 203–240.

Chandler, A., 'The Prevalence and Epidemiology of Hookworm and Other Helminth Infection in India, *Indian Journal of Medical Research*, 15, Pt. XII, 1928, 695–743.

Chen, M.A., *Coping with Seasonality and Drought*, New Delhi: Sage, 1991.

Chhabra, R., 'Reaping Rewards of Social Development,' *People and the Planet*, 3, 3, 1994, 16–20.

Chowdhury, A.M.K., S.L. Huffman, and L.C. Chen, 'Agriculture and Nutrition in Matlab Thana, Bangladesh,' in R. Chambers, R. Longhurst, and A. Pacey, eds., *Seasonal Dimensions to Rural Poverty*, London: Frances Pinter Publ., 1981, 52–66.

Christophers, S.R., 'On Malaria in the Punjab,' *Proceedings of the Imperial Malaria Conference held at Simla in October 1909*, 29–47.

———, 'Malaria in the Punjab,' *Scientific Memoirs by Officers of the Medical and Sanitary Departments of the Government of India* (New Series), No. 46, Calcutta: Superintendent Govt Printing, 1911.

———, 'Malaria: Endemiology and Epidemiology,' in W. Byam, and R.G. Archibald, eds., *The Practice of Medicine in the Tropics*, vol. 2, London: Henry Frowde, Hodder, and Stoughton, 1922, 1546–1554.

———, *Enquiry on Malaria, Blackwater-fever and Ankylostomiasis in Singhbhum. Report No. 1*, Behar and Orissa: Govt Publ., Jan. 1923, 363–407.

———, 'The Mechanism of Immunity against Malaria in Communities Living under Hyper-Endemic Conditions,' *Indian Journal of Medical Research*, 12, 2, Oct. 1924, 273–294.

———, 'What Disease Costs India: A Statement of the Problem Before Medical Research in India,' *Indian Medical Gazette*, Apr. 1924, 196–200.

———, 'Note on Malaria Research and Prevention in India,' 11–26, in *Report of the Malaria Commission on its Study Tour of India*, Geneva: League of Nations, 1930, 11–26.

———, 'Commentary,' in C.A. Gill, 'Some Points in the Epidemiology of Malaria Arising out of the Study of the Malaria Epidemic in Ceylon in 1934–35,' *Transactions of the Royal Society of Tropical Medicine and Hygiene*, 29, 5, Feb. 1936, 427–480.

———, 'Measures for the Control of Malaria in India,' *Journal of the Royal Society of Arts*, Apr. 30, 1943, 285–295.

———, 'Sydney Price James,' *Obituary Notice of Fellows of the Royal Society*, 5, 1945–48, 507–523.

———, 'Endemic and Epidemic Prevalence,' in M.F. Boyd, ed., *Malariology*, Philadelphia: W.B. Saunders Co. 1949, 698–721.

———, 'Policy in Relation to Malaria Control,' *Indian Journal of Malariology*, Dec. 1955, 297–303.

273

Christophers, S.R., and C.A. Bentley, 'Black-water Fever: Being the First Report to the Advisory Committee Appointed by the Government of India to Conduct an Enquiry Regarding Black-water and other fevers prevalent in the Duars,' *Scientific Memoirs by Officers of the Medical and Sanitary Departments of the Government of India* (New Series), no. 35, 1908.

———, *Malaria in the Duars*. Being the Second Report to the Advisory Committee Appointed by the Government of India to Conduct an Enquiry Regarding Black-water and Other Fevers Prevalent in the Duars, Simla: Government Monotype Press, 1909.

———, 'The Human Factor,' in W.E. Jennings, ed., *Transactions of the Bombay Medical Congress, 1909*, Bombay: Bennett, Coleman & Co., 1910, 78–83.

Christophers, S.R., J.A. Sinton, and G. Covell, 'How to take a malaria survey,' *Health Bulletin*, No. 14, Calcutta: GOI, 1928.

Cleaver, H., 'Malaria and the political economy of public health,' *International Journal of Health Services*, 7, 4, 1977, 557–579.

Coale, A.J., E.M. Hoover, *Population Growth and Economic Development in Low Income Countries: A Case Study of India's Prospects*, Princeton: Princeton University Press, 1958.

Cohn, E.J., 'Assessing the Costs and Benefits of Anti-Malarial Programs: The Indian Experience,' *American Journal of Public Health*, 63, 12, Dec. 1973, 1086–1096.

Coluzzi, M., 'Malaria and the Afrotropical Ecosystems: Impact of Man-Made Environmental Changes,' *Parassitologia*, 46, 1–2, 1994, 223–227.

———, 'The Clay Feet of the Malaria Giant and its African Roots: Hypotheses and Inferences About Origin, Spread and Control of *Plasmodium falciparum*,' *Parassitologia*, 41, 1999, 277–283.

Cornish, W.R., *Report of the Sanitary Commissioner for Madras for 1877*, Madras: Govt Press, 1878.

Cotton, A., *The Madras Famine*, London: Simpkin, Marshall [1878]; reprinted in A. Cotton, *Famine in India*, New York: Arno Press, 1976.

Covell, G., and J.D. Baily, 'The Study of a Regional Epidemic of Malaria in Northern Sind,' *Records of the Malaria Survey of India*, 3, 2, Dec. 1932, 279–321.

Croll, E., *The Family Rice Bowl: Food and the Domestic Economy*, London: UNRISD/Zed Press, 1983.

Cueto, M., 'The Cycles of Eradication: The Rockefeller Foundation and Latin American Public Health, 1918–1940,' in P. Weindling, ed., *International Health Organisations and Movements, 1918–1939*, Cambridge, Cambridge University Press, 1995, 222–243.

———, *Cold War, Deadly Fevers: Malaria Eradication in Mexico, 1955–1975*, Baltimore: Johns Hopkins University Press, 2007.

Cueto, M., and S. Palmer, *Medicine and Public Health in Latin America: A History*, New York: Cambridge University Press, 2015.

Cullumbine, H., 'The Influence of Environment on Certain Anthropomorphic Characters,' *Ceylon Journal of Medical Science* (D), 6, 3, 1949, 164–170.

———, 'An Analysis of the Vital Statistics of Ceylon,' *Ceylon Journal of Medical Science*, Dec. 1950, 134–135.

Davis, K., 'The Population Specter: Rapidly Declining Death Rate in Densely Populated Countries: The Amazing Decline of Mortality in Underdeveloped Areas,' *American Economic Review*, 46, 2, 1956, 305–318.

Davis, K.S., 'Deadly Dust: The Unhappy History of DDT,' *American Heritage*, 22, Feb. 1971, 44–47.

De Silva, K.M., *A History of Sri Lanka*, Delhi: Oxford University Press, 1981.

Deb Roy, R., *Malarial Subjects: Empire, Medicine and Nonhumans in British India, 1820–1909*, Cambridge: Cambridge University Press, 2017.

Deb Roy, R., and G.N.A. Attewell, eds., *Locating the Medical: Explorations in South Asian History*, New Delhi: Oxford University Press, 2018.

Dickson, R.M., 'The Malaria Epidemic in Ceylon, 1934–35,' *Journal of the Royal Army Medical Corps*, 1935, 85–90

Digby, W., *'Prosperous' British India: A Revelation from Official Records*, London: T. Fisher Unwin, 1901.

Dobson, M.J., M. Malowany, and R.W. Snow, 'Malaria Control in East Africa: The Kampala Conference and Pare-Taveta Scheme: A Meeting of Common and High Ground,' *Parassitologia*, 42, 2000, 149–166.

Drèze, J., 'Famine Prevention in India,' in J. Drèze, and A. Sen, eds., *The Political Economy of Hunger*, vol. 2, Oxford: Clarendon Press, 1990, 13–122.

Drèze, J., and A. Sen, *An Uncertain Glory: India and its Contradictions*, Princeton: Princeton University Press, 2013.

Dubin, M.D., 'The League of Nations Health Organisation,' in P. Weindling, ed., *International Health Organisations and Movements, 1918–1939*, New York: Cambridge University Press, 1995, 56–80.

Dunn, C.L., *Malaria in Ceylon: An Enquiry into its Causes*, London: Bailliere, Tindall and Cox, 1936.

Dutt, R.C., *Open Letter to Lord Curzon on Famines and Land Assessment in India*, London: Paul Kegan, 1900.

———, *The Economic History of India under Early British Rule*, London: Kegan Paul & Co., 1906.

Dy, F.J., 'Present Status of Malaria Control in Asia,' *Bulletin of the WHO*, 11, 1954, 725–763.

Dyson, T., 'The Historical Demography of Berar, 1881–1980,' in T. Dyson, ed., *India's Historical Demography: Studies in Famine, Disease and Society*, London: Curzon, 1989, 150–196.

———, 'On the Demography of South Asian Famines,' *Population Studies*, 45, 1991, Pts. 1 & 2, 5–25, 279–297.

———, 'Infant and Child Mortality in the Indian Subcontinent, 1881–1947,' in A. Bideau, B. Desjardins, and H. Brignoli, eds., *Infant and Child Mortality in the Past*, Oxford: Clarendon Press, 1997, 109–135.

Dyson, T., and A. Maharatna, 'Excess Mortality during the Bengal Famine: A Reevaluation,' *Indian Economic and Social History Review*, 28, 3, 1991, 281–297.

Dyson, T., and C. Ó Gráda, 'Introduction,' in T. Dyson, and C. Ó Gráda, eds., *Famine Demography: Perspectives from the Past and Present*, Oxford: Oxford University Press, 2002, 1–18.

Dyson, T., and M. Das Gupta, 'Demographic Trends in Ludhiana District, Punjab, 1881–1981: An Exploration of Vital Registration Data in Colonial India,' in Ts'ui-jung Liu, et al., eds., *Asian Population History*, Oxford: Oxford University Press, 2001, 79–104.

Dyson, T., and M. Murphy, 'Macro-level Study of Socioeconomic Development and Mortality: Adequacy of Indicators and Methods of Statistical Analysis,' in

J. Cleland, and A. Hill, eds., *The Health Transition: Methods and Measures*, Canberra: Australian National University, 1991, Health Transition Series No. 3, 147–164.

Editorial, 'Dietary and Nutritional Standards in India,' *Indian Medical Gazette*, July 1936, 405–406.

Editorial, 'The Economic Factor in Tropical Disease,' *Indian Medical Gazette*, 57, Sept. 1922, 341–343.

Ettling, J., *The Germ of Laziness: Rockefeller Philanthropy and Public Health in the New South*, Cambridge, MA: Harvard University Press, 1981.

Evans, H., 'European Malaria Policy in the 1920s and 1930s: The Epidemiology of Minutiae,' *ISIS*, 80, 1989, 40–59.

Farid, M.A., 'The Malaria Programme – from Euphoria to Anarchy,' *World Health Forum*, 1, 1–2, 1980, 8–33.

Farley, J., *Bilharzia: A History of Imperial Tropical Medicine*, Cambridge: Cambridge University Press, 1991.

———, 'Mosquitoes or Malaria? Rockefeller Campaigns in the American South and Sardinia,' *Parassitologia*, 36, 1994, 165–173.

———, *To Cast Out Disease: A History of the International Health Division of the Rockefeller Foundation, 1913–1951*, New York: Oxford University Press, 2004.

———, *Brock Chisholm, the World Health Organization, and the Cold War*, Vancouver: University of British Columbia Press, 2008.

Fayrer, Sir J., *On the Climate and Fevers of India*, Croonian Lecture, London: J&A Churchill, 1882.

Fernando, D.F.S., 'Health Statistics in Sri Lanka, 1921–80,' in S.B. Halstead, et al., eds., *Good Health at Low Cost*, New York: Rockefeller Foundation, 1985.

Finer, S.E., *The Life and Times of Sir Edwin Chadwick*, New York: Barnes and Noble, 1952.

Fisher, D., 'Rockefeller Philanthropy and the British Empire: The Creation of the London School of Hygiene and Tropical Medicine,' *History of Education*, 7, 2, 1978, 129–143.

Fischer-Walker, C.L., et al., 'Global Burden of Childhood Pneumonia and Diarrhea,' *Lancet*, 381, 9875, 2013, 1405–1416.

Floate, H.F.G., 'The Mauritian Malaria Epidemic 1866–1868: Geographical Determinism one Hundred Years Ago,' *Journal of Tropical Geography*, 29, 1969, 10–20.

Floud, R., R. Fogel, B. Harris, and S.C. Hong, eds., *The Changing Body: Health, Nutrition, and Human Development in the Western World since 1700*, Cambridge: Cambridge University Press, 2011.

Fogel, R., 'Second Thoughts on the European Escape from Hunger: Famines, Chronic Malnutrition, and Mortality Rates,' in S.R. Osmani, ed., *Nutrition and Poverty*, Oxford: Clarendon Press, 1992, 243–280.

Fontaine, R.E., A.E. Najjar, and J.S. Prince, 'The 1958 Malaria Epidemic in Ethiopia,' *American Journal of Tropical Medicine and Hygiene*, 10, 795–803.

Fosdick, R., *History of the Rockefeller Foundation*, New York: Harper Bros, 1952.

Franco-Agudelo, S., 'The Rockefeller Foundation's Antimalarial Program in Latin America: Donating or Dominating?' *International Journal of Health Services*, 13, 1, 1983, 51–67.

Frederiksen, H., 'Malaria Control and Population Pressure in Ceylon,' *Public Health Reports*, 75, 10, Oct. 1960, 865–868.

————, 'Determinants and Consequences of Mortality Trends in Ceylon, *Public Health Reports*, 76, 8, Aug. 1961, 659–663.

————, 'Economic and Demographic Consequences of Malaria Control in Ceylon,' *Indian Journal of Malariology*, 16, 4, Dec. 1962, 370–391.

————, 'Dynamic Equilibrium of Economic and Demographic Transition,' *Economic Development and Cultural Change*, 14, 1, Oct. 1965, 316–322.

————, Book Review of P. Newman, 'Malaria Eradication and Population Growth, 1965,' *American Journal of Tropical Medicine and Hygiene*, 15, 2, 1966, 262–264.

————, 'Determinants and Consequences of Mortality and Fertility Trends,' *Public Health Reports*, 81, 8, Aug. 1966, 715–727.

————, 'Malaria Eradication and the Fall of Mortality: A Note,' *Population Studies*, 24, 1, Mar. 1970, 111–113.

Fulton, J.D, and B.G. Maegraith, 'The Physiologic Pathology of Malaria,' in M.F. Boyd, ed., *Malariology: A Comprehensive Survey of All Aspects of This Group of Diseases from a Global Standpoint*, Philadelphia: W.B. Saunders, 1949.

Galdston, I., 'Humanism and Public Health', *Bulletin of the History of Medicine*, Jan. 1940, 1032–1039.

Gandhi, M.K., *Diet and Diet Reform*, Ahmedabad: Navajivan Publ. House, 1949.

Gangulee, N., *Health and Nutrition in India*, London: Faber and Faber, 1939.

Garenne, M., et al., 'The Demographic Impact of a Mild Famine in an African City: The Case of Antananarivo, 1985–87,' in T. Dyson, and C. Ó Gráda, eds., *Famine Demography: Perspectives from the Past and Present*, Oxford: Oxford University Press, 2002, 204–217.

George, S., How the Other Half Dies: The Real Reasons for World Hunger, Hammondsworth: Penguin, 1977.

Gill, C.A., 'Epidemic or Fulminant Malaria Together with a Preliminary Study of the Part Played by Immunity in Malaria,' *Indian Journal of Medical Research*, 2, 1, Jul. 1914, 268–314.

————, *Report on Malaria in Amritsar, Together with a Study of Endemic and Epidemic Malaria and an Account of the Measures Necessary to Their Control*, Lahore: Punjab Govt, 1917.

————, Gill, 'The Relationship of Malaria and Rainfall,' *Indian Journal of Medical Research*, 7, 3, 1920, 618–632.

————, 'The Role of Meteorology in Malaria,' *Indian Journal of Medical Research*, 8, 4, 1921, 633–693.

————, *The Genesis of Epidemics and Natural History of Disease*, London: Bailliere, Tindall and Cox, 1928.

————, *Report on the Malaria Epidemic in Ceylon in 1934–35*, Colombo: Ceylon Govt Press, Sept. 1935.

Gillespie, J.A., 'Social Medicine, Social Security and International Health, 1940–60,' in E. Rodríguez-Ocaña, ed., *The Politics of the Healthy Life: An International Perspective*, Sheffield: European Association for the History of Medicine and Health, 2002, 219–239.

————, 'International Organisations and the Problem of Child Health, 1945–1960,' *Dynamis: Acta Hispanica ad Medicinae Scientiarumque Historiam Illustrandam*, 23, 2003, 115–142.

Govt, India, *Statistical Abstract Relating to British India*, London: HMSO, 1840–1920.

———, *Report of the Commissioners Appointed to Inquire into the Sanitary State of the Army in India, Parliamentary Papers*, vol. I, London: HMSO, 1863.

———, *Proceedings of the Imperial Malaria Conference Held at Simla in October 1909*, Simla, 1910.

———, *Proceedings of the Imperial Malaria Committee Held in Bombay on 16th and 17th November 1911, in Paludism*, no. 4, 1911, 110–111.

———, *Proceedings of the Third Meeting of the General Malaria Committee Held at Madras, Nov. 18–20, 1912*.

———, *Indian Sanitary Policy, 1914: Being a Resolution Issued by the Governor General in Council on the 23rd of May 1914*, Calcutta, 1914.

———, *Proceedings of the Third All-India Sanitary Conference, Held at Lucknow, January 1914*.

———, *Annual Report of the Sanitary Commissioner with the Government of India (1867–1921)*, continued as *Annual report of the Public Health Commissioner with the Government of India (1922–46)*.

———, *Report of the Assam Labour Enquiry Committee, 1921–22*.

———, *Report of the Indian Fiscal Commission, 1921–22*, Simla, 1922.

———, *Report of the Royal Commission on Agriculture in India*, London: HMSO, 1928.

———, *Report of the Royal Commission on Labour in India*, vol. 1, Calcutta: GOI Central Publication Branch, 1931.

———, *Famine Inquiry Commission: Final Report*, New Delhi: Govt Press, 1945.

———, *Famine Inquiry Commission: Report on Bengal*, New Delhi: GOI, 1945.

———, *Report of the Health Survey and Development Committee*, vols. 1 & 2, New Delhi: GOI, 1946.

———, Ministry of Labour, *Agricultural Labour in India, Intensive Family Survey*, New Delhi: Ministry of Labour, Govt of India, 1955.

———, Ministry of Food and Agriculture, *Report of the Foodgrains Enquiry Committee*, New Delhi: GOI, 1957.

———, Directorate of the National Malaria Eradication Programme, *Malaria and Its Control in India*, vol. 1, 1986.

Goodman, N., *International Health Organizations and their Works*, London: J & A Churchill, 1952.

Govt, Madras, *Annual Report of the Sanitary Commissioner for Madras*, 1877, 1878.

Govt, Punjab, *Annual Report, Public Works Dept., Irrigation Branch*.

———, *Gazetteer of the Gurgaon District, 1883–84* (Lahore: Govt Press, 1884).

———, *Famine Commission Report* (Punjab), 1900, vol. I.

———, *Report of the Land Revenue Administration of the Punjab*.

———, *Report on the Sanitary Administration of the Punjab*, 1867–1921, continued as *Report on the Public Health Administration of the Punjab*, 1922–47.

Graboyes, M., *The Experiment Must Continue: Medical Research and Ethics in East Africa, 1940–2014*, Athens, OH: Ohio University Press, 2015, 155–186.

Grant, H.E., *The Indian Manual of Hygiene being King's Madras Manual*. Revised, Madras: Higginbotham & Co., 1894.

Gray, R.H., 'The Decline of Mortality in Ceylon and the Demographic Effects of Malaria Control,' *Population Studies*, 28, 2, Jul. 1974, 205–229.

Guha, S., 'Mortality Decline in Early Twentieth Century India: A Preliminary Inquiry,' *Indian Economic and Social History Review*, 28, 4, 1991, 371–392.

———, The Importance of Social Intervention in England's Mortality Decline: The Evidence Reviewed,' *Social History of Medicine*, 7, 1, 1994, 89–113.

———, 'Mortality Decline in Early Twentieth Century India: A Preliminary Enquiry,' in S. Guha, ed., *Health and Population in South Asia: From Earliest Times to the Present*, London: Hurst, 2001.

Guilmoto, G., 'Towards a New Demographic Equilibrium: The Inception of Demographic Transition South India,' *Indian Economic and Social History Review*, 28, 3, 1992, 247–289.

Guntupalli, A.M., and J. Baten, 'The Development and Inequality of Heights in North, West, and East India 1915–1944,' *Explorations in Economic History*, 43, 2006, 578–608.

Hackett, L., *Malaria in Europe: An Ecological Study*, London: Oxford University Press, 1937.

Halstead, S.B., J.A. Walsh, and K.S. Warren, *Good Health at Low Cost*, New York: Rockefeller Foundation, 1985.

Hamlin, C., 'Predisposing Causes and Public Health in Early Nineteenth-Century Medical Thought', *Society for the Social History of Medicine*, 5, 1, Apr. 1992, 43–70.

———, 'Could You Starve to Death in England in 1839? The Chadwick-Farr Controversy and the Loss of the "Social" in Public Health,' *American Journal of Public Health*, 85, 6, 1995, 856–866.

———, 'State Medicine in Great Britain,' in D. Arnold, ed., *Warm Climates in Western Medicine: The Emergence of Tropical Medicine, 1500–1900*, Amsterdam: Rodopi, 1996.

———, *Public Health and Social Justice in the Age of Chadwick*, Cambridge: Cambridge University Press, 1998.

———, 'William Pulteney Alison, the Scottish Philosophy, and the Making of a Political Medicine,' *Journal of the History of Medicine and Allied Sciences*, 61, 2, 2006, 144–186.

———, *More Than Hot: A Short History of Fever*, Baltimore: Johns Hopkins University Press, 2014.

———, *Cholera: The Biography*, Oxford: Oxford University Press, 2009.

Harden, V.A., 'Typhus, Epidemic,' in K.F. Kiple, ed., *The Cambridge World History of Human Disease*, Cambridge: Cambridge University Press, 1993, 1080–1084.

Hardy, A., *The Epidemic Streets: Infectious Disease and the Rise of Preventive Medicine, 1856–1900*, Oxford: Clarendon Press, 1993.

Hardy, A., and E.M. Tansey, 'Medical Enterprise and Global Response, 1945–2000,' in W. Bynum, et al., eds., *The Western Medical Tradition*, Cambridge: Cambridge University Press, 2006.

Harrison, G., *Mosquitoes, Malaria and Man: A History of the Hostilities since 1880*, New York: E. P. Dutton, 1978.

Harrison, M., *Public Health in British India: Anglo-Indian Preventive Medicine 1859–1914*, Cambridge: Cambridge University Press, 1994.

———, ' "Hot Beds of Disease": Malaria and Civilization in Nineteenth-century British India,' *Parassitologia*, 40, 1–2, 1998, 11–18.

———, *Climates and Constitutions: Health, Race Environment and British Imperialism in India*, Delhi: Oxford University Press, 2002, 173–176.

Hay, D., 'War, Dearth and Theft in the Eighteenth Century: The Record of the English Courts,' *Past and Present*, 95, 117–160.

Hehir, P., *Prophylaxis of Malaria in India*, Allahabad: Pioneer Press, 1910.

———, *Malaria in India*, London: Humphrey Milford, 1927.

Hewa, S., 'The Hookworm Epidemic on the Plantations in Colonial Sri Lanka,' *Medical History*, 38, 1994, 73–90, at 84–87.

Hicks, E.P., and S. Abdul Majid, 'A Study of the Epidemiology of Malaria in a Punjab District,' *Records of the Malaria Survey of India*, 7, 1, 1937, 1–43.

Holt-Giménez, E., and R. Patel, *Food Rebellions: Crisis and the Hunger for Justice*, Cape Town: Pambazuka Press, 2009.

Horrocks, S.M., 'The Business of Vitamins: Nutrition Science and the Food Industry in Inter-war Britain,' in H. Kamminga, and A. Cunningham, eds., *The Science and Culture of Nutrition, 1840–1940*, Amsterdam: Rodopi, 1995.

Hooton, A., Letter to the *Indian Medical Gazette*, Apr. 14, 1909, in W.E. Jennings, ed., *Transactions of the Bombay Medical Congress, 1909*, Bombay: Bennett, Coleman & Co., 1910, 93.

Howard-Jones, N., *International Public Health between the Two World Wars – The Organizational Problems*, Geneva: World Health Organization, 1978.

Hume, J.C., 'Colonialism and Sanitary Medicine: The Development of Preventive Health Policy in the Punjab, 1860 to 1900,' *Modern Asian Studies*, 20, 4, 1986, 703–724.

Indian Famine Emergency Commission, *India's Hunger: Report of the American Famine Mission to India*, New York, 1946.

Irudaya Rajan, S., and P. Mohanachandran, 'Estimating Infant Mortality in Kerala,' *Economic and Political Weekly*, 34, 12, Mar. 20–26, 1999, 713–716.

Isenman, P., 'Basic Needs: The Case of Sri Lanka,' *World Development*, 8, 1980, 237–258.

Iyengar, M.O.T, 'Studies on Malaria in the Deltaic Regions of Bengal,' *Journal of the Malaria Institute of India*, Dec. 1942, 435–446.

Jackson, J., 'Cognition and the Global Malaria Eradication Programme,' *Parassitologia*, 40, 1998, 193–216.

James, S.P., 'Malaria in Mian Mir,' in W.E. Jennings, ed., *Transactions of the Bombay Medical Congress, 1909*, Bombay: Bennett, Coleman & Co., 1910, 84–93.

———, 'The Disappearance of Malaria from England,' *Proceedings of the Royal Society of Medicine*, 23, 1929–30, 71–87.

———, Commentary, in R. Briercliffe; 'Discussion on the Malaria Epidemic in Ceylon 1934–35,' *Proceedings of the Royal Society of Medicine*, 29, 1936, 537–562.

———, 'Advances in Knowledge of Malaria since the War,' *Transactions of the Royal Society of Tropical Medicine and Hygiene*, 31, 1937, 263–280.

James, S.P., and S.R. Christophers, 'Malaria. General Etiology,' in W. Byam, and R.G. Archibald, eds., *The Practice of Medicine in the Tropics*, vol. 2, London: Henry Frowde and Hodder and Stoughton, 1922, 1509–1515.

Jamison, D.T., and A. Piazza, 'China's Food and Nutrition Planning,' in J.P. Gittinger, J. Leslie, and C. Hoisington, *Food Policy: Integrating Supply, Distribution, and Consumption*, Baltimore: Johns Hopkins Press, 1987, 467–484.

Jeffrey, Roger, *Politics of Health in India*, Berkeley: University of California Press, 1988.

Jennings, W.E., ed., *Transactions of the Bombay Medical Congress, 1909*, Bombay: Bennett, Coleman & Co., 1910, 84–93.

Jha, P., and A. Mills, *Improving Health Outcomes of the Poor: The Report of Working Group 5 of the Commission on Macroeconomics and Health*, Geneva: World Health Organization, 2002.

Jones, M., *Health Policy in Britain's Model Colony: Ceylon, 1900–1948*, New Delhi: Orient Longman, 2004.

Jones, W.H.S., *Malaria: A Neglected Factor in the History of Greece and Rome*, London: Macmillan, 1907.

Kamminga, H., and A. Cunningham, 'Introduction,' in H. Kamminga, and A. Cunningham, eds., *The Science and Culture of Nutrition, 1840–1940*, Amsterdam: Rodopi, 1995.

Kavadi, S.N., *The Rockefeller Foundation and Public Health in Colonial India, 1916–1945, A Narrative History*, Pune, Mumbai: Foundation for Research in Community Health, 1999.

———, ' "Wolves Come to Take Care of the Lamb": The Rockefeller Foundation Hookworm Campaign in the Madras Presidency, 1920–29,' in E. Rodríguez-Ocaña, ed., *The Politics of the Healthy Life: An International Perspective*, Sheffield: European Association for the History of Medicine and Health, 2002, 89–111.

Kazi, I., *Historical Study of Malaria in Bengal, 1860–1920*, Dhaka: Pip International Publs., 2004.

Kennedy, P., *Preparing for the Twenty-first Century*, New York: Random House, 1993.

King, W., 'Sanitation in Politics,' *Science Progress [in the twentieth century]*, 18 (1923/24), 113–125.

Kinkela, D., *DDT and the American Century: Global Health, Environmental Politics, and the Pesticide That Changed the World*, Chapel Hill: University of North Carolina Press, 2011.

Kligler, I.J., *The Epidemiology and Control of Malaria in Palestine*, Chicago: University of Chicago Press, 1928.

Klein, I., 'Malaria and Mortality in Bengal, 1840–1921,' *Indian Economic and Social History Review*, 9, 2, 1972, 132–160.

———, 'Death in India,' *Journal of Asian Studies*, Aug. 1973, 639–659.

———, 'When the Rains Failed: Famine, Relief, And Mortality in British India,' *Indian Economic and Social History Review*, 21, 2, 1984, 185–214.

———, 'Population Growth and Mortality in British India Part I: The Climacteric of Death,' *Indian Economic and Social History Review*, 26, 4, 1989, 387–403.

———, 'Population Growth and Mortality in British India Part II: The Demographic Revolution,' *Indian Economic and Social History Review*, 27, 1, 1990, 33–63.

———, 'Development and Death: Reinterpreting Malaria, Economics and Ecology in British India,' *Indian Economic and Social History Review*, 38, 2, 2001, 147–179.

Knight, H., *Food Administration in India 1939–47*, Stanford: Stanford University Press, 1954.

Krieger, N., *Epidemiology and the People's Health: Theory and Context*, Oxford: Oxford University Press, 2011.

Kumar, B.G., 'Quality of Life and Nutritional Status: A Reconsideration of Some Puzzles from Kerala,' in P. Bardhan, M. Datta-Chaudhuri, and T.N. Krishnan, eds., *Development and Change: Essays in Honour of K.N. Raj*, Bombay: Oxford University Press, 1993, 318–340.

Kumar, S.K., 'Impact of Subsidized Rice on Food Consumption and Nutrition in Kerala,' International Food Policy Research Institute, Research Report, No. 5, Jan. 1979.

Kunitz, S.J., 'Mortality since Malthus,' in R. Scofield, and D. Coleman, eds., *The State of Population Theory: Forward from Malthus*, Oxford: Basil Blackwell, 1986, 279–302.

Lal, D., *The Hindu Equilibrium*, Oxford: Clarendon Press, Oxford, 2005.

Lal, R.B., and S.C. Seal, *General Rural Health Survey, Singur Health Centre, 1944*, Calcutta: All-India Institute of Hygiene and Public Health, Govt of India Press, 1949.

Langford, C., 'Reasons for the Decline in Mortality in Sri Lanka Immediately after the Second World War: A Re-examination of the Evidence,' *Health Transition Review*, 6, 1996, 3–23, 15.

League of Nations, 'The Problem of Nutrition,' *Interim Report of the Mixed Committee on the Problem of Nutrition*, vol. 1, Geneva: League of Nations, 1936.

———, *Final Report of the Mixed Committee of the League of Nations on The Relation of Nutrition to Health, Agriculture and Economic Policy*, Geneva: League of Nations, 1937.

League of Nations Health Organisation, 'The Most Suitable Methods of Detecting Malnutrition due to the Economic Depression, Conference held at Berlin from December 5th to 7th, 1932,' in *Quarterly Bulletin of the Health Organisation*, 2, 1, Mar. 1933, 116–129.

———, 'Report on an International Conference of representatives of health services of African Territories and British India,' *Quarterly Bulletin of the Health Organisation of the League of Nations*, II, 1933.

League of Nations Malaria Commission, *Report on its Tour of Investigation in Certain European Countries in 1924*, Geneva: League of Nations, 1925.

———, *Principles and Methods of Antimalarial Methods in Europe*, Geneva: League of Nations, 1927.

———, *Report of the Malaria Commission on its Study Tour of India*, Geneva: League of Nations, 1930.

———, *Report on The Method of Forecasting the Probable Incidence of Malaria in the Punjab*, Geneva: League of Nations, 1938.

Learmonth, A.T.A., 'Some Contrasts in the Regional Geography of Malaria in India and Pakistan,' *Transactions and Paper*, Institute of British Geographers, 23, 1957, 37–59.

Lee, S., 'WHO and the Developing World: The Contest for Ideology,' in B. Andrews, and A. Cunningham, eds., *Western Medicine as Contested Knowledge*, Manchester: Manchester University Press, 1997, 24–45.

Levenstein, H., *Paradox of Plenty: A Social History of Eating in Modern America*, New York: Oxford University Press, 1993.

Litsios, S., *The Tomorrow of Malaria*, Wellington, NZ: Pacific Press, 1996.

————, 'Malaria Control, the Cold War, and the Postwar Reorganization of International Assistance,' *Medical Anthropology*, 17, 1997, 255–278.

————, 'Malaria Control and the Future of International Public Health,' in E. Casman, and H. Dowlatabadi, eds., *The Contextual Determinants of Malaria*, Washington, D.C.: Resources for the Future, 2002, 292–328.

Lobo, L., *Malaria in the Social Context: A Study in Western India*, New Delhi: Routledge, 2010.

Macdonald, G., 'Community Aspects of Immunity to Malaria,' in L.J. Bruce-Chwatt, and V.J. Glanville, eds., *Dynamics of Tropical Disease: The Late George Macdonald*, London: Oxford University Press, 1973, 77–84.

————, 'The Analysis of Malaria Epidemics,' in L.J. Bruce-Chwatt, and V.J. Glanville, eds., *Dynamics of Tropical Disease: The Late George Macdonald*, London: Oxford University Press, 1973, 146–160.

Macdonald, G., and J. Abdul Majid, 'Report on an Intensive Malaria Survey in the Karnal District, Punjab,' *Records of the Malaria Survey of India*, 2, 3, Sep. 1931, 423–477.

Macdonnell, A.P., *Report of the Indian Famine Commission 1901*, Calcutta: Government Printing Office, 1901.

Macleod, R., 'Introduction,' in R. Macleod, and M. Lewis, eds., *Disease, Medicine and Empire*, London: Routledge, 1988.

Mackenzie, S., 'The Powers of Natural Resistance, or the Personal Factor in Disease of Microbic Origin,' The Annual Oration, May 26, 1902, *Transactions of the Medical Society of London*, 25, 302–318.

Maharatna, A., 'Regional Variation in Demographic Consequences of Famines in Late Nineteenth and Early twentieth Century India,' *Economic and Political Weekly*, Jun. 4, 1994, 1399–1410.

————, *The Demography of Famines: An Indian Historical Perspective*, Delhi: Oxford University Press, 1996.

————, 'Famines and Epidemics: An Historical Perspective,' in T. Dyson, and C. Ó Gráda, eds., *Famine Demography: Perspective from the Past and Present*, Oxford: Oxford University Press, 2002, 113–141.

Mankodi, K., 'Political and Economic Roots of Disease: Malaria in Rajasthan,' *Economic and Political Weekly*, Jan. 27, 1996, PE-42–48.

Manson, P., *Tropical Diseases: A Manual of the Diseases of Warm Climates*, London: Cassell and Co., 1898.

Marshall, P.J., *Bengal: The British Bridgehead: Eastern India 1740–1838*, Cambridge: Cambridge University Press, 1987.

Martorell, R., and T.J. Ho, 'Malnutrition, Morbidity and Mortality,' in H. Mosley, and L. Chen, eds., *Child Survival: Strategies for Research*, Supplement to vol. 10, *Population and Development Review*, 1984, 49–68.

Mathur, J., and N. Gopal Jayal, *Drought Policy and Politics in India*, Delhi: Sage, 1993.

Mazumdar, P.M.H., 'Immunity in 1890,' *Journal of the History of Medicine and Allied Sciences* 27, 3, 1972, 312–324.

McCarrison, R., *Studies in Deficiency Diseases*, London: Henry Frowde, Hodder & Stoughton, 1921.

283

————, 'Memorandum on Malnutrition as a Cause of Physical Inefficiency and Ill-Health among the Masses in India,' in *Report of the Royal Commission on Agriculture in India*, vol. 1, London: HMSO, 1928, Pt. II, 100.

————, 'Problems of Nutrition in India,' *Nutrition Abstracts and Reviews*, 2, 1932, 1–2.

McCarrison, R., and R.V. Norris, 'The Relation of Rice to Beri-beri in India,' *Indian Medical Research Memoir*, No. 2, Calcutta: Thacker, Spink & Co, 1924, reprinted in H.M. Sinclair, *The Work of Sir Robert McCarrison*, London: Faber and Faber, 1953.

McCay, D., *Investigations on Bengal Jail Dietaries: With Some Observations on the Influence of Dietary on the Physical Development and Well-Being of the People of Bengal*, Calcutta: Superintendent Govt. Print., 1910.

McConnell, J., 'Barefoot No More,' *Lancet*, 341, 8855, 1993, 1275.

McGregor, I.A., 'Malaria and Nutrition,' in W.H. Wernsdorfer, and I.A. McGregor, eds., *Malaria: Principles and Practice of Malariology*, Edinburgh: Churchill Livingstone, 1988, 754–777.

————, 'Specific Immunity: Acquired in Man,' in W.H. Wernsdorfer, and I.A. McGregor, eds., *Malaria: Principles and Practice of Malariology*, Edinburgh: Churchill Livingstone, 1988, 559–619.

McKeown, T., *The Modern Rise of Population*, London: Edward Arnold, 1976.

————, *The Role of Medicine*, Oxford: Basil Blackwell, 1979.

McNeill, W., *Plagues and People*, Garden City, NY: Anchor Press, 1976.

Meade, M.S., 'Beriberi,' in F. Kiple, ed., *Cambridge World History of Human Disease*, Cambridge: Cambridge University Press, 1993, 606–611.

Meade, T.W., 'Medicine and Population,' *Public Health*, 82, 3, 1968, 100–110.

Meegama, S.A., 'Malaria Eradication and Its Effect on Mortality Levels,' *Population Studies*, 21, 3, Nov. 1967, 207–237.

————, 'The Decline in Maternal and Infant Mortality and its relation to Malaria Eradication,' *Population Studies*, 23, 2, 1969, 289–302.

Meyer, E., 'L'Épidémie de malaria de 1934–1935 à Sri-Lanka: Fluctuations Économiques et fluctuations climatiques,' *Cultures et Développement*, 14, 2–3, 1982, 183–226; 14, 4, 589–638.

Millman, S., and R.W. Kates, 'Toward Understanding Hunger,' in L.F. Newman, ed., *Hunger in History: Food Shortage, Poverty, and Deprivation*, Cambridge, Massachusetts: Blackwell, 1990, 3–24.

Mohanty, B., 'Orissa Famine of 1866: Demographic and Economic Consequences,' *Economic and Political Weekly*, 28, Jan. 2–9, 1993, 55–66.

Mohapatra, P., 'Assam and the West Indies, 1860–1920: Immobilizing Plantation Labour,' in D. Hay, and P. Craven, eds., *Masters, Servants and Magistrates in Britain and the Empire, 1562–1955*, Chapel Hill and London: University of North Carolina Press, 2004, 455–480.

Molineaux, L., 'The Epidemiology of Human Malaria as an Explanation of Its Distribution, Including Implications for Its Control,' in W.H. Wernsdorfer, and I.A. McGregor, eds., *Malaria: Principles and Practice of Malariology*, Edinburgh: Churchill Livingstone, 1988, 913–998.

Morgan, D., *Merchants of Grain*, New York: Viking Press, 1979.

Morley, D., *Paediatric Priorities in the Developing World*, London: Butterworth-Heinemann, 1973.

Mosby, I., *Food Will Win the War: The Politics, Culture, and Science of Food on Canada's Home Front*, Vancouver: University of British Columbia Press, 2014.

Mukherjee, A., 'Scarcity and Crime: A Study of Nineteenth Century Bengal,' *Economic and Political Weekly*, 28, Feb. 6, 1993, 237–243.

Mukharji, P.B., 'Verncularizing Political Medicine: Locating the Medical betwixt the Literal and the Literary in Two Texts on the Burdwan Fever, Bengal c. 1870s,' in R. Deb Roy, and G.N.A. Attewell, eds., *Locating the Medical: Explorations in South Asian History*, New Delhi: Oxford University Press, 2018, 235–263.

Mukherjee, N., and A. Mukherjee, 'Rural Women and Food Insecurity: What a Food Calendar Reveals,' *Economic and Political Weekly*, Mar. 12, 1994, 597–599.

Mukherjee, R., *Changing Face of Bengal: A Study in Riverine Economy*, Calcutta: University of Calcutta, 1938.

Munro, H.N., 'Historical Perspective on Protein Requirement: Objectives for the Future,' in K. Blaxter, and J.C. Waterlow, eds., *Nutritional Adaption in Man*, London: John Libby, 1985, 155–168.

Muraleedharan, V.R., 'Diet, Disease and Death in Colonial South India', *Economic and Political Weekly*, Jan. 1–8, 1994, 55–63.

Muraleedharan, V.R., and D. Veeraraghavan, 'Anti-malaria Policy in the Madras Presidency: An Overview of the Early Decades of the Twentieth Century,' *Medical History*, 36, 1992, 290–305.

Nájera, J.A., 'The Control of Tropical Diseases and Socioeconomic Development, with Special Reference to Malaria and Its Control,' *Parassitologia*, 36, 1–2, Aug. 1994, 17–33.

———, *Malaria Control: Achievements, Problems and Strategies*, Geneva: World Health Organization, 1999, 10–31.

———, 'Malaria Control: Achievements, Problems and Strategies,' *Parassitologia*, 43, 1–2, 1–89, 2001.

Nandi, J., et al., 'Anthropophily of Anophelines in Duars of West Bengal and Other Regions of India,' *Journal of Communicable Disease*, 32, 2, 2000, 95–99.

National Nutrition Monitoring Bureau (NNMB), *Report of the NNMB-NNSO Linked Survey, 1983–84*. Hyderabad, n.d.

———, *Report of the First Repeat Rural Surveys* [1988–90], Hyderabad, n.d.

———, *Report of Repeat Surveys: 1988–90*, Hyderabad, 1991.

Nestle, M, *Food Politics: How the Food Industry Influences Nutrition, and Health*, Berkeley: University of California Press, 2007.

Newman, L.F., ed., *Hunger in History: Food Shortage, Poverty, and Deprivation*, Cambridge, Massachusetts: Blackwell, 1990.

Newman, P., *Malaria Eradication and Population Growth with Special Reference to Ceylon and British Guiana*, Bureau of Public Health Economics, Research Series No. 10, School of Public Health, Ann Arbor: University of Michigan, 1965.

———, 'Malaria Eradication and Its Effects on Mortality Levels: A Comment,' *Population Studies*, 23, 2, 1969, 285–288.

———, 'Malaria Control and Population Growth,' *Journal of Development Studies*, 6, 2, Jan. 1970, 133–158.

———, 'Malaria and Mortality,' *Journal of the American Statistical Association*, 72, 358, 1977, 257–263.

Newnham, H.E., *Report on the Relief of Distress due to Sickness and Shortage of Food, September 1934 to December 1935*, Colombo: Ceylon Government Press, Mar. 1936.

Nicholls, L., and A. Nimalasuriya, 'A Nutritional Survey of the Poorer Classes in Ceylon,' *Ceylon Journal of Science* (D), IV, Pt. 1, Apr. 30, 1936, 1–70.

————, 'Rural Dietary Surveys in Ceylon,' *Ceylon Journal of Science* (D), V, Pt. D, Nov. 12, 1941, 59–110.

Niven, J., 'Poverty and Disease,' Presidential Address, Epidemiology Section, Oct. 22, 1909, *Proceedings of the Royal Society of Medicine*, 3, 1910, 1–44.

Notestein, F.W., and Chi-ming Chiao, 'Population,' in J.L. Buck, ed., *Land Utilization in China*, Chicago: University of Chicago Press, 1937, vol. 1, 358–399.

Onori, E., and B. Grab, 'Indicators for the Forecasting of Malaria Epidemics,' *Bulletin of the WHO*, 58, 1, 1980, 91–98.

Opie, E.L., 'Tuberculosis of First Infection in Adults from Rural Districts of China,' *Chinese Medical Journal*, 56, 3, 1939, 216–224.

Ortega Osona, J.A., 'The Attenuation of Mortality Fluctuations in British Punjab and Bengal, 1870–1947,' in Ts'ui-jung Liu, et al., eds., *Asian Population History*, Oxford: Oxford University Press, 2001, 306–349.

Packard, R., and P. Gadehla, 'A Land Filled with Mosquitoes: Fred L. Soper, the Rockefeller Foundation, and the *Anopheles gambiae* Invasion of Brazil,' *Parassitologia*, 36, 1–2, 1994, 197–213.

Packard, R., and P.J. Brown, 'Rethinking Health, Development, and Malaria: Historicizing a Cultural Model in International Health,' *Medical Anthropology*, 17, 1997, 181–194.

Packard, R.M., 'Maize, Cattle and Mosquitoes: The Political Economy of Malaria Epidemics in Colonial Swaziland,' *Journal of African History*, 25, 1984, 189–212.

————, 'Malaria Dreams: Postwar Visions of Health and Development in the Third World,' *Medical Anthropology*, 17, 1997, 279–296.

————, 'Visions of Postwar Health and Development and Their Impact on Public Health Interventions in the Developing World,' in F. Cooper, and R. Packard, eds., *International Development and the Social Sciences: Essays on the History and Politics of Knowledge*, Berkeley: University of California Press, 1997, 93–115.

————, ' "No Other Logical Choice": Global Malaria Eradication and the Politics of International Health in the Post-War Era,' *Parassitologia*, 40, 1998, 217–229.

————, *The Making of a Tropical Disease: A Short History of Malaria*, Baltimore: Johns Hopkins University Press, 2007.

————, ' "Roll Back Malaria, Roll in Development"? Reassessing the Economic Burden of Malaria,' *Population and Development Review*, 35, 1, 2009, 53–87.

Pampana, E., and E.J. Pampana, 'Malaria Research and the Malaria Commission of the League of Nations,' *Annals of Tropical Medicine and Parasitology*, 28, 1, 1934, 63–65.

————, 'Malaria as a Problem for the World Health Organization,' *Proceedings of the Fourth International Congress on Tropical Medicine and Malaria*, Washington, D.C., 2, May 10–18, 1948, 940–946.

————, 'Lutte antipaludique par les insecticides à action rémanents: résultats des campagnes antipaludiques,' *Bull. Org. Mond. Santé*, 3, 1951, 557–619.

————, *A Textbook of Malaria Eradication*, London: Oxford University Press, 1969.

Panikar, P.G.K., and C.R. Soman, *Health Status of Kerala: Paradox of Economic Backwardness and Health Development*, Trivandrum: Center for Development Studies, 1984.

Parkes, E.A., *A Manual of Practical Hygiene, Prepared Especially for Use in the Medical Service of the Army*, London: John Churchill, 1866.

Passmore, R., and T. Sommerville, 'An Investigation of the Effect of Diet on the Course of Experimental Malaria in Monkeys,' *Journal of the Malaria Institute of India*, 3, 4, Dec. 1940, 447–455.

Pati, B., and M. Harrison, *Health, Medicine and Empire: Perspectives on Colonial India*, London: Sangam Books, 2001.

Paton, D.N., and L. Findlay, *Child Life Investigations. Poverty, Nutrition and Growth. Studies of Child Life in Cities and Rural Districts in Scotland*, Medical Research Council Special Report Series, no. 101, 1926.

Patterson, T., *On Every Front: The Making and Unmaking of the Cold War*, New York: W.W. Norton, 1992.

Peiris, W.A.A.S., *Socio-Economic Development and Fertility Decline in Sri Lanka*, New York: United Nations, Dept. International Economic and Social Affairs, 1986.

Pelling, M., *The Common Lot: Sickness, Medical Occupations and the Urban Poor in Early Modern England*, London: Longman, 1998.

Perkins, J.H., *Geopolitics and the Green Revolution: Wheat, Genes, and the Cold War*, Oxford: Oxford University Press, 1999.

Perry, E.L., *Recent Additions to Our Knowledge of Malaria in the Punjab*. A paper read before the Punjab Branch of the British Medical Association at Simla, on July 17, 1914, Simla: Thacker, Spink & Co, 1914.

Petty, C., 'Food, Poverty and Growth: The Application of Nutrition Science, 1918–1939,' *Bulletin of the Society for the Social History of Medicine*, 1987, 37–40.

Piazza, A., *Food Consumption and Nutritional Status in the PRC*, Boulder: Westview Press, 1986.

Polu, S., *Infectious Disease in India, 1892–1940: Policy-Making and the Perceptions of Risk*, London: Palgrave Macmillan, 2012.

Porter, D., 'Social Medicine and the New Society: Medicine and Scientific Humanism in mid-Twentieth Century Britain,' *Journal of Historical Sociology*, 9, 2, June 1996, 168–187.

Poser, C.M., and G.W. Bruyn, *An Illustrated History of Malaria*, New York: Parthenon Publ., 1999.

Preston, S., 'The Changing Relationship between Mortality and Level of Economic Development,' *Population Studies*, 29, 2, July 1975, 231–248.

———, 'Causes and Consequences of Mortality Declines in Less Developed Countries during the Twentieth Century,' in R.A. Easterlin, ed., *Population and Economic Change in Developing Countries*, Chicago: University of Chicago Press, 1980.

Qadeer, I., K, Sen, and K.R. Nayar, eds., *Public Health and the Poverty of Reforms*, New Delhi: Sage, 2001.

Rajendram, S., and S.H. Jayewickreme, 'Malaria in Ceylon,' Pt. 1, *Indian Journal of Malariology*, 5, 1, Mar. 1951, 1–73.

Ramanna, M., 'A Mixed Record: Malaria Control in Bombay Presidency, 1900–1935,' in D. Kumar, and R. Sekhar Basu, eds., *Medical Encounters in British India*, New Delhi: Oxford University Press, 2013, 208–231.

Ramasubban, R., *Public Health and Medical Research in India: Their Origins under the Impact of British Colonial Policy*, SAREC report R4, Stockholm: SIDA, 1982.

———, 'Imperial Health in British India, 1857–1900,' in R. Macleod, and M. Lewis, eds., *Disease, Medicine and Empire*, London: Routledge, 1988, 38–60.

Ray, P.C., 'The Problem of Nutrition in India,' *The Indian Review*, 42, Apr. 1941, 209–212.

Rao, M., *Disinvesting in Health: The World Bank's Prescriptions for Health*, Delhi: Sage, 1999.

———, *From Population Control to Reproductive Health: Malthusian Arithmetic*, New Delhi: Sage, 2004.

Rieff, D., *A Bed for the Night: Humanitarianism in Crisis*, New York: Simon & Schuster, 2003.

Riley, J.C., *Low Income, Social Growth, and Good Health: A History of Twelve Countries*, Berkeley: University of California Press, 2008.

Robb, P., 'New Directions in South Asian History,' *South Asia Research*, 7, 2, Nov. 1987, 133.

Ross, R., 'Malaria Prevention at Mian Mir, *Lancet*, Jul. 3, 1909, 43–45.

———, 'The Practice of Malaria Prevention,' in W.E. Jennings, ed., *Transactions of the Bombay Medical Congress*, Bombay: Bennett, Coleman & Co., 1910, 67–74.

———, *The Prevention of Malaria*, London: John Murray, 1910.

———, *Memoirs: The Great Malaria Problem and its Solution*, London: John Murray, 1923.

———, 'Malaria and Feeding,' *Journal of Tropical Medicine and Hygiene*, May 1, 1929, 132.

Rotberg, R.I., 'Nutrition and History,' *Journal of Interdisciplinary History*, 14, 3, 1983, 199–204.

Rowlands, M.G.M, et al., 'Seasonality and the Growth of Infants in a Gambian Village,' in R. Chambers, R. Longhurst, and A. Pacey, eds., *Seasonal Dimensions to Rural Poverty*, London: Frances Pinter, 1981.

Russell, P.F., 'Malaria in India: Impressions from a Tour,' *American Journal of Tropical Medicine*, 16, 6, 1936, 653–664.

———, 'Malaria Due to Defective and Untidy Irrigation,' *Journal of the Malaria Institute of India*, 1, 4, 1938, 339–349.

———, 'Some Social Obstacles to Malaria Control,' *Indian Medical Gazette*, Nov. 1941, 681–690.

———, 'A Lively Corpse,' *Tropical Medicine News*, Jun. 5, 1948, 25.

———, *Malaria: Basic Principles Briefly Stated*, Oxford: Blackwell Scientific Publs., 1952.

———, *Man's Mastery of Malaria*, London: Oxford University Press, 1955.

Russell, P.F., and M.K. Menon, 'A Malario-economic Survey in Rural South India,' *Indian Medical Gazette*, 77, Mar. 1942, 167–180.

Russell, P.F., F.W. Knipe, and T.R. Rao, 'Epidemiology of Malaria with Special Reference to South India,' *Indian Medical Gazette*, 77, 1942, 477–479.

Russell, P., L.S. West, and R.D. Manwell, *Practical Malariology*, Philadelphia: W.B. Saunders, 1946.

Russell, P., L.S. West, R.D. Manwell, and G. Macdonald, *Practical Malariology*, London: Oxford University Press, 1963.

Ruzicka, L.T., and H. Hansluwka, 'Mortality in Selected Countries of South and East Asia,' in WHO, ed., *Mortality in South and East Asia: A Review of Changing Trends and Patterns, 1950–1975*, Manila: World Health Organization, 1982, 83–155.

Salaff, J., Mortality Decline in the People's Republic of China and the United States,' *Population Studies*, 27, 1973, 551–576.

Samanta, A., *Malaria Fever in Colonial Bengal, 1820–1939: Social History of an Epidemic*, Kolkata: Firma KLM, 2002.

Sami, L., 'Starvation, Disease and Death: Explaining Famine Mortality in Madras, 1876–1878,' *Social History of Medicine*, 24, 3, 2011, 700–719.

Sarkar, K.N., *The Demography of Ceylon*, Colombo: Govt Press, 1958.

Sathyamala, C., 'Nutrition as a Public Health Problem (1990–1947)', International Institute of Social Studies, Working Paper No. 510, Dec. 2010.

Schüffner, W., 'Notes on the Indian Tour of the Malaria Commission of the League of Nations,' *Records of the Malaria Survey of India*, 11, 3, Sept. 1931, 337–347.

Scrimshaw, N.S., 'The Phenomenon of Famine,' *American Review of Nutrition*, 7, 1987, 1–21.

Scrimshaw, N.S., C.E. Taylor, and J.E. Gordon, *Interactions of Nutrition and Infection*, Geneva: World Health Organization, 1968.

Seal, S.C., 'Diet and the Incidence of Disease in India', *Indian Medical Gazette*, May 1938, 291–301.

Sen, A., *Poverty and Famines: An Essay on Entitlement and Deprivation*, Oxford: Oxford University Press, 1981.

Sen, S., *Women and Labour in Late Colonial India: The Bengal Jute Industry*, Cambridge: Cambridge University Press, 1999.

Sen, S.R., *Growth and Instability in Indian Agriculture*, New Delhi: Ministry of Food and Agriculture, 1967.

Senior White, R., *Studies in Malaria as It Affect Indian Railways*, Indian Research Fund Association, Technical Paper, No. 258, Calcutta: Central Publications Branch, 1928.

Sewell, E.P., 'The Results of the Campaign Against Malaria in Mian Mir,' *British Medical Journal*, Sept. 1904, 635–636.

Sharma, S., *Famine, Philanthropy and the Colonial State*, Delhi: Oxford University Press, 2001.

Sharma, V.P., 'Determinants of Malaria in South Asia,' in E.A. Casman, and H. Dowlatabadi, eds., *The Contextual Determinants of Malaria*, Washington, D.C.: Resources for the Future, 2002, 110–132.

———, 'Malaria and Poverty,' *Current Science*, 84, 2003, 513–515.

Sharma, V.P., and K.N. Mehotra, 'Malaria Resurgence in India: A Critical Study,' *Social Science Medicine*, 22, 1986, 835–845, 836.

Shorten, J.A., 'The Role of Vitamins in Tropical Diseases,' *Indian Medical Gazette*, May 1922, 164–169.

Siddiqui, J., *World Health and World Politics: The World Health Organization and the UN System*, London: Hurst, 1995.

Sinclair, H.M., *The Work of Sir Robert McCarrison*, London: Faber and Faber, 1953.

Singh, J., 'Malaria and Its Control in India,' *Perspectives in Public Health*, 72, 1952, 515–525.

Sinha, R.P., *Food in India: An Analysis of the Prospects for Self-Sufficiency By 1975–76*, Bombay: Oxford University Press, 1961.

Sinton, J.A., 'Rice Cultivation in Spain, with Special Reference to the Conditions in the Delta of the River Ebro,' *Records of the Malaria Survey of India*, 3, 3, June 1933, 495–506.

——, 'What Malaria Costs India, Nationally, Socially and Economically,' *Records of the Malaria Survey of India*, 5, 3, Sept. 1935, 223–264; 4, 4, Dec. 1935, 413–489; 6,1, Mar. 1936, 91–169.

Smith, D.F., ed., *Nutrition in Britain: Science, Scientists and Politics in the Twentieth Century*, London: Routledge, 1997.

Smith, D.F., and M. Nicolson, 'Nutrition, Education, Ignorance and Income: A Twentieth-Century Debate,' in H. Kamminga, and A. Cunningham, eds., *The Science and Culture of Nutrition, 1840–1940*, Amsterdam: Rodopi, 1995.

Snowdon, F.M., *The Conquest of Malaria: Italy, 1900–1962*, New Haven: Yale University Press, 2006.

Snowden, F.M., and R. Bucala, eds., *The Global Challenge of Malaria: Past Lessons and Future Prospects*, Hackensack, NJ: World Scientific Publ., 2014.

Solomon, S.G., L. Murard, and P. Zylberman, eds., *Shifting Boundaries of Public Health: Europe in the Twentieth Century*, Rochester: University of Rochester Press, 2008.

Sotiroff-Junker, J., *Behavioural, Social and Economic Aspects of Malaria and its Control*, Geneva: World Health Organization, 1978.

Staples, A.L.S., *The Birth of Development: How the World Bank, Food and Agriculture Organization, and World Health Organization Changed the World, 1945–1965*, Kent, OH: Kent State University Press, 2006.

Stephens, J.W.W., and S.R. Christophers, 'The Malaria Infection in Native Children,' in *Reports of the Malaria Committee of the Royal Society*, 3rd series, London: Harrison and Sons, 1900.

Stone, I., *Canal Irrigation in British India: Perspectives on Technological Changes in a Peasant Economy*, Cambridge: Cambridge University Press, 1984.

Sur, S.N., *Malaria Problem in Bengal*, Calcutta: Bengal Public Health Department, 1929, 188.

Sweet, W.C., 'Irrigation and Malaria,' *Proceedings of the National Academy of Sciences, India*, 4, 1938, 185–189.

Swellengrebel, N.H., 'Malaria in the Kingdom of the Netherlands,' Geneva: League of Nations, Mar. 1924, 15–17.

——, 'Some Aspects of the Malaria Problem in Italy,' in League of Nations Malaria Commission, *Report on its Tour of Investigation in Certain European Countries in 1924*, C.H. 273, Geneva, March 26, 1925, Annex 11, 168–171.

Szreter, S., 'The Importance of Social Intervention in Britain's Mortality Decline,' *Social History of Medicine*, 1, 1, 1988, 1–37.

——, *Health and Wealth: Studies in History and Polity*, Rochester: University of Rochester Press, 2005.

Topley, W.W.C., 'The Biology of Epidemics,' Croonian Lecture, *Proceedings of the Royal Society of London. Series B, Biological Sciences*, 130, 861, May 8, 1942, 337–359.

Terroine, E.F., 'Report on the Protein Component of the Human Diet,' *Quarterly Bulletin of the Health Organisation*, 4, 1935.

Tyssul Jones, T.W., 'Deforestation and Epidemic Malaria in the Wet and Inter-mediate Zones of Ceylon,' *Indian Journal of Malariology*, 5, 1, Mar. 1951, 135–161.

———, 'Malaria and the Ancient Cities of Ceylon,' *Indian Journal of Malariology*, 5, 1, Mar. 1951, 125–133.

United Nations Conference, 'Final Act of the United Nations Conference on Food and Agriculture, Hot Springs, Virginia, United States of America, 18th May – 3rd June 1943,' reproduced in *American Journal of International Law*, 37, 4, Supplement: Official Documents (Oct. 1943), 159–192.

United States, Department of State. 'Address of Welcome by the Honorable George Marshall, Secretary of State,' *Proceedings of the Fourth International Congresses on Tropical Medicine and Malaria*, Washington, D.C., 2, May 10–18, 1948, 1–4.

Venkat Rao, V., 'Review of Malaria Control in India,' *Indian Journal of Malariology*, 3, 4, Dec. 313–326.

Vernon, J., *Hunger: A Modern History*, Cambridge, MA: Belknap Press of Harvard University Press, 2007.

Vine, M.J., The Malarial Campaign in Greece,' *Bulletin of the WHO*, 1, 1947, 197–204.

Viswanathan, D.K., 'Activities of the Bombay Province Malaria Organization, 1942–47, in *Proceedings of the Fourth International Congresses on Tropical Medicine and Malaria*, Washington, D.C., May 10–18, 1948, 873–880.

———, 'A Study of the Effects of Malaria and of Malaria Control Measures on Population and Vital Statistics in Kanara and Dharwar Districts as Compared with the Rest of the Province of Bombay', *Indian Journal of Malariology*, 3, 1, Mar. 1949, 69–99.

———, *The Conquest of Malaria in India: An Indo-American Co-operative Effort*, Madras: Law Institute Press, 1958.

Wakimura, K., 'Epidemic malaria and "Colonial Development": Reconsidering the Cases of Northern and Western India,' Economic History Congress XIII, Buenos Aires, Argentina, July 2002, mimeo.

Waterlow, J.C., and P.R. Payne, 'The Protein Gap,' *Nature*, 258, 113–115.

Watson, M., 'The Lesson of Mian Mir,' *Journal of Tropical Medicine and Hygiene*, July 1, 1931, 183–189.

Watts, S., 'British Development Policies and Malaria in India 1897-c.1929,' *Past and Present*, 165, 1999, 141–181.

Webb, J.L.A., *Humanity's Burden: A Global History of Malaria*, New York: Cambridge University Press, 2009, 27–41.

———, 'The First Large-Scale Use of Synthetic Insecticide for Malaria Control in Tropical Africa: Lessons from Liberia, 1945–1962,' *Journal of the History of Medicine and Allied Sciences*, 66, 3, July 2011, 347–376.

———, *The Long Struggle Against Malaria in Tropical Africa*, New York: Cambridge University Press, 2014.

Weindling, P., 'Social medicine at the League of Nations Health Organisation and the International Labour Office compared,' in P. Weindling, ed. *International Health Organisations and Movements, 1918–1939*, New York: Cambridge University Press, 1995, 134–153.

———, 'The Role of International Organizations in Setting Nutritional Standards in the 1920s and 1930s,' in A. Kamminga, and A. Cunningham, eds., *The Science and Culture of Nutrition, 1840–1940*, Amsterdam: Rodopi, 1995, 319–332.

———, 'American Foundations and the Internationalizing of Public Health,' in S.G. Solomon, L. Murard, and P. Zylberman, eds., *Shifting Boundaries of Public Health: Europe in the Twentieth Century*, Rochester: University of Rochester Press, 2008, 63–85.

Wernsdorfer, W.H., 'Social and Economic Aspects,' 1434, in W.H. Wernsdorfer, and I.A. McGregor, eds., *Malaria: Principles and Practice of Malariology*, vol. 2, Edinburgh: Churchill Livingstone, 1988, 1422–1471.

Whitcombe, E., *Agrarian Conditions in Northern India*, Berkeley: University of California Press, 1972.

———, 'Famine Mortality,' *Economic and Political Weekly*, 28, Jun. 5, 1993, 1169–1179.

———, 'The Environmental Costs of Irrigation in British India: Waterlogging, Salinity, Malaria,' in D. Arnold, and R. Guha, eds., *Nature, Culture, Imperialism: Essays on the Environmental History of South Asia*, Delhi: Oxford University Press, 1995, 237–259.

Wigglesworth, V.B., 'Malaria in Ceylon,' *Asiatic Review*, 32, 1936, 611–619.

Woodbridge, G., *UNRRA: The History of the United Nations Relief and Rehabilitation Administration*, New York: Columbia University Press, 1950.

Worboys, M., 'The Discovery of Colonial Malnutrition Between the Wars,' in D. Arnold, ed., *Imperial Medicine and Indigenous Societies*, Manchester: Manchester University Press, 1988, 208–225.

———, 'Germs, Malaria and the Invention of Mansonian Tropical Medicine: From "Diseases in the Tropics" to "Tropical Diseases",' in D. Arnold, ed., *Warm Climates in Western Medicine: The Emergence of Tropical Medicine, 1500–1900*, Amsterdam: Rodopi, 1996, 181–207.

———, 'Colonial Medicine,' in R. Cooter, and J. Pickstone, eds., *Medicine in the Twentieth Century*, Amsterdam: Harwood Academic Publishers, 2000.

———, *Spreading Germs: Disease Theories and Medical Practice in Britain, 1865–1900*, Cambridge: Cambridge University Press, 2000.

———, 'Before McKeown: Explaining the Decline in Tuberculosis in Britain, 1880–1930,' in F. Condrau, and M. Worboys, eds., *Tuberculosis Then and Now: Perspectives on the History of an Infectious Disease*, Montreal: McGill-Queen's University Press, 2010, 148–170.

World Bank, *The Economic Development of Ceylon*, Baltimore: Johns Hopkins Press, 1952.

———, *China: The Health Sector*, Washington, D.C., 1984.

World Health Organization, Extract from the Report on the First Session, Note by the Secretariat, *Bulletin of the World Health Organization*, 1, 1, 1948, 21–28.

———, *Official Records of the World Health Organization*, No. 2, 4, 5, 7, 8, 9.

———, *World Malaria Report*, 2009.

World Health Organization, Expert Committee on Malaria, *Report on the First Session*, Geneva, 22–25 April 1947, WHO.IC/Mal./4

———, 'Summary Minutes of the First Session,' 22–25 April 1947, WHO.IC/Mal./6, 1–45.

————, WHO *Technical Report Series*, No. 8, ECM, Report on the Third Session, 10–17 Aug. 1949.

Yacob, M., and S. Swaroop, 'Malaria and Spleen Rate in the Punjab,' *Indian Journal of Malariology*, 1, 4, 1947, 469–489.

Zhang, D., and P. Unschuld, 'China's Barefoot Doctor: Past, Present, and Future,' *Lancet*, 372 (9653), 2008, 1865–1867.

Zurbrigg, S., 'Hunger and Epidemic Malaria in Punjab, 1868–1940,' *Economic and Political Weekly*, Jan. 12, 1992, PE 2–26.

————, 'Re-thinking the "Human Factor" in Malaria Mortality: The Case of Punjab, 1868–1940,' *Parassitologia*, 36, 1–2, 1994, 121–136.

————, 'Did Starvation Protect from Malaria? Distinguishing Between Severity and Lethality of Infectious Disease in Colonial India,' *Social Science History*, 21, 1, 1997, 27–58.

————, *Epidemic Malaria and Hunger in Colonial Punjab: Weakened by Want*, London and New Delhi: Routledge, 2019.

# INDEX

Abdul Majid, J. 32–33
Ackerknecht, E. 144, 232
Acton, H. W. 21
Africa, holoendemic malaria in 15n34, 29, 67, 145, 161n13, 183–184, 217
aggregation of labour (tropical, migrant) 68, 39n46, 73n61, 238
Alison, W. P. 115, 229–230, 250, 261n149
All-India Conference of Medical Research Workers 81, 144, 154, 165n69
All-India Institute of Hygiene and Public Health 80, 149, 154, 239
All-India Labour Enquiry 122
All-India Sanitary Conference (1911) 122, 129n49
Amrith, Sunil 154, 165n72, 185, 193n65, 195n86, 88, 202, 205, 221n40
Amritsar, analysis of epidemic malaria in 30, 71n22, 124, 185
*An. culicifacies* 9, 34, 201; Ceylon (Sri Lanka) 43, 45, 48, 61, 62
*An. gambiae* 15n34, 74n87, 183, 196n104
anophelism without malaria 201–202
*An. philippinensis* 236
*An. stephensi* 28, 159
Antananarivo, Madagascar 247
Arnold, David 6, 22, 84, 101, 138n30, 165n69, 218n8
Assam Labour Enquiry Committee (1922) 24
Aykroyd, W. R. 85–99 *passim*; influence on policy 98, 234; LNHO 88; malnutrition as technical problem 93, 98; milk protein focus 88–90, 98; *Nutritive Value of Indian Foods* 90; *see also* Bhore Report (*Report of the Health Survey and Development Committee*); *Report on Bengal* (1945)

Balfour, Andrew 67, 143, 163n40, 164n60, 198n122
Bamber, C. J. 129–130
Bellew, H. W. 126–128, 130
Bengal 1943–44: Burdwan fever 27, 39n56, 140n57, 152, 236, 267n3; famine 84–86; Permanent Settlement (1793) 27, 39n55, 104n36; *see also Malaria in the Duars* (1909)
Bentley, C. A. 16n42, 19, 21–23, 43, 145, 186, 229, 249, 253n33; Burdwan fever analysis inverted 147; nutrient 'imbalance' queried 81–83, 86
Bhore Report (*Report of the Health Survey and Development Committee*) 97–99
biomedical model of infective disease, epistemic significance of 1–6, 44, 57, 87, 148, 156, 216; contest, truce 122–125; epistemic community 173–174; *see also* Human Factor
Birn, Anne-Emanuelle 164n55, 191n34
Biswas, A. 39n56
blackwater fever 19
Bombay (municipality), malaria vector control in 16n42, 28, 159
Bombay Medical Congress (1909) 18–19, 134; *see also* Human Factor; Mian Mir vector control trial
Bombay Textile Labour Union 90

294

For Product Safety Concerns and Information please contact our EU
representative GPSR@taylorandfrancis.com
Taylor & Francis Verlag GmbH, Kaufingerstraße 24, 80331 München, Germany